The Health Services – Administration, Research and Management

The Health Services – Administration, Research and Management

EDITED BY

H.P. FERRER

M.B., Ch. B. Ed., D.P.H. (Distinc.)

*County Medical Officer of
Health and Principal School
Medical Officer, Westmoreland
County Council; formerly
Lecturer, Department of Social
and Preventive Medicine,
University of Manchester*

London: Butterworths

ENGLAND: BUTTERWORTH & CO. (PUBLISHERS) LTD.
                LONDON: 88 Kingsway, WC2B 6AB

AUSTRALIA: BUTTERWORTH & CO. (AUSTRALIA) LTD.
                SYDNEY: 586 Pacific Highway, 2067
                MELBOURNE: 343 Little Collins Street, 3000
                BRISBANE: 240 Queen Street, 4000

CANADA   BUTTERWORTH & CO. (CANADA) LTD.
                TORONTO: 14 Curity Avenue, 374

NEW ZEALAND: BUTTERWORTH & CO. (NEW ZEALAND) LTD.
                WELLINGTON: 26–28 Waring Taylor Street, 1

SOUTH AFRICA: BUTTERWORTH & CO. (SOUTH AFRICA) (PTY.) LTD.
                DURBAN: 152–154 Gale Street

Suggested UDC No. 362·1:65·01
ISBN 0 407 19920 9

Printed by Redwood Press Ltd., Trowbridge & London.

Contents

CONTENTS

CONTENTS

Contributors

DAVID M. BOSWELL, MA, MPhil (Sociology)   (*Chapter 13*)
Lecturer in Sociology. The Open University,
Milton Keynes

H.P. FERRER, MB, ChB (Ed.) DPH (Distinc.)   (*Chapters 1, 4 and 7*)
County Medical Officer of Health and Principal
School Medical Officer, Westmorland County
Council; formerly Lecturer, Department of
Social and Preventive Medicine University of
Manchester

F.J. GLEN, BSc, FRSH   (*Chapter 12*)
Senior Lecturer in Applied Psychology,
Department of Behaviour in Organizations,
University of Lancaster

ANTHONY HINDLE, PhD   (*Chapters 9 and 10*)
Research Director, Unit for Operational Research
in the Health Services, Department of Operational
Research, University of Lancaster

PATRICIA MORTON, SRN, HV, Diploma in Social *(Chapter 5)*
    Studies, Nursing Administration (Public Health)
    Certificate (RCN).
Chief Administrative Nursing Officer, City of
Nottingham Health Services; formerly Lecturer
in Nursing, Department of Social and Preventive
Medicine, University of Manchester

R.M. POLLOCK, BA, MB, BChir, MRCS, LRCP   *(Chapter 3)*
Deputy Senior Administrative Medical Officer,
Oxford Regional Hospital Board

ALWYN SMITH, MB, ChB, PhD, MSc, DPH, FRCP   *(Chapter 8)*
Professor of Social and Preventive Medicine,
University of Manchester

D.H. VAUGHAN, MB, ChB, DPH   *(Chapter 2)*
Senior Lecturer, Department of Social and
Preventive Medicine, University of Manchester

R.W. WALLIS, BCom., AIMTA   *(Chapter 11)*
Lecturer in Accounting and Tutor to the
Faculty of Economic and Social Studies,
University of Manchester

B. WATKIN, SRN, BSc (Econ.)   *(Chapter 6)*
Senior Tutor in Hospital Administration,
University of Manchester

Foreword

'It is proposed that throughout the new administrative structure there should be a clear definition and allocation of responsibilities; that there should be maximum delegation downwards matched by accountability upwards; and a sound management structure should be created at all levels ... The aim will be to set clear objectives and standards and measure performance against them.'
National Health Services Reorganisation Consultative Document.

May 1971.

Management and evaluation are keynotes of the Consultative Document on National Health Service Reorganisation and, indeed, of much discussion that there has been during the last twenty years concerning our health services. It is hardly surprising that there should be much discussion of management in relation to an enterprise which spends more than five million pounds every day. However, the problems of management in the National Health Service are in a number of important ways different from the problems of management in many other enterprises. Perhaps the most important difference lies in the difficulty and complexity of the problem of formulating appropriate objectives.

Hitherto, this key question has been conspicuously neglected. It has seemed generally sufficient to provide an efficient administrative context in which doctors and nurses might identify and tackle such problems of individual patients as were brought to their attention. Only in the preventive field, and only in that part of it which has been the responsibility of the local health authorities, has there been much evidence of the conscious formulation of health objectives.

To some extent this situation has arisen because the part to be played by administrators with a medical and nursing background has been confused, limited and fragmented, and the involvement of the health professionals within the health services management team has been somewhat peripheral. This is partly because the only body of appropriately trained health professions have been the Medical Officers of Health whose isolation within the local health authorities has severely limited their opportunity to contribute to the effective management of the National Health Service as a whole. The proposed reorganization of the National Health Service will end this isolation.

However, if the new organization is to achieve the more efficient and therefore more integrated management that is required it will be necessary for an understanding of management to be much more widely disseminated than has hitherto been the case. This knowledge must embrace not only those techniques that have been developed in the context of other enterprises but also the techniques as well as the theoretical background of public health as it has developed both in the field and in the university departments. Public health has always consisted of the identification of population health problems and the organization of the means for their solution. In the early and triumphant days the problems were mainly those of communicable disease and the solutions involved the deployment of whatever techniques were required to interrupt the transmission of micro-organisms. The solution of these early problems has left us with a range of new problems which although various and complex have generally in common the likelihood that their solution will lie in a more effective deployment of existing medical and health care resources. The management of these resources and their specific direction to the general and specific objectives which will need to be formulated will require the concerted action of a multi-professional managerial team. The present volume is intended to provide an initial basis for such teams' collaborative discussions.

ALWYN SMITH

1– Introduction

H.P. Ferrer

During recent years there has been increasing interest in the application of the skills of management to the health services. To many people this is a new departure and it is inevitable that it should sometimes be misunderstood. Although the application of the skills of management in the health services presents problems different to those encountered in industry, there are many parallels with the situation that occurred when management skills were first applied in the multiplying business schools during the 1930s and 1940s in the United States of America and in Britain. This is not the place to discuss whether or not management can be taught as a university academic subject. Many people will still claim that managers in any sphere of activity are born and not made. However, there is little doubt that the presence of the appropriate skill, at birth, can alleviate many of the complications and hasten what might, for some, be a rather tedious process.

This work is intended as an introduction for personnel in the health services who may find the approach to management unusual after many years as administrators within the service. It should be emphasized that each section is an introduction, and at the end of each bibliography and reference lists are available which may be useful for those who wish to delve deeper. Many management appreciation courses are being set up for health services personnel. Unfortunately, these courses have largely concentrated on the administrators in the hospital services. As

1

yet there has been no uniform and systematic approach to bring these skills to the notice of those in the community services which form such an important part of the health services. The reason is partly financial, as the ever increasing cost of the hospital services (approx. 55 per cent of the total expenditure on the health services) has made concentration in this particular field inevitable. It is certain that at least 90 per cent of the use of the health services, in terms of patient encounter, takes place outside the hospital setting, and it is probable that it is within the community in future years that increasing use will be made of management skills.

MEDICAL MANAGEMENT AND TRAINING

There is no systematic in-service training for medical personnel who wish to make a career in medical management. Several centres (including London and Manchester) have introduced some degree of management training in modifications of the traditional Diploma in Public Health type of course. As yet there has been no continuous training of the medical administrator and manager along the lines indicated for nurses in the Salmon Report. It would seem that there are two lines along which training in medical management can be done.

(1) Continuous training in short management courses combined with appropriate in-service experience.

(2) An initial long period of training which concentrates on the reorientation in management thinking of medically trained personnel over a period of two years, and which is followed up by short repeated courses of training during progressive stages of in-service experience.

A combination of these types of training may be necessary during the transitional period, but it should be possible for medically trained personnel to opt for a career in management and administration at a comparatively early stage in their postgraduate experience.

The question of the status of the medical manager and administrator in the profession is one which has still not been resolved. Various solutions put forward in the last few years do not seem to tackle the problem of the high degree of skill needed in modern management. It is not sufficient that management expertise should be annexed only to the end of a distinguished clinical career, although there must be a place for the experience and wisdom of the most senior clinicians in the advice given to the medical manager and administrator. There is a particular danger that the medical manager can lose touch with the insight that his basic medical training gave him. It is essential that he should be able, at all times, to discuss with his clinical colleagues problems confronting them in their work situation. It is equally false to assume that a clinician with great experience can assume the mantle of medical management without the up-to-date knowledge of the skills which are an essential part of the manager's armamentarium.

Although at the present time a committee (the Hunter Committee) is sitting from which it is hoped a new and more comprehensive career structure for the medical manager will be adopted, there needs to be a much greater degree of flexibility between the existing career structures in medical management. In particular, there needs to be a greater understanding between community and hospital services administrators. There should be a possibility of interchange between the two spheres, giving comprehensive in-service training with experience in all branches of the present health services. Undoubtedly, in a reorganized health service the differences will be less marked, and in time the distinction between the community services manager and administrator and the hospital-orientated administrator will become less. It is from this combined experience that the new type of medical manager may emerge. Undoubtedly, the medical manager of the future will need to be a highly skilled person indeed. He will have to hold his own alongside highly trained nursing and general administrators and work in harmonious co-operation with them. Until such time as a comprehensive and radical reappraisal of the role of the medical manager and administrator has been made, medical services may well find that their voice in the management and administration of the health services impaired.

USE OF MANAGEMENT IN HEALTH SERVICES

Unlike most management considerations the health services do not have a recognizable end-product. Therefore, the consideration of marketing techniques does not enter the discussion. The main objective of the health services is a delicate balance between the welfare of the patients within the services and the optimum use of the resources within the service. In any system of comprehensive medical care it is to be expected that the resources will not be unlimited. Balancing of priorities within the services, however, is closely related to the needs of the service. This means an objective assessment of the needs of the health services in relationship to the community which they serve. Needs may be divided into two overlapping groups.

(1) The apparent needs of the health services. ·
(2) The actual needs of the community.

Apparent needs may be made up of various subjective assessments made by personnel within the services, which have a great deal of value in so far as they represent the subjective assessment in clinical (or other) terms of the needs of patients as they are presented to the health services for treatment or other kinds of health service processing. The *actual needs* of the health services are based closely on the monitoring of the community need, in which various types of technique may be used. As will be discussed in a later section of this book, epidemiology forms the basis of the study of the community in this field. Whatever the function of the future community physician, it seems that a large part of his work will be concerned with this monitoring of the community need. His training will have to be orientated towards the epidemiology of disease within the community in relationship to the needs of the health services. Unfortunately, most management courses provided for nurses and general administrators have not, to date, taken in the full implications of the epidemiologist's expertise and functions in relationship to management. Until monitoring of community need has been fully explored management within the health services can do little more than cope with short-term expediency. Forward planning, as such, has to be based on the apparent or subjective needs of the health services which, in turn, are based on retrospective experience or present apparent demand. At times some personnel may object that revolutions in medical care may make much of forward planning redundant, and even superfluous. However, revolutions of this nature are comparatively infrequent. It should be possible for the community physician to be very much more aware of the actual needs of the community concerning demands for health care, in relation with forward planning.

LIMITATIONS OF HEALTH SERVICES MANAGERS

It is sometimes expected that, by the application of a certain technique in management to a particular problem, the health services manager will be able to cope with the many conflicting demands made on the services. Disappointment frequently results from this attitude of mind, and administrators within the health services have been bitterly disappointed in that the appropriate department of a university may fail to come up with the solution to a problem. This is partly because of a misapprehension of the way in which management techniques may be applied within the health services' setting. Until we have highly trained and skilled health service managers, this use of management techniques as a sort of diagnostic aid must inevitably make administrators rather suspicious of the whole field of application of management. Equally, the experienced operations researcher, or financial manager, may hold up his hands in despair at the lack of appreciation shown towards a particular solution that he has presented. It is the writer's opinion that management appreciation courses may be partly responsible for these mutual misunderstandings. In the same way that medical personnel use their training almost unconsciously to approach clinical problems, it is important that management skills are used instinctively. The very least that can be expected from the health services manager is that he should have a deep appreciation of the techniques available to him and of the many solutions that may present themselves. He may find it difficult, for example, to balance the real needs of the community as discussed above with the apparent needs of the health services. It may not be possible to implement fully the expected future needs in a particular area because of the conflict of these with the apparent needs in relation to other health services within the area. The balancing of these conflicts goes far deeper, and demands a far higher degree of expertise, and a skilful balancing of personalities who may clash over apparently rival claims within the immediate administrative situation, than superficial appreciation of management can give.

At the present time the comprehensive feedback mechanism and the interchange at different levels of the health service have tended to make for expedient solutions to long-term problems. Within the necessarily limited resources of the health services this kind of imbalance will always persist, but the worst effects can be minimized at local level by blending the conflicting aims within the service. Although some may consider that the health services are subject too much to pressures which cannot be evaluated in the long term, the training of the health services manager, whether he be a medical, nursing, or general administrator, will undoubtedly present one of the most fascinating challenges and evolutions within the health services over the next ten years. As yet, we are only beginning to see some of the implications which this kind of evolution can bring about. It is perhaps especially relevant at present, when there is so much discussion regarding the reorganization of the administrative structure of the health services, that the consideration of the development of the health services manager must form an essential part of the health services of the future. Those at present at the top of the administrative levels of health services may have to look with more than benign tolerance at the emergence of the highly skilled manager. The use they can make now of the trained medical manager will say much for their wisdom and skill learned over long years of experience within the services. However, there is a great deal of scope for cross-fertilization of ideas which should produce interesting, if not dramatic, results.

These broader considerations may seem rather remote from the day-to-day problems which clinicians, both in the community and the hospital services, experience. The bridging of this gap between those with the higher administrative and managerial responsibilities within the services forms one of the most important considerations of the health services manager. The single-handed general practitioner can benefit by his appreciation of management skills not only in understanding the general direction of the health services as a whole, but also in the more immediate problems which beset him in the management of his practice. Those working in larger units of group practice or health centres are presented with problems to which some of the skills outlined in this book may be usefully applied. If the practitioner is as aware of the limitations of applying a diagnostic managerial skill as he is of applying one skill alone in the diagnosis of a patient's condition, good use may be made of management advisory services that are available to the local or area health authority. Advisory services of this nature have not so far been discussed in relation to the reorganization of the health services. At the highest level, management advisory services are available in the Department of Health and Social Security. It is to be hoped that some kind of management advisory unit will be available at the area or regional level which will be of use to those concerned with the day-to-day functioning of the health services.

As a last resort it may be objected that efficient health services management often conflicts with the basic humanitarian needs of the patient. This should not occur provided those responsible for the health services and their management and administration are deeply aware of the overriding need to provide a humanitarian service. Those personnel in the health services trained in the basic problems of patient care are never likely to lose sight of the humanitarian considerations. Much skill is required, sometimes, to resolve conflict between the apparently efficient use of the health services and the patient's comfort and health care needs. This problem, of course, is already with us in the consideration of selection for certain types of therapy (for example, the provision of renal dialysis). How far the resources are to be distributed between the strident and conflicting demands of different types of patient care would require the wisdom of Solomon and the judgement of an angel. Nevertheless, it is hoped that this book will bring a deeper appreciation of the use of quantitative techniques in the skills of management, and will provide a channel for those who wish to delve much more deeply into a very fascinating field. Several volumes would be needed to discuss in depth some of the problems raised. However, it is hoped that sufficient interest will be aroused to help personnel to realize that management and the health services have passed beyond the realm of academic considerations and must play an increasing part at every level of our health services. If at times we seem to have stated the obvious then we must beg the indulgence of those with many years' experience and wisdom in health services administration. However, as the application of management skills is so new within the health services, there is a comparative scarcity of literature on the subject and most has to be adapted from other fields where management skills have been applied for some time. A constructive approach to the more advanced literature on management and, in particular, its relationship to the health services, will provide the experienced administrator with a great deal which is fruitful and thought provoking. Until such a time as the backlog of more introductory courses in management has been completed it is unlikely that many centres will be found where this kind of study can be carried out and integrated with the experienced administrator's in-service experience and skill. In these situations both teacher and pupil provide the stimulus and information for each other. The accumulated experience of such a teaching centre will provide one of the most useful keystones for the whole range of management training in future years.

ACKNOWLEDGEMENTS

The Editor wishes to acknowledge the invaluable help received from the following.

Professor John Butterfield for the original inspiration.

Professor Alwyn Smith and staff of the Department of Social and Preventive Medicine, University of Manchester, for criticisms and help.

Dr A. Hindle, of Lancaster University, without whom it would have been impossible to produce this work.

To Miss H. Moore for continuous help with typing and checking of the work.

BIBLIOGRAPHY

Drucker, P.F. (Ed.) (1969). *The Practice of Management.* London ; Prentice-Hall

Kempner, T. (Ed.) (1969). *A Guide to the Study of Management.* Oxford; Blackwell

Logan, R.F.L. (1969). 'Some Problems in Medical Care.' In *The Medical Annual.* Bristol; John Wright and Sons

Milne, J.F. and Chaplin, N.W. (Eds.) (1969). *Modern Hospital Management.* London; The Institute of Hospital Administrators

Peters, R.J. and Kinnaird, J. (Eds.) (1965). *Health Services Administration.* Edinburgh; Livingstone

White, K.L. and Murnaghan, J.H. (1969). *Vital and Health Statistics.* (Series 2, No. 33.) Washington D.C.; U.S. Dept of Health, Education and Welfare

2–The Administrative Structure of the Health Services and Future Developments

D.H. Vaughan

The National Health Service Today

The National Health Service Act 1946, section 1 made it the duty of the Minister of Health to '. . . promote the establishment in England and Wales of a comprehensive health service designed to secure improvement in the physical and mental health of the people of England and Wales, and the prevention, diagnosis, and treatment of illness, and for that purpose to provide or secure the effective provision of services . . .' The new service was one part of the plan introducing our modern welfare state in the phase of reconstruction after World War II. To enable him to carry out this ambitious and difficult plan the Minister was given control, either directly or indirectly, over most of the existing health facilities of the country. Important areas not included in the service were the occupational health services for schoolchildren and for workers, medical research and the services related to the hazards of the environment. The services thus brought under the Minister's control were placed in three groups: (1) hospital and specialist services; (2) services provided by local authorities; and (3) general, medical, dental, pharmaceutical and ophthalmic services.

THE NATIONAL HEALTH SERVICE TODAY

HISTORY

The Ministry of Health was created in 1919 to act as the central government office responsible for the health of the country. These duties had previously been exercised largely by the Local Government Board, and the separation resulted from the increasing disenchantment with the board as an agency for the care of the nation's health. The Ministry did not, however, have responsibility for mental illness, for industrial health services or for research. During its existance the Ministry has been responsible for other matters as well as those particularly relating to health. These have included housing and a general responsibility for local government affairs, but both are now placed in the care of a separate government department. The Ministry of Health was amalgamated in 1968 with the Ministry of Pensions and National Insurance, to become the Department of Health and Social Security which, thus, to some extent resembles the Local Government Board at the end of the nineteenth century.

In the 1930s, the hospitals of this country could be divided into two main groups: (1) the voluntary hospitals, maintained by voluntary subscriptions; and (2) the hospitals run by local authorities who had taken over responsibilities from the Poor Law Boards of Guardians after 1929. Nation wide enquiries into our hospitals prior to World War II revealed that the facilities varied greatly in different parts of the country, and in some areas were deplorably poor. The voluntary hospitals, apart perhaps from those in London, could no longer rely on receiving enough money to provide the services demanded, and many local authorities could not afford the rate expenditure necessary to maintain their hospitals. It was not only the physical facilities which varied, the number and quality of the staff were also affected. The National Health Service Act 1946 took over almost all the hospitals in order to 'provide effective services'.

It could be said that local authorities have been providing services of a kind for the inhabitants of their areas for centuries, but it was not until the nineteenth century that anything like the present system evolved. Before that, the services could only be provided by such authorities as municipal corporations and parish councils, and were limited to safeguarding the environment. In the absence of other authorities, or in the face of indifference and inefficiency, these services were often provided by private water companies, improvement companies and the like.

Last century the network of authorities that we know today was built up step by step, and dealt in the first place with the control of the environment. However, by the early years of the present century, concern for personal health led to the development of services for particular groups, such as mothers and young children, and school-children, because no other appropriate services were readily available. This aspect of the local authorities' activity developed greatly in the 1920s and 1930s, but the services were being provided by different types of authority, the smaller of which were finding it difficult to provide the range of services which their inhabitants were beginning to expect.

Curative services outside the hospital could be said to have become organized after the 1911 National Health Insurance Act. This enabled workers whose income was below a certain level to insure themselves for medical care and insurance benefit during illness. It did not cover their dependants, nor did it cover most hospital care, for which they had to rely on the voluntary hospitals or poor law infirmaries.

The essential administrative feature of this care was that it was operated by local insurance committees, which were separate from both the hospitals and the local authorities and upon which there was considerable professional representation. This system, as it developed, also had the incidental effect of crystallizing the different groups of doctors – those who worked in hospital and those who did not. From it arose the process of referral from one doctor to another and to the hospital out-patient department.

Present Administrative Structure

The Department of Health and Social Security is organized along lines similar to those of other government ministries. The Secretary of State for Social Services heads a small group of politicians, he is by tradition, responsible to Parliament for all the decisions made by the Department. The large civil service element is somewhat unusual among ministries in that a fairly high number of its members have professional qualifications – doctors, nurses, social workers for example. The various areas of interest are grouped into divisions and sections, each with the appropriate grades of civil servants. The non-professional civil servants have an orthodox bureaucratic hierarchy leading up to the Permanent Secretary, whose functions include that of advising the political head. The professionals have their own parallel systems under the Chief Medical Officer. At each level the professionals are regarded, in the main, as advisers who must work through the ordinary civil service channels, but there are many professional and semi-professional matters in which these are not necessarily appropriate.

The Department is concerned with many aspects of health in this country which are not directly related to the National Health Service (N.H.S.). These include, for example, environmental services, international aspects of health and medical education. However, much of the work is concerned with the running of the three main branches of the Service.

The hospital and specialist services are administered by the 15 Regional Hospital Boards. These Boards have 20–25 members including their chairmen, which are appointed by the Secretary of State. The members are appointed on a personal basis and do not represent any particular body or organization, although the Secretary of State is obliged to consult various local interests before making the appointments. One of these interests is the local medical school around which the region is organized. Thus, the area and size of the regions was originally determined by the distribution of medical schools, emphasizing the connection between the service and medical education. London was regarded, as in so many other fields, as a special case, and the four Metropolitan Regions each relate to several schools. Paradoxically, the teaching hospitals related to the medical schools are not administered by the Regional Boards, but by separate Boards of Governors.

The hospitals of the regions are further grouped on an area basis, and each group is administered by a Hospital Management Committee whose members and chairman are appointed by the Regional Hospital Board after appropriate local consultation. Most of the groups contain hospitals with a wide range of specialties which provide most of the services required by an area, but a few groups consist mainly of one type of hospital, often a psychiatric one which is so large or so isolated, or both, that it requires a group of its own for satisfactory management.

The staff employed by the Boards and Committees in their own offices are those appropriate to their functions, which can be summarized briefly as planning in the case of the Boards, and day-to-day administration in the case of the Committees. Apart from its secretarial and financial staff the Board has many professional personnel, for example engineers and architects, who are actively engaged on the plans for new hospitals, as well as dealing with the obsolescence of many of the existing hospitals. A fairly recent development is the formation of organizations and methods or research and development groups which are engaged in the study of existing hospitals as well as plans for new ones. Each Board has a small number of medically qualified staff to deal with the medical problems of the present and future service, and a similarly small number of nurses.

The Hospital Management Committee have secretarial and financial staff and engineers to deal with the many day-to-day maintenance problems of a modern hospital, but no medical staff; and they have only recently begun to appoint nurses with responsibility for the nursing services of the group as a whole.

A similar reduction in the number of authorities concerned occurred in 1948 in the services provided by the local authorities. Here, the county councils and county borough councils were designated Local Health Authorities and given responsibilities for a wide range of services. The councils discharge their responsibilities through a health committee whose chief officer, the Medical Officer of Health, is at the same time its adviser and chief executive. He has working with him an appropriately-sized staff with a variety of qualifications, for example, doctors, nurses, chiropodists and ambulance officers.

The administrative structure of the Local Health Authority may be complicated in a number of ways. Between a third and half are integrated with the welfare services provided mainly under the National Assistance Act 1948. In the county boroughs the environmental work carried out mainly by public health inspectors is closely related, although' lying outside the National Health Service. In both counties and county boroughs the school health service has a similar close but separate relationship, and many of the doctors, nurses and others may work in both. Some of the larger counties have formed area or divisional committees to concern themselves with parts of the county, advised by a medical officer who is then usually the Medical Officer of Health of the constituent county districts (municipal borough, urban or rural district). A further complication is that county districts with a population of 60,000 or over may have had powers delegated to them from the county council to administer certain Local Health Authority services as their own. The Health Committee, like other committees of the council, consists largely of council members, but usually co-opts one or two other members; these will often be doctors working in the area.

Executive councils

The successors to the former Insurance Committees are called Executive Councils, and are now responsible for general medical, general dental, pharmaceutical and ophthalmic services in areas corresponding to those of Local Health Authorities. In a number of instances, however, one Executive Council may cover, for example, a small county borough and its neighbouring county. Alone among the major administrative committees of the Health Service, the size and composition of the Executive Councils are laid down. They consist of 30 members, and so balanced that none of the three major interests involved – the Local

Health Authority, the professions providing the services and the interested persons appointed by the Secretary of State – can, on their own, control the decisions of the Council. In addition to the Council, there exist local committees representative of each of the professions involved, and these have the responsibility of examining the problems related to their particular profession and preparing advice for the Council.

The Councils are responsible for maintaining an adequate and appropriate service in their areas. The professional persons providing the service are not employees but, for the most part, contract to give their services. Before they give care to patients under the N.H.S. they have to fulfil certain obligations and provide the Council with information regarding such things as their premises and hours of availability. Much of the day-to-day work of the Council is concerned with these matters and with ensuring that appropriate payments are made.

Responsibilities

Thus it can be seen that three or four authorities are responsible for different aspects of patient care in the N.H.S. The general area for which each is responsible is fairly easy to establish, but the borders inevitably are vague. These divisions, in what was supposed to be one service, came under attack at an early stage, but the Guillibaud Committee (Report, 1956) were not inclined to suggest any changes before the new system had had time to settle down. However, the maternity services came under special criticism because of the dangers to mothers who were cared for within a short space of time by staff working for two or three different authorities. Another committee (Ministry of Health, 1959) suggested that maternity liaison committees should be set up in each area so that common practices could be established to ensure continuity of care. This idea of liaison has been extended in some areas by the establishment of committees or councils to encourage joint working arrangements in other fields. Such bodies have, of course, no statutory existence and can only make recommendations to those more directly concerned.

Problems of Today

ISOLATION

This isolation of authorities which has been referred to can be seen as one of the big problems of the Service today. In the past, some staff have worked in two different fields, for example, as general practitioners and hospital specialists. Local authorities were responsible for running hospital services and also services for those outside hospital. In this way staff, both professional and administrative, were able to see their particular day-to-day problems from different angles in a way which is difficult, if not impossible today, when the various career structures effectively preclude any worthwhile experience in more than one branch of the service.

It is not, perhaps, the different administrative detail which is important, but the differences in outlook and attitudes which detract from the notion of one service. The expectations which one branch has of another may be so unrealistic as to prejudice the care of the patients. The divisions are perhaps made more acute by the separate professional groupings which have developed, and do not encourage contact between those working in different fields.

The need for closer working arrangements has been recognized in recent years, and there are many instances where workers from two or even three branches of the Service have been drawn together into a team to care for particular types of patient (Anderson, 1969). These arrangements are more common in some specialties − psychiatry, paediatrics and geriatrics − than in others, and this is determined, perhaps more than anything else, by the recognition that specialist care outside hospital is of the greatest benefit to many of the patients. Often these teams were brought into being, despite administrative and even legal difficulties*, by a few determined and far-seeing people who happened to be working in the same place at the same time.

A particular type of this arrangement is the attachment of local authority staff (mainly health visitors and home nurses) to general practices. Before 1948, it was envisaged that the service would be provided from health centres where the Executive Council, Local Health Authority and possibly, even some of the hospital services would have accommodation. For various reasons such a network of centres was not built, and the medical profession became antagonistic to the idea of such buildings which would be owned and administered by the local authorities. Due to a change in the financial arrangements for general practice, and a gradual acceptance by practitioners that the centres have advantages to offer the patients and themselves, many more have been built in recent years (Curwen and Brookes, 1969). One of the original advantages put forward for health centres was that staff from the different parts of the Service would be brought together, and

*Nurses employed by Local Health Authorities are now able to work in places other than the patient's home as a result of various sections of the Health Services and Public Health Act, 1968.

this expectation is fulfilled when a centre is working well. Attachment of local authority staff to general practices can occur in the absence of a health centre, but in this case the isolation may be reduced without the accommodation being suitable for co-ordinated working arrangements to be made.

Isolation in the working of the Service can be overcome if the staff are sufficiently determined and the various authorities are not actively opposed to the idea, but it has to be admitted that the developments are piecemeal. At the official level, co-ordination is expected to be ensured by cross-representation on the various committees — various local interests on Regional Hospital Boards and Hospital Management Committees; local doctors co-opted to the Health Committees of local authorities; the Local Health Authority representation on Executive Councils — but in practice the voices do not appear loud enough to do more than pay lip service to the ideal.

PLANNING

Nowhere is this isolation so evident as in the field of planning. New developments may proceed before the possible repercussions are studied by the other branches concerned. Indeed, in some instances the other branches may not even be informed.

The concept of overall planning presupposes an authority which is able to review activities in all the appropriate fields and come to rational decisions regarding the most suitable allocation of staff and resources. The most obvious fields where this deficiency may be seen are in the care of the old and mentally disturbed. The allocation of beds and staff often proceeds independently in the local authority and hospital fields. Each may have a different view of its own responsibilities in terms of the kind of person for whom they should provide care. It is true that in some areas co-ordinated planning is carried out, but this remains the exception. As a result of the different ways the developments are financed, it is usually not possible to consider the overall benefits to be derived from some increased expenditure in one field.

FINANCE

The need to plan the most economical use of resources is perhaps made more necessary by the limited finance available for the health service. Most of the money comes directly or indirectly from general taxation, the only other major sources being the local authority rates and the contributions of those using some parts of the Service*. The original thinking about a national health service (Report, 1942) included the idea that, after an initial period to overcome current deficienties, the expenditure would be likely to fall. The reverse has proved to be the case. This is not the place to suggest reasons for this, but they are related to increased medical knowledge, different patterns of disease, different expectations of a hospital, and changing demands for medical care.

Current expenditure on all aspects of the Service is estimated to be £1,853 million (1969/70), and this represents 4.75 per cent of the gross national product (Public Expenditure, 1969). This is a lower proportion than many other 'Western' countries spend on health, but it has been steadily increasing in the past ten years. There is virtually no limit to the amount which could be spent on health services, but there are two problems involved. Is it an appropriate amount, having regard to the general pattern of disease and the other calls on the national income? Is it being allocated in the way most likely to produce most benefit? No-one, however, can adequately define the benefit to be sought nor describe a way to compare the needs of health, housing, education and defence.

On the one hand the decisions are political ones, and on the other they are determined by the need to keep the existing Service going while changes are bein planned and put into effect.

INFORMATION

It is often said that change ought to occur after analysis of information about current patterns, but one of the sad things about the first 20 years of the Health Service is the paucity of information available regarding its operation. Other sections in this book are devoted to the subject, but it is significant that almost all the important information comes from the Hospital Service. This is appropriate in the sense that the hospitals spend 55 per cent of the budget and are the most highly organized, but they deal with only 10 per cent of all the episodes of illness for which treatment is sought. Each local health authority prepares an annual report which gives information about some aspects of their services, but very little is known on a routine basis of the services of the Executive Councils. As a result, information about services outside hospital has to be sought by special investigations, and this is particularly the case where the interaction of two or more branches is to be studied.

---

*The details for each year are contained in the Annual Report of the Department of Health and Social Security. These, and other statistics, now appear in an annual *Digest of Health Statistics for England and Wales,* London; H.M.S.O.

Experiment or Uniformity

The lack of detailed local information may have had the effect of establishing national policies in the Service which do not take much account of major local variables. There is no way for a local area to establish a convincing case. On paper, however, the administrative structure is remarkably uniform, except in the autonomous local authorities. With detailed control of expenditure by the central department, opportunity for experimentation in the provision of services has been lacking. This is all the more unfortunate when one considers the different quantity and quality of buildings and staff which areas inherited in 1948. The result has been a stifling of initiative and differences between areas in terms of buildings and practices which reflect the old patterns.

Prevention

A problem which cuts across all branches of the Service is the low priority given in practice to prevention, despite the importance suggested for it in the last 60 years*. Although it has been the special responsibility of the Local Health Authorities, the other branches could be involved. The usual difficulties of time, space and money are involved even though most practitioners admit the potential value of preventive measures for persons of all ages. As always, in Britain and other countries, care takes precedence in most cases over prevention, and the resources are allocated accordingly. The problem is to know the extent to which this depends on the structure of the Service, and how much to professional attitudes. Is it appropriate to have one authority responsible for both aspects or should there be a separate service devoted to health education and screening? Would this, in fact, be more effective?

Expectations and Aims of the Service

NATIONAL

The N.H.S. was devised by Beveridge (Report, 1942) and the governments of the 1940s as an integral part of the social welfare provisions of the

---

*The National Health Insurance Act 1911 contained provisions for the active work of general practitioners in the detection of insanitary conditions and the prevention of disease, but in practice little developed from this.

country. It was necessary to provide a service to restore to health those who became ill and were unable to work. The unrealistic idea that the need for such a service would soon decrease has already been mentioned. The existence of the Service is now taken so much for granted that it is difficult, today, to define what the national expectations are. 'The best possible care for all' is clearly inappropriate as an expectation in the face of two-year delays for hernia repairs and the scarcity of kidney machines. Nevertheless the care available to all has improved, and the differences between areas is now less than in 1948.

Four fundamental principles for the N.H.S. have been stated — a national service, financed by taxation, giving clinical freedom for doctors, and centred on the family doctor team (Department of Health and Social Security, 1970). The country, as a whole, is beginning to understand the decisions involved and, perhaps, to question some of the underlying assumptions (Owen, 1968).

PROFESSIONAL

The staff working in the Service expect it to provide not only care for patients, but to provide them with an environment within which they may practice their skills. Their assessment of the Service is often coloured by the extent to which their requirements are met. The administrative structure may be seen as opposing 'professional activity', because it is unable to provide more equipment or staff.

The expectation of the professional to do the best for his patient conflicts with the needs of the Service as a whole, and compromise is necessary. The involvement of professionals in the administrative process is one way of making the decisions more acceptable. Their presence on committees at all levels not only ensures their expert contributions, but involves them in the running of the Service and the harsh decisions which must be taken. The inability of the Service to provide everything for everybody is accepted as inevitable by some, and rejected as interference by others. (see, for example, the series 'Unheard Voices' – Br. med. J. (1970) (1) 358, 421, 492, 559, 624, 685, 748, 813 (2) 45, 171. These give the views of consultants from different specialties).

INDIVIDUAL

For many, if not most, people the N.H.S. is something they pay for and which will be there when they require it. But slowly it has been found that this is not always the case (that is, a period of waiting may be involved), and it may not be what was expected. Almost all the population uses some part of the Service, but more and more are finding it worthwhile to insure for private hospital care (Crossman, 1969). This is designed to ensure that care is available when it is required, and is from whom the patient chooses. The implications of this movement will be discussed later.

Dissatisfaction with the Service has shown itself in the rise of national pressure groups seeking better facilities in hospitals and elsewhere — improvement of maternity services, improved visiting of children in hospital, facilities for cervical cytology and better care for the aged. Such groups owe their existence, in part, to the feeling that the present structure in which appointed committees are responsible for the services, is too remote from the population as a whole and too susceptible to suggestion from higher authority.

Recent disclosures about conditions of care in certain hospitals (Department of Health and Social Security, 1969b) have brought a demand for more appropriate facilities to enquire into complaints by patients and staff. At the moment complaints, other than the most serious, are dealt with by procedures within the Service. It has been suggested that an independent Health Commissioner (Ombudsman) should be appointed. Along the same lines the Department of Health has created a Hospital Advisory Service* which has responsibility of examining and advising on professional practices within the hospital (but not individual complaints). This service is starting with psychiatric hospitals and its work will extend to others.

The emergence of these official and unofficial groups is perhaps indicative of the insensitivity of the existing structure to the general welfare of patients, and the need for more formal channels through which complaints may be made. The existing channels are not well publicized, and complaints can be fairly easily lost sight of. The public on the whole accept the care given to them, and expect it to be the best available. Despite increasing awareness and outspokenness there is not the same level of 'litigation-mindedness' which has been reached in other countries, for example the United States of America.

INTERNATIONAL

The administration of the health services of a country must be seen in the wider context of the administration of other services. In Eastern Europe, for example, it is accepted that health is a community

---

*H.M. (70) 17 Department of Health and Social Security accompanies a document giving details of this Service.

responsibility, and it is financed from taxes along with other such services directed and controlled by elected representative councils at different levels.

In much of Western Europe and Scandinavia the finance for health services comes largely from insurance contributions in various forms, and the services are provided by a mixture of state, private and charitable organizations. Britain is alone in this group, where a high proportion of finance and provision is supplied directly by the state. Apart from a small number of payments for particular services treatment is free.

The other extreme in the provision of health services is seen in the United States of America where, until recently, there was virtually no federal provision of curative services. States provided services for a few groups, but for the majority of the population health care came from private sources and payment was aided by insurance benefits. Difficulties in this system have led to federal aid for certain groups of people – particularly the aged, and those on low wages. This aid is in the form of financial contributions to existing organizations and does not extend to the direct provision of services on any sizable scale. The administration of services is very largely on an independent basis, and it is only in a few large towns that any overall planning is possible.

Green Papers

The first decade of the N.H.S. was a period of adjustment and consolidation, during which the main emphasis was on making the Service work and on correcting, as far as possible, the major inequalities and deficiencies. It was a period of general financial stringency for the country as a whole, and the money which could be devoted to the health services was limited. In the early 1960s, however, the situation began to change, and attention was paid to the need for the expansion of services and the replacement of buildings. The length of time required to plan and build a major hospital was found to be about 10 years, and this meant that future financial commitments had to be made so that realistic planning could take place. Regional Hospital Boards were asked to prepare plans giving priority to the most urgent tasks. These plans were published, and formed the basis of the present hospital building programme (Ministry of Health 1962; 1966a). Local Health Authorities were also asked to prepare plans for their 10-year development programmes (Ministry of Health, 1963; 1964; 1966b). The two authorities were expected to consult each other and co-ordinate their plans, but it soon became fairly clear that difficulties would be experienced in keeping the two programmes in step.

These attempts at forward planning reawakened interest in the idea of changing the administrative structure of the Service, with a view to integrating the three branches. This idea had been rejected by the Guillibaud Committee (Report, 1956) but had been suggested by the Porritt Committee's report (Report, 1964). This committee had been set up by various medical professional bodies and, because it tended to propose a greater degree of professional control in the service, it did not receive much support at the time.

In 1968 the Government issued a Green Paper (indicating that it was put forward for discussion and did not represent Government policy as a White Paper does) (Ministry of Health, 1968). This clearly stated the advantages which would follow from the unification of administration, and suggested the formation of 40–50 Area Boards, each with 15–16 appointed members and a strong internal organization with appropriate staff. All the health services in the area would be transferred to the Boards, with the exception of environmental services which would remain with local authorities. At the time a Royal Commission was considering the future of local government in England and Wales, and the Green Paper made it clear that some of its proposals might require revision after the commission had reported.

The Green Paper was criticized by many individuals and organizations, most strongly perhaps by the British Medical Association. The criticisms could be grouped into three main areas: (1) the size of the areas involved and the small number of people on the Board with little representation of public or professions; (2) possible domination by the hospital service; and (3) the absence of regional planning.

The Government, as a result, issued a second Green Paper early in 1970 (Department of Health and Social Security, 1970). In the interim the Royal Commission on Local Government had issued its report (Report, 1969b) which had been largely accepted by the Government (Reform of Local Government in England, 1970). Certain firm decisions were made by the Government in relation to the health services. These were that it would not be administered by local authorities, but that the new health authorities would match the new unitary authorities suggested by the Royal Commission, and that the division of health and social services between the two authorities would depend on the main skills required to provide each service.

The idea of area health authorities was retained, but the number increased to approximately 90, in line with the Royal Commission's report. In addition, Regional Councils and District Councils were proposed, in each case without much executive authority. The regions would be responsible for overall planning, post-graduate education, deployment of staff, blood transfusion and ambulance services. They would cover areas similar to the present Regional Hospital Boards but would not in any way supervise or control the Area Health Authorities which would have a direct relationship with the central Department.

It was envisaged that the central Department would need re-organization, and have strengthened regional offices. It would allocate available funds, satisfying itself that the money was spent to the best advantage, and concern itself more closely than in the past with the efficiency of local administration. There was a need to maintain a balance between the main areas of expenditure, and the Department would require powers of guidance and possibly direction.

This apparent increase in the controlling powers of the central government was criticized by some, but the Secretary of State was at some pains to point out that already he had more or less unlimited powers.

One-third of the members of the Area Health Authority would be appointed by the health professions; one-third by the local authority, and one-third, and the Chairman, by the Secretary of State. This attempt to broaden the basis of local participation in the Service is also seen in the proposals for District Committees. These would cover areas covered by District General Hospitals and would have half their membership drawn from the Area Health Authority and half from those living and working in the district. The committee would have no budget or powers delegated by statute, but would be used to supervise the running of services in the district.

The Area Health Authorities would be able to develop and plan the unified services in its area within the budget allocated. They would require close relations with the local authority, which would retain responsibility for certain environmental health problems – control of communicable disease, food hygiene, and port health, among others. Close contact, also, would have to be maintained with the Social Services Department of the local authorities which would be responsible for social work, day care of children and adults, and residential accommodation where the main skills required are social rather than medical. Report (1968b) discusses the question in greater detail.

In order to safeguard the status of family practitioners as independent contractors, it was proposed to establish a statutory committee of the Area Health Authority with which the practitioners would enter into contract. They would thus closely resemble the existing Executive Councils.

The proposals made for the internal organization of the Authority were regarded as tentative. One of the main functions would be to formulate requirements for health services and plan their organization and use. Co-ordination of this function would be a major responsibility of a chief administrative medical officer, but he would work closely with other medical bodies and the other professions involved. Co-ordination of other activities would also be the responsibility of a chief administrative officer, and other professional groups would each have a principal officer on the Authority's staff. Each of these officers would have others working under their direction and be responsible for different aspects of the Authority's work.

The part to be played by doctors in the new administrative arrangements was put forward in some detail. In each area there would be a corps of administrative medical staff serving the new authorities and the local authorities. They would take over the work of the Medical Officer of Health, and of the administrative medical staff of Regional Hospital Boards, and be able to survey the pattern of health-care in the whole area.

Reactions to the second Green Paper tended to centre around the distribution of power between the Department, the regions, the areas and the districts. Despite official denials there was a general feeling that more central control was inevitable, and that the districts were not likely to be in a position to have much influence. The doctors working in hospitals felt strongly that a regional organization must be retained.

DISTRICT GENERAL HOSPITAL

One of the basic concepts which matured during the 1940s and 1950s was that of the District General Hospital. It received official blessing in the hospital plan of 1962 (Ministry of Health, 1962). The idea, in its simplest terms, is to provide under one roof in-patient and out-patient facilities for the population of a district, including all but a few specialties which require to be provided for a larger population. There are two points of view to be balanced in putting this idea forward; (1) the economy of size (including the economy of staff); and (2) accessibility for the patient. The hospital plan suggested hospitals of 600–800 beds serving a population of 100,000–150,000. It was thought that separate hospitals would continue for some long-stay cases and in some peripheral towns.

A recent report (Department of Health and Social Security, 1969a) has criticized some of these older views. It was suggested that two other factors were important – that long-stay patients required the facilities of the 'acute' hospital to be available to them, and such patients should be cared for by members of the professions also caring for more acute cases; and that consultant medical staff should not be expected to work in isolation from colleagues in the same specialty. It was therefore proposed that the hospitals should be larger and serve a population of 200,000–300,000 unless geographical problems were too great. Each hospital should include enough beds to supply the needs of all long-stay patients of the district. Even with these larger hospitals some specialties would not be represented in them because of the requirement that at least two consultants from each specialty should work in each hospital. Small hospitals in peripheral towns could be retained in a limited role.

The recommendations of this report would take time to implement for a number of reasons. The future pattern of services is under review and many hospital plans are in the process of development. Larger hospitals would require not only larger sites but accessible ones, and these are not easy to find in the expanding towns today.

CONSULTANTS

One of the major changes brought about by the N.H.S. has been in the distribution for consultants. Nevertheless there are still considerable differences between regions, which may be related to the number of beds available. From time to time difficulties arise as a result of imbalance between the number of consultants and the numbers in training. As a result, some who may be said to have finished their training do not obtain a consultant post. There are further difficulties in the delegation of work to junior staff and the availability of junior staff.

A working party (Department of Health and Social Security, 1969c) has looked at this problem, and put forward the idea of one permanent career grade of consultant who would undertake full responsibility for the clinical care of his patients. The implications of this, apparently, simple idea produced a storm of protest in the profession (Report, 1969a). The staffing structure of the hospital would require to be changed, with more consultant posts and fewer juniors. This implies that future consultants would be obliged to do work now thought suitable for juniors, and the same amount of private practice would have to be shared among more consultants.

Some of the hospital work could be carried out by general practitioners working in part-time posts (Oxford Regional Hospital Board, 1969). A small proportion of general practitioners already do so, but a considerable increase is sometimes envisaged. The main problem is whether they work in hospital caring for their own patients and being wholly responsible for them, or work as part of a team under the consultant.

MEDICAL EDUCATION

Today, many of those in general practice have worked in hospitals for years developing a skill in a particular specialty. They therefore have something to contribute to the working of a consultant-led team. They are also very well able, on their own, to look after patients with many conditions who are in hospital because they cannot be nursed at home. The Royal Commission on Medical Education (Report, 1968a) recommended changes which might affect this situation. After a more general education, newly qualified doctors would embark on general and special professional training orientated to a particular speciality — one of which would be general practice. At the end of the training they would be eligible to be placed on a specialist register. Only those on the appropriate register would be eligible for appointment as a consultant. The idea is that each specialty has appropriate knowledge, which can best be obtained by following a particular series of training posts. These implications for the staffing of the whole service are not entirely clear, and the idea of specialist registration has encountered a good deal of opposition within the profession.

'COGWHEEL'

The changes in the pattern of care in hospitals, envisaged in the last few sections, directs attention to the internal management problems involved. The need for effective management of these complex institutions is made more obvious by the high proportion — about two-thirds — of the total Health Service expenditure which they absorb, and by the evidence that there are big differences in efficiency between regions and between this country and others. Much has been written, for example, on differences in length of stay, and on the cost of treating cases (Forsyth, Thomas and Jones, 1970). Studies of this kind can demonstrate bottle-necks in operating theatres or laboratories which impede the smooth treatment of cases; but sometimes the problems are more obscure.

The need for a more integrated management structure in hospitals to overcome these problems was put forward in a report, now usually known as the Cogwheel Report, from the design on its cover, (Ministry of Health, 1967). This suggested that allied specialties within a hospital should be grouped in divisions, with the doctors concerned forming a group responsible for organizing the care of patients within their own division. Work within the hospital would be co-ordinated by an executive committee comprising the chairmen of the divisions. The chairman of the executive committee was envisaged as having a part-time management function for which he should be paid.

25

The need for medical management within a hospital, or hospital group, has not been accepted by all, and not many groups appear to have put these ideas into practice. One problem which has to be faced is the need for co-ordination with other groups within the hospital — for example, nurses and administrators. The nurses are developing their own management structure (*see* Chapter 5), and at least one hospital group has described a way in which this further integration may be carried out (Sleight, Spencer and Towler, 1970). The developing management structure within the hospital would fit fairly easily into the broader framework of the Area Health Authority.

SEEBOHM

One of the firm decisions already made in connection with the future of health and social services is that those services which do not have a large medical component will remain with the local authority and will be brought under the control of a Social Services Committee, and an appropriate staff under a Director of Social Services. This arrangement was suggested by the Seebohm Committee (Report, 1968b) and incorporated in a Bill introduced into Parliament early in 1970 (Local Authority Social Services Act 1970). Some of these services were previously run by Local Health Authorities, and division of the responsibilities for patient care will still remain. The welfare of the patient will depend on the administrative links and working arrangements which are developed in the future.

The Future

RELATIONS WITH LOCAL GOVERNMENT

The second Green Paper said unification was the first main objective of reorganization of the N.H.S. The proposals bring together many of the services which require predominantly medical skills, but there are two main areas where an arbitrary division has been made. Both concern relationships between the Area Health Authority and the new local authorities.

The first is in the environmental field, where the local authorities will have responsibility and employ certain kinds of staff (for example, public health inspectors) but will be expected to obtain medical advice from doctors employed by the Area Health Authority. These doctors may well spend all their time on such work, and their exact working relationships may take time to evolve. There is at least the danger that they will be out of the main stream of the Area Health Authority's work. It is also possible that the local authority could obtain medical advice from other sources. Divided responsibilities for the prevention and cure of communicable disease might also lead to difficulties between the authorities.

No doubt such problems will be quickly resolved when the two authorities are working together, but this may not be the case in the other difficult area which is in relation to the social services.

There are, at the moment, difficulties between the branches of the health services (mainly the hospitals and Local Health Authorities) in the care of aged or mentally disordered patients. These difficulties are not so much in professional practice, although this is affected, as in the provision of hostels and day centres. It is not always possible to plan the smooth transfer of patients to the type of accommodation best suited to their needs. Such facilities will remain with local authorities under the provisions of the Local Authority Social Services Act 1970 unless the patients need primarily the services of the health professions. Under the existing arrangements these services are provided by health or welfare or combined health and welfare departments of local authorities, either directly under the supervision and control of the Medical Officer of Health, or in circumstances where his advice can be easily obtained; there may be difficulties in seeking such advice from a doctor who is employed by a different authority. The existing division of responsibilities may be accentuated by a clear separation from the N.H.S., although there are cogent professional reasons for the proposal (Report, 1968b). The difficulties may be related more to policies, with regard to the provision of facilities, than to the differing professional outlooks. The separation may affect the continuity of care for the patient.

THE COMMUNITY PHYSICIAN

The term Community Physician has been increasingly used in the last 10 years to describe a doctor who is expected to have a broader outlook than the present Medical Officer of Health (Morris, 1969; McGregor, 1970; Gooding, Reid and Yule, 1970). Those who use the term do not always agree on what it stands for, and the second Green Paper proposed setting up a working party to look at the scope and nature of his work. There is, however, general agreement now that the 'community' concerned is not that part of medical work which takes place outside a hospital but all the health services provided for the population of an area.

He would thus be informed on the working of the health services in the area, and act as adviser to the Area Health Authority and the local authority – including the work now carried out by the Medical Officer of Health. In each area there may be a number of community physicians working on different aspects in this field and, as has been noted the chief administrative medical officer of the Area Health Authority would be responsible for the planning, provision and use of the services.

This type of skill is limited, at the moment, to the Local Health Authorities and the Regional Hospital Boards, and a big deficiency is its absence at hospital level (Morrison, 1967). This would be available under the Green Paper proposals. One of the criticisms of both Green Papers made by the medical profession was that the chief administrative officer of the proposed Area Health Authority would not necessarily be medically qualified. The important need of the Health Service is for managerial capacity rather than the predominance of any one of professions making a contribution, and it may be that co-ordination of the many activities of the Area Health Authority will benefit by a trained administrator rather than someone whose primary skills are those of a doctor, nurse, or engineer.

FINANCE

Expenditure on the N.H.S. has been rising steadily, and is planned to reach £2,002 million by 1972 (Public Expenditure, 1969). This represents 5 per cent of the gross national product, and is felt to be not enough. Of this money 85 per cent is provided by general taxation or rates, and there is some agreement that the level of taxation could not be raised – despite the fact that we are by no means the highest taxed nation in the world; nor do we spend the highest proportion of our resources on health; and it would be possible to reallocate the money raised by taxes among the various competing interests.

Other sources of revenue have been explored. One of these – increased charges by patients using the service – has been rejected on the grounds that it would be difficult to raise as much as an extra 10 per cent in this way (Crossman, 1969). Another source suggested has been the increased reliance on private insurance schemes. In the last few years these have become an important part of the health scene; about 800,000 people are thought to be registered as members. Crossman (1969) put it bluntly when he said that such schemes buy a name and buy time, add nothing in terms of skill and resources, and introduce two standards into the Health Service.

The British Medical Association (1970) commissioned a report from an advisory panel which strongly supported the use of voluntary insurance schemes to provide the extra £500 million needed to make the services adequate for the time being. It suggested that certain expenditure for long-term patients, preventive medicine, education, research and all capital expenditure should come from taxation, and that the cost of general medical and hospital care should come from insurance contributions. The schemes would be of two kinds, compulsory and voluntary (with higher premiums), into which the insured person could opt. All would have to be insured, but those voluntarily paying a higher rate would be taking an opportunity of increasing the amount of benefit.

This explicit provision of two standards of care is defended on the grounds that any claim that there is now equality is an illusion. Two levels of contribution presume that those paying are able to judge the standard being provided. It is by no means certain that this is true as far as health is concerned. The administration of such a scheme would be complex and probably cumbersome.

EXPECTATIONS

Some of the increasing costs of the health services are due to general inflation, some to equalization of services within the country, some to an increased proportionate rise in salaries and costs within the Service compared with those outside, but much of it is due to the increased complexity of the medical care provided and the increased expectations of patients.

These expectations include not only that a doctor be available for fairly minor conditions, but that appropriate investigation and treatment be available for all. The standards thought to be appropriate are steadily becoming higher nor is this all. The provision of expensive services is not solely the result of demand, but itself creates a demand. This has been seen in the provision of intermittent dialysis for patients with kidney disease. It has been suggested (Leach, 1970) that the community must face up to the problem and decide, perhaps as a result of some advanced cost-benefit analysis, what it is able to provide for all, and what it cannot provide with the present limited staff, resources and money.

Training

The three branches of the Health Service have gradually come to realize the importance of training for all types of staff employed in an administrative capacity. Those working in the central Department are civil servants, and those working in the Local Health Authorities are local government employees. Both participate in the appropriate general training and promotional schemes. In the hospital service schemes for lay administration have been developed over the last 10–12 years, and allied with appropriate courses.

The situation is different for those coming to administration from professional fields. Medical Officers of Health must have special training, and the courses for the Diploma in Public Health have recently been concerned with all the health problems of an area, and with techniques of management. Doctors working in the administration of hospitals or the central Department need not have any special training, although some have a Diploma in Public Health. Nurses, too, are now having special courses provided and appropriate training given (Chapter 5).

Great changes in the administrative structure of the services, such as those proposed, will throw a great strain on those involved in planning the change. There are very few people who are conversant with the problems of all three branches which are to be integrated, and perhaps fewer still who.have been trained to look at the health problems of a community as a whole. Despite frequent statements to the contrary, the number of people involved in administrating the health services is small in relation to the expenditure and activity involved.

What is required as an urgent priority is the establishment of an organizational structure and training programme for the proposed new Area Health Authorities, and much more realization that team-work is needed. The King Edward Fund has run joint professional courses of the kind envisaged, but these are needed at all levels if the ideals of the second Green Paper are to be realized. 'Both the members and the officers must view the service which they are administering as an integrated service, and base their plans upon the total health needs of the patients for whom the services are provided and of the communities in which they are providing them'.

References

Anderson, J.A.D. (1969). 'The Health Team in the Community.' *Lancet* 2, 679

British Medical Association (1970). *Report of an Advisory Panel on Health Services Financing.* London; H.M.S.O. (Summary appears in *Br. med. J. suppl.* (1970) 2, 86)

Crossman, R.H.S. (1969). *Paying for the Social Services.* (Fabian Tract 399.) London; Fabian Society

Curwen, M. and Brookes, B. (1969). 'Health Centres: Facts and Figures.' *Lancet* **2**, 945

Department of Health and Social Security (1969a). *Report of the Committee on the Functions of the District General Hospital.* (Central Health Services Council.) London; H.M.S.O.

— (1969b). *Report of the Committee of Inquiry into Allegations of Ill-treatment of Patients and Other Irregularities at the Ely Hospital, Cardiff.* London; H.M.S.O.

— (1969c). *Report of the Working Party on the Responsibilities of the Consultant Grade.* London; H.M.S.O.

— (1970). *The Future Structure of the National Health Service.* London; H.M.S.O.

Forsyth, G., Thomas, R.G. and Jones, S.P. (1970). 'Planning in Practice.' In *Problems and Progress in Medical Care.* (Fourth Series.) Ed. by G. McLachlan. Oxford; University Press for Nuffield Provincial Hospitals Trust, London

Gooding, D.G., Reid, J.J.A. and Yule, I.G. (1970). 'The Community Physician's Work.' *Lancet* **1**, 711

Leach, G. (1970). *The Biocrats.* London; Cape

McGregor, A. (1970). 'The Community Physician.' *Med. Offr.* **123**, 95

Ministry of Health (1959). *Report of the Maternity Services Committee.* London; H.M.S.O.

— (1962). *The Hospital Plan for England and Wales.* Cmnd. 1604. London; H.M.S.O.

— (1963). *Health and Welfare: the Development of Community Care.* Cmnd. 1973. London; H.M.S.O.

— (1964). *Health and Welfare: the Development of Community Care.* Revision to 1973–74. London; H.M.S.O.

— (1966a). *The Hospital Building Programme:* a Revision of the *Hospital Plan for England and Wales.* Cmnd. 3000. London; H.M.S.O.

— (1966b). *Health and Welfare: the Development of Community Care.* Revision to 1975–76. Cmnd. 3022. London; H.M.S.O.

— (1967). *First Report of the Joint Working Party on Organization of Medical Work in Hospitals.* London; H.M.S.O.

— (1968). *The Administrative Structure of the Medical and Related Services in England and Wales.* London; H.M.S.O.

Morris, J.N. (1969). 'Tomorrow's Community Physician.' *Lancet* **2**, 811

Morrison, S.L. (1967). 'Social Medicine and Management.' *Lancet* **2**, 1295

Owen, D. (Ed.) (1968). *A Unified Health Service.* Oxford; Pergamon Press

Oxford Regional Hospital Board (1969). *The General Practitioner and the Hospital Service in the 1970s*

Public Expenditure (1969). Report covering period 1968–69 to 1973–74 Cmnd. 4234. London; H.M.S.O.

Reform of Local Government in England (1970). Cmnd. 4276. London; H.M.S.O.

Report (1942). *Social Insurance and Allied Services* (by Sir William Beveridge). Cmd. 6404. London; H.M.S.O.

– (1956). *The Committee of Inquiry into the Cost of the National Health Service*. Cmd. 9663. London; H.M.S.O.

– (1964). *A Review of the Medical Services of Great Britain*. London; Social Assay.

– (1968a). *The Royal Commission on Medical Education 1965–68*. Cmnd. 3569. London; H.M.S.O.

– (1968b) *The Committee on Local Authority and Allied Personal Social Services*. Cmnd. 3703. London; H.M.S.O.

– (1969a). Meeting of the Central Committee for Hospital Medical Services. *Br. med. J. suppl.* **4**, 77

– (1969b). *The Royal Commission on Local Government in England, 1966–1969*. (Volume 1.) Cmnd. 4040. London; H.M.S.O.

Sleight, P., Spencer, J.A. and Towler, E.W. (1970). 'Oxford and McKinsey: Cogwheel and Beyond.' *Br. med. J.* **1**, 682

3—The Medical Practitioner and Management

R.M. Pollock

Management and Administration

The use of both terms management and administration in the title of this section is not tautology; it underlines that there is a fundamental difference between these two activities, which it is essential to recognize in defining the role of doctors in the management of the Health Service. To define management itself is a substantial task which would require a chapter of its own to do it justice, and there are in common use a number of differing formal definitions of the word. Nevertheless, no matter what definition is accepted, it is recognized as a cyclical pattern of interrelated activities, which conventionally are categorized as **planning, motivation, innovation and control**. These functions, and the techniques which contribute to them, comprise the mechanisms by which a group of people decide what they are going to do and how they are going to do it (Draper, 1970). In some circumstances implementation of management decisions is in the hands of those who make them, and in such cases the terms manager and administrator are synonymous. In most instances, however, the implementation of management decisions is in the hands of people other than those responsible for making them; that is of administrators. It is in recognizing this that we, *pari passu,* recognize the importance of communication in effective management, for management must not only be convinced of what it wants to do it must also convey the desired effect to all those who are part of the operation (Falk, 1970). In the N.H.S. it is particularly critical to clarify this difference between policy making and management on the one hand and administration on the other, for we see it to be important that doctors are involved in policy making and yet, because of the scarcity of medical manpower resources, we wish to spare them where possible from assuming tasks which will sever them from their clinical responsibilities. Indeed, until relatively recently, doctors themselves have been extremely reluctant to enter the management arena. 'We are clinicians not managers,' was a frequently expressed attitude. However, the recognition that Health Services management is largely concerned with the allocation and use of resources, and that every clinical decision has effects such as the disposition of people and things and the expenditure of money (that is, the use of resources), has accelerated the readiness of clinicians to involve themselves in the management of these services. This commitment to managerial decision making is especially important because of the key position clinicians hold in the Service. As the result of this commitment by clinicians the likely effectiveness of implementation of decisions is increased. It cannot be too strongly emphasized that involvement of medical men in management and decision making should not be seen as the exclusive preserve of the professional medical administrator, but that it necessarily involves all clinicians.

THE DOCTOR AS MANAGER

We can usefully consider separately the role of the doctor as manager and administrator at a number of different levels within the Health Service, and in doing this it is convenient to consider principally the hospital service, as it is the part of the Health Service which has the most complex organizational pattern and which absorbs the majority of the resources of the service, but the conclusions are equally applicable to all branches of the service.

It would be all too easy to discard from the consideration of medical involvement in management any consideration of management at the level of the individual patient and yet, as we have already indicated, it is at this level that decisions are taken which may have far reaching consequences on the use of resources. The individual clinician has responsibility to his patient to give him the best possible care, and the traditional training of the clinician teaches him to do this without respect for cost-benefit considerations. Increasingly, however, the clinician is coming to recognize his responsibilities to the organization, whether it be his department or hospital, to ensure that he is not

34

profligate with the use of its resources, and he is now having to recognize the effect which the clinical decisions he makes about an individual patient may have on the availability of resources for the treatment of other patients, both his own and those of his colleagues. In addition, the management role of the individual clinician must embrace his responsibility to train and to teach his subordinates, to assess their performance, and to counsel them on their progress and prospects.

The association of numbers of individual clinicians produces the second level of management, at departmental level, or at the level of divisions of like clinical disciplines such as proposed in the Cogwheel Report. The problems posed at this level are more complex and so the management information and management skills required are necessarily more sophisticated. At this level we can begin to see where benefit is to be derived by the separation of management decision making from the administrative implementation of the decision. The Cogwheel Report illustrates this by reference to the surgical disciplines. Here the aggregation of different surgical disciplines into a division of surgery forms a group with common interests and common problems, the solution to many of which can be achieved without involving the whole hospital system. Thus the operating theatres are used in common by all the surgical disciplines, and the problems of staffing, timetabling of operating lists and engineering maintenance, are common to all members of the division. The management policies for operating theatres must be determined by the clinicians who form the division, and in these circumstances they are acting as medical managers. But the implementation of their policy need not involve them, and it would indeed be a waste of their time and skill if it did so. It is, as the Cogwheel Report phrases it, 'the stuff of general administration' (Report, 1967a).

EXISTING ORGANIZATIONAL PATTERNS

The form of organizational patterns for departments and divisions is inextricably bound up with the organizational structure which is selected for the whole hospital or group, so that consideration of possible alternative patterns for these levels can be given together. But before turning to an examination of alternative patterns of organization it is appropriate to review the existing pattern. Hospitals are organized under three heads, medical, nursing and administrative; of these, the nursing and administrative channels have hierarchical patterns; the medical channel, by contrast, is a non-hierarchical association of equals. This has been the pattern hitherto in the hospital organization in which medical policy is supposed to evolve as the consensus view of the medical staff expressed through medical staff committees or medical advisory committees. The more recent trend in the organization of medical work in hospitals has been to formalize the medical representative arrangements, and in effect create a hierarchical pattern within this sphere in parallel with those existing within nursing and administration. While the various proposed changes are more or less effective in doing this, they do nothing to affect the position at the point where the three channels, medical nursing and administrative, converge. This failure underlines further that management at this level is by an ill-defined coalition between the chief officers, without any definition of where executive responsibility lies. The deficiences inherent in this system of 'fractured management' have long been recognized, and both the King's Fund Working Party on the Future Pattern of Management (Report, 1967b) and the Farquharson–Lang Report (Scottish Home and Health Department, 1966) proposed to solve the problem by the creation of a new role of general manager, who would be the chief executive of the group and to whom all three hierarchies would be responsible. The analogy with the chief executive officer of local authorities and of commercial organizations is evident. Certainly the most obvious and startling fact which emerges when beginning a study of hospital management organizations is that there is no individual who is responsible for that organization, and that there is no *single* position where one can seek answers on the performance of that organization. The conventional answer to this criticism is that the group itself is the management. But because of the fragmentation of responsibility at lower level it is not uncommon to see the group committee operating in an administrative capacity and acting to put into effect the consequences of its policy decisions. Group committees (Hospital Management Committees and Boards of Governors) are served by loyal and industrious people, but is evident that their skills, and the time they are able to devote to this work are not sufficient to do this task efficiently.

PROBLEMS OF THE GENERAL MANAGER ROLE

Is then the creation of a general manager the solution to the problem? In purely organizational terms there is a good deal of evidence to suggest that it probably is. Nevertheless two difficulties in this solution are evident. One may be only transient, but the other is likely to be long-term. The first is the acceptability of a general manager at this time to the three channels of hospital activity, each of which has operated autonomously, and in which there would probably be reluctance to give up their freedom. While it is evident that there would be immediate difficulties in overcoming this attitude, it is also clearly likely that this problem would disappear with the emergence of candidates of the appropriate calibre. The second, more persistant problem is that in establishing a general manager role we must seek an individual who is knowledgeable across the range of medical, nursing and administrative activities (and has a considerable depth of knowledge in some of these areas) who is skilled in management matters, and who is capable of formulating new lines of policy. These assets clearly do exist to some extent, or can be evolved; but we may ask whether there are sufficient persons of the requisite degree of skill to fill this role within the present pattern of organization, and more so with the revisions in the organizational structure such as were proposed in the Green Papers (1970a and 1970b). Further, given the large number of managers which would be required are we prepared to pay adequate salaries, bearing in mind that the qualities demanded are likely to obtain, in other spheres, salaries of an altogether higher order than those available now to our chief administrators, both medical and lay. If, for either of these reasons, we are unable at present to create a new role of general manager, how are we to overcome the problem of the fractured management situation? In answering this it would be useful to look first at the proposals outlined in the Cogwheel Report. These recommend the formation of a medical executive committee formed by the chairmen of Clinical Divisions, with the Chairman of the Medical Executive (that is, the chairman of chairmen) as the medical voice on the managing committee of the group (Hospital Management Committee or Board of Governors). The major weakness of these proposals is that a medical executive committee so constructed is not in the fullest sense executive but simply advisory, for while the Cogwheel proposals will in effect be creating a system which formalizes the flow of medical advice, they do nothing to co-ordinate the three channels of activity, and would not contribute to filling the general manager void. A limited degree of executive activity is of course envisaged, and has been outlined in the example from the report quoted earlier in which it is seen that the aim is to create a forum for decisions at limited levels, as in the example at division level. The weakness of the proposals is that there is no indication of what executive authority divisions would have to impose their decisions and, further, there is no sanction apparent which would be available if the decisions were disregarded.

AN ALTERNATIVE TO THE GENERAL MANAGER ROLE

The committee structure which has been evolved at the United Oxford Hospitals following the study of the organization by McKinsey and Company does, however, present a solution to the fractured management problem and to the difficulties of filling the general manager role. The Oxford pattern is, in a simplified form, as follows. Apart from the Board itself and the statutorily necessary Finance Committee, all other committees have been disbanded and replaced by a single Executive Committee to which the Board has delegated the executive authority for running the group. The entire clinical medical organization is grouped into three sections – medicine, surgery and laboratory medicine. Each section elects a chairman by secret ballot and these three, together with the chairman of the Medical Staff Council (the entire consultant medical staff) who is also elected by secret ballot, comprise the medical representation on the Executive Committee. These four medical personnel are paired with four lay members of the Board: the Chairman; the Vice-chiarman; the Chairman of the Finance Committee; and one other, preferably a woman, with an interest in nursing affairs. The committee is completed by the three chief officers – the administrator, the treasurer and chief nursing officer.

It will at once be apparent that, by virtue of their membership of the Executive Committee, the elected medical chairmen form not only a truly executive medical group, but one which cannot fall into the trap of offering medical advice unconstrained by financial or other administrative considerations. The most outstanding feature of the Executive Committee, however, is that it acts as a corporate general manager, and in so doing unifies the otherwise disparate medical, nursing and lay administrative channels. Furthermore, the fact that the chairman of each section has to be elected by a ballot, requiring more than half the membership of the section to support him, ensures clear support for executive action within and on behalf of the section.

Within this almost federal system the work of the sections is aided by the appointment of section administrators. Although, as yet, the full section mechanism has not come into action, the sanction so markedly lacking in other proposals for control of the newly created medical hierarchy appears to exist in the Oxford structure. It is intended that each of the sections shall be allocated its own budget, and will be responsible for operating it. The sections themselves, therefore, can be either rewarded or penalized in subsequent allocations of funds. In this way there is an incentive for clinicians to conform with the pattern which their elected organization has decided upon, and there is a stick with which to beat those who do not conform.

This system, we believe, is an effective way of creating medical managerial input into hospital group management. It also fills, at this stage, the apparently unfillable role of general manager. Whether it will totally obviate the need for a general manager is a matter that time and the operation of the system will determine. Ideally, however, it should eliminate the need for a full-time medical adviser or medical administrator at this level. Whether it can do so will ultimately depend on the demands the system makes on the clinicians who assume this executive role part-time, and the relief which good administrative support can give them.

It would be most desirable if this formation could release administrators to operate on a wider scale at regional and national levels, for it seems unlikely that there will ever be sufficient medical administrators at every level. Changes in the organizational pattern resulting in the creation of a number of units of a size midway between groups and regions – as foreshadowed in the Green Paper proposals – might, initially at any rate, require full-time medical administrative effort. But, management training of the clinicians who can undertake an executive role advances, the need for a purely medical administrative position at this level should decline.

One of the criticisms levelled at this system has been that it creates an organizational difficulty in that the chairman of the sections are representative of their sections and yet, as employees of the Board, must themselves be subject to the decisions that the Board's executive committee make. These two situations are not irreconcilable, for this is after all the pattern of Parliamentary government. Members of Parliament are elected as constituency representatives, and themselves select some of their number to form an executive committee, the Cabinet, from whose decisions they are not exempt.

A more general involvement of doctors at unit and group level in medical management should, if successful, markedly diminish or eliminate the need for full-time medical administrative commit·nent. But at regional and national level there is a continuing and increasing need for specialist medical administrative skills (although, from a consideration of their activities, these roles would be more accurately described as medical managers).

THE SPECIALIST MEDICAL ADMINISTRATOR

The role of the medical administrator is described briefly as 'the organization of medical services'. Clearly this description embraces activities undertaken by both individual clinicians and organizations at section and group level. What is it then which distinguishes the role of the medical administrator at regional and national level? It is the span and the scale of his activities. Basically, of course, the problems at these levels are similar to those further down the organization. They revolve chiefly around the determination of objectives, and the conservation and allocation of resources. The optimum scale for the determination of decisions in certain fields is, however, very large. Thus, for instance, while discussions about the allocation of manpower resources may properly be the concern of group and section management organizations, their decisions and those of regional authorities must necessarily be made within the framework of a national policy. Many relevant facts will have gone into the making of a national policy, such as the total availability of doctors, the rate of creation of new doctors, the rate of wastage, the distribution of doctors and specialties, as well as evaluations of factors such as population trends and morbidity patterns.

It is a self-evident feature of decision making at regional level and above that, as in the above examples, it involves the collection and assessment of a large amount of complex information. All the principle problems to be encountered at these levels — the provision and planning of hospital facilities, both new and existing; the allocation of manpower and financial resources; the development of new trends in the services — require a vast amount of data to assess needs and estimate requirements. The role of the medical administrator at these levels is, therefore, principally concerned with acquiring the appropriate information, assessing it, devising policies on that assessment, and considering the various options available to implement the chosen policy within existing constraints. To do this he must be skilled in management techniques, in statistics, and in epidemiology. He must also be able to co-ordinate the results of these various studies and communicate them to his clinical colleagues. It is obvious that it is useless to devise well constructed plans on the basis of sound information if the desirability of the proposals, their benefits, and the conditions for their achievement, are not communicated to the clinicians and others who must by their actions bring them about, and if the full and willing co-operation of clinicians is not obtained. An important part, therefore, of the role of the regional or national medical administrator lies in co-ordination and co-operation with, and persuasion of, his clinical colleagues.

It is vital also that management at this level should concern itself with innovation. We should be concerned that such a mammoth organization as the N.H.S. should not become paralysed, and that its activities should not become sanctioned by custom, so that it is incapable of reacting flexibly to challenges from unexpected directions. Any organization which matures solely by acquiring more firmly established ways of doing things is heading for stagnation. What is important is to ensure that there is a maturing framework within which continuous innovation and renewal can occur. Development, the assessment of the services being given, and the specification of desirable change (Kogan, 1970), is the essential function of a living organization. Clearly, boards and committees carry a responsibility to be ready to meet new challenges, but it is an important special role of the medical manager to have anticipated changing circumstances and to have initiated innovations to take account of them. From this basis, he must be in a position to advise his board comprehensively on the appropriate courses of action.

Many of the skills described as being necessary for the medical administrator are ones which are equally requisite for the lay administrator. It may be asked, therefore, whether there is some special requirement for medical skills in this role. This is a question about which it is foolish to be dogmatic for, when individual situations are examined, it is often difficult to highlight a particular one which could not be dealt with by a lay administrator and which specifically demands a medical man. Nevertheless, some desirable consequences do flow from the commitment of doctors in this role. Co-ordination with, and persuasion of, clinical colleagues is certainly facilitated by an intimate knowledge of the problems they will face in implementing a proposed policy, and an appreciation that proposals for change are made with the real knowledge of the background against which they must be set certainly increases the likelihood of their being accepted.

TRAINING OF THE MEDICAL ADMINISTRATOR

What should then predominate in the training of the medical administrator? Firstly, and of profound importantance, he should be a good clinician with a depth of experience in medicine, preferably in one of the major specialties. He should not, therefore, be seeking to enter medical administration too early in his career - certainly not until he has acquired a sufficient depth of experience of his clinical field in the registrar grade. In this grade he will acquire some knowledge of the problems of medical management at firm and section level. His early formal management training should embrace experience of management problems at the hospital and group level, and later at regional and national level. He must also acquire familiarity with the tools of his trade through a study of statistics, operational research methods, and epidemiology. As a manager he must be fully conversant with organizational theory and management techniques. Some of this education will be acquired by in-service training, but it will also require a substantial period of full-time study and research, which should lead to a higher degree in the specialty.

A programme of training along these lines is being introduced experimentally at Oxford where the Regional Hospital Board and the Board of Governors, together with the University, have set up a four-year senior registrar training programme. The first year in a hospital admissions officer role, and as a lecturer in the Department of the Regius Professor of Medicine, allows the interested young clinician to become involved in medical management in a way which does not inevitably commit him to specializing in that field. If he does not do so, his training will be valuable to him in his division or group management role; if he does go on in the specialty his second year of training will continue his lectureship and also place him in a number of training situations with the Regional Hospital Board. Subsequently, in the third and fourth years he will undertake full-time study and research on the course being organized by the London School of Hygeine and Tropical Medicine, leading eventually to an M.Sc. degree.

Management Techniques

A short synopsis of some of the simpler management techniques may be an appropriate ending to this section. This clearly cannot in any way be exhaustive, and this chapter does no more than point the way to those techniques which the clinician, as manager at hospital or firm level, will find helpful in defining and solving his problems. It should give some appreciation of the management tools which are applicable in this field.

In the interests of brevity it will be convenient to consider techniques as they are appropriate to the identifiable phases of the management process, that is, planning, motivation, innovation and control.

PLANNING

Trend chart

This is a simple graphic display which is useful in measuring change and in bringing attention to bear on relevant parts of a large problem. A common example of the planning trend chart is the standard type of waiting list graph. (*Figure 3.1*).

The total waiting list, though showing an upward trend, is relatively steady. This overall picture, however, conceals that the three individual disciplines, which form the bulk of the waiting list, are performing in quite different ways. But for the steadily decreasing gynaecology numbers, the rising trend in the total waiting list would be much more marked because of the sharp rises in ear, nose and throat cases, and surgery.

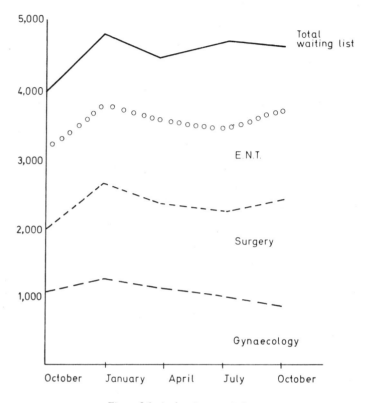

Figure 3.1. A planning trend chart

The 80/20 chart

The 80/20 chart is a useful technique based on the observation that in a complex situation causes and effects are not usually of a comparable magnitude. Thus a very large expenditure of effort does not necessarily produce a very large change. The name of the technique is derived from the observation that about 20 per cent of the total effort usually results in about 80 per cent of the resulting change. In practice, these proportions are rarely quite so precise.

Figure 3.2 is an 80/20 chart used in an investigation into prescribing costs. It is seen that only 8 per cent of the prescribers account for 70 per cent of the costs. In an attempt to reduce costs, therefore, it would be likely that the impact of an examination of the practices of the 8 per cent would yield better results than the dissipation of effort over the remaining 92 per cent who, together, account for only a small proportion of the total cost.

Number of
prescribers
(150)

Cost of
prescriptions
(£10,000)

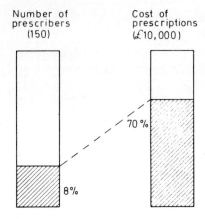

70 %

8%

Figure 3.2. The 80/20 chart

Sensitivity analysis technique

The sensitivity analysis technique allows the manager to assess the comparative effects of proposed changes. Its value again lies in concentrating his attention on areas of greatest pay-off. From such an analysis (Table 3.1) the determination of the effects of a change become

TABLE 3.1

Sensitivity Analysis Technique

Factors to be considered	Possible percentage reduction	Effect of change (saving)
Reduction in staff	5	£50,000
Reduce expenditure on drugs	8	£35,000
Reduce pathology tests	12	£30,000

clear and the choice between options is facilitated. Here, if it were possible to select only one course in pursuance of economy one would choose the first. It is noteworthy that a very much larger and possibly more restricting change in pathology tests is seen to have a substantially smaller effect, an observation which might not have been so apparent without the application of a sensitivity analysis.

Analysis of differences

As an example *Figure 3.3* shows the analysis of differences technique applied to the comparative lengths of stay of patients with a particular condition in a number of hospitals. Analyses of this kind would probably

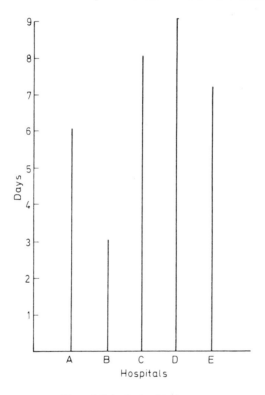

Figure 3.3 Analysis of differences

lead the medical manager to investigate more deeply the reasons for the large difference in performance between hospital B and hospital D. It should be emphasized that the sensitivity analysis itself allows no judgement such as that hospital D is less efficient than hospital B. Factors may exist which fully explain the observed difference, but all this technique does is draw attention to the need for further scrutiny.

Motivation

Two simple techniques which aid motivation are the organization chart and the job description. The organization chart may be so simple a device as hardly to merit the description technique at all, yet it is of unique value in relating the individual in the organization and in graphically displaying his organizational relationships with superiors, subordinates and collaterals. The job description, by clarifying to the individual the purpose and scope of his job, allows him to identify himself more closely with objectives, and thus motivates him to carry out his job more effectively. It should contain a list of the principal duties of the post, a statement of the working relationships of the post, and an account of how the holder's performance will be assessed. The job description should be fully discussed and agreed by the holder of the job and, ideally, he should write the final version himself.

Innovation

Converting a decision into effective action requires that the responsibilities of each of the individuals who will be involved be defined and that a timetable of implementation be drawn up.

TABLE 3.2

Implementation chart

Main tasks	Responsibility	April	May	June	July	Aug.
Identify remaining problems in transferring children to Ward 4	Planning officer	—				
Resolve these with (1) Paediatricians (2) Principal Nurse	Planning officer	—	—			
Liaise with architects over alterations and finalization of drawings	Assistant secretary			—		
Preparation of Bills of Quantity	Quantity surveyors				—	

An implementation chart (Table 3.2) can be quite simple, but it should list each of the activities to be undertaken, the persons responsible for undertaking them, and the timetable for completion.

The procedure having been implemented, the chart becomes an instrument of control allowing measurement of success or failure in achieving established targets.

Control

A further useful control technique is the performance measurement chart.

In Table 3.3 is seen a measure of the performance in accepting patients for out-patient appointment with three degrees of urgency as measured by the general practitioner. Most consultants achieve the desired objective but consultant D is failing to satisfy the desired standard. Again it should be noted that there is no indication from this technique why his performance is below the aimed-for standard. That would have to be the subject of a further investigation, and the establishment of a new action programme.

TABLE 3.3

Performance Measurement Chart

Consultant	Number of days between requesting and being given appointment		
	3–4 days	10–14 days	14 + days
A	5	18	28
B	3	16	21
C	1	8	28
D	7	56	120
E	3	15	50

References

Draper, P. (1970). 'The Development of Management and Participation.' in The N.H.S., Three Views. London; Fabian Society

Falk, R. (1970). The Business of Management. Harmondsworth; Penguin

Green Paper (1970a). *The Administrative Structure of the Medical and Related Services in England and Wales.* London; H.M.S.O.
— (1970b). *The Future of the N.H.S.* London; H.M.S.O.
Kogan, M. (1970). 'Hospital Management and Administration.' In *The N.H.S., Three Views.* London; Fabian Society
Report (1967a). *The First Report of the Joint Working Party in the Organisation of Medical Work in Hospitals.* London; H.M.S.O.
— (1967b). *The Shape of Management in the 1980's.* London; King's Fund and Institute of Hospital Administrators
Scottish Home and Health Department (1966). *The Administrative Practice of Hospital Boards in Scotland.* Edinburgh; H.M.S.O.

4—Role of the Community Physician within the Health Services

H.P. Ferrer

Introduction

The public health service has a long and honourable history of adaptation to change. The most recent demand that has been made upon it is that of transmuting or, rather, evolving the medical officer of health into the community physician. The role of the community physician, however, has so far not been defined, but one of the major contributions he can make towards the management of the health services will undoubtedly be concerned with the monitoring of community need.

The position at present puts him in a unique position to be sensitive to this community need because he is concerned with many community services. Not only would he have to look at the demands made upon the hospital services within the area, but he would also be in a position to assess the needs of the community in relationship to the prevalence and incidence of disease within it.

Sensitive areas

The two areas in which disease can occur most insidiously, and which require continuous monitoring, are those of community paediatrics and old age. Both these groups have certain factors in common. They

49

are less likely to present themselves when something is wrong which could, by early intervention, have been alleviated with the appropriate treatment. With the right kind of organization both groups are available for continuous monitoring. In particular, the child health service have had long experience of systematic examination of the child from the moment of birth. Parallel methods could be used on the elderly population with the reservation that this is a more delicate operation requiring some degree of tact in the approach to otherwise well elderly persons.

Community Paediatrics

A complete reorganization of the present tripartite system has already been initiated in many areas where the general practitioner, community services and hospital specialist paediatric services are working in much closer co-operation than was the case a few years ago. The community physician has a unique opportunity of bringing his expertise in the field to help in the compilation of adequate peadiatric records. However, despite fears of confidentiality of such centrally based records the undoubted benefit in the paediatric field of systematic and centralized records is widely recognized.

The West Sussex scheme, in particular, has shown how it is possible to bring back children for routine immunization procedures. It is a short step involving some degree of reorganization to bring the child back at the same time for continuous assessment of his development. Although large areas will undoubtedly need the aids that the electronic computer can bring, many centralized records for smaller areas can be carried out using appropriate card indexing systems. The central record may consist of the following, either separately or in combination.

(1)   A call/re-call follow-up system, which brings the child back at certain agreed intervals for immunization and/or developmental assessment.

(2)   A paediatric record of the child's progress in health and disease which brings together all the information available from the general practitioner, community services and the consultant paediatrician.

VULNERABLE CHILDREN

Much has been written about the concept of the 'at risk' child. There is little doubt that the administrative system for implementing this invaluable concept is, in many cases, imperfect. The quality of history available from obstetric sources is not yet geared to the quality of child that may be produced at the end of a sequence of events between conception and final discharge from hospital. Even were it possible to assess accurately the degree of disorder during the pre- and perinatal and postnatal periods which are required to produce a discernible impairment in the child's development, there are still considerable administrative problems in bringing together the appropriate records which will guide in prospect those children selected for careful monitoring.

DYNAMIC AT RISK REGISTERS

It has been thought that it is more useful to consider those children at risk of handicapping conditions as those who consistently fail to match up to the performance – social, psychological or physical – of the rest of their fellows during the first two years of life. Continuous developmental assessment during the first two years of life can clearly show whether a child is matching up to those children who otherwise are meeting the performance that is expected in a similar age-structured group. Much more detailed assessment is needed to assess how this performance is affected by social class, parity of the mother, position in the family, mother's education and so on. All that such a system can do at present is bring to light those children who for any reason are failing to match the performance of their fellows. The assessment of the reasons for this failure in performance can then be carried out in a diagnostic situation. This is the kind of process the administrative outline for which was considered in a report on child welfare centres.* Unfortunately, there is still a delay in the setting up of regional diagnostic centres.

This kind of continuous monitoring of the child in the first two years of life can provide valuable information, not only for the health services but also for the associated services primarily concerned with education and other aspects of welfare. As an example, spina bifida used to be a usually fatal condition in the first months of life. Modern treatment has changed the pattern, and many children affected by this condition are now surviving to school age and beyond. Rather than taking a short-term expediency, by which provision for their health and education was discussed when the need arose, a continuous child monitoring system such as that outlined above could have provided early warning of what was needed in terms of facilities within the health and education services. Other examples may be quoted but this kind of continuous monitoring has enormous implications when it comes to spotting early outbreaks of congenital defects and deformities. Although there is at present a system of notification of these defects which is monitored

*Sheldon (1967) Report on Child Welfare Centres. London; H.M.S.O.

centrally, minor defects are not readily noticed at birth, and may only become apparent during the first two years of life. This type of defect can have equally serious implications for the child. A scheme of examination is suggested here as being a practical means by which the health of the child can be continuously assessed. Those who are consistently failing to meet the norms of the group could, of course, be piloted in a sub-system which included more frequent examination or more specialized intervention.

The Community Physician and the Elderly

Problems of the aged population present the health services with one of the major challenges of the present time. Unfortunately, medical training in the past has tended to concentrate mainly on the exciting clinical manifestations of disease. The manifestations of chronic and insidious disease have received less attention, and at times the practitioner may find that his training and management of these cases is outside the scope of the medical practice for which he was prepared. There is little doubt, however, that the continuous monitoring of the aged population can provide detection of what are apparently insidious conditions which could, by their presence in such a population, result in serious demands being made upon the health services. An effective monitoring system could possibly have prevented such a deterioration. The monitoring of aged persons in their homes is at once essential and delicate. The able-bodied aged person who is able to attend his medical practitioner, or other types of screening clinic, is often the one in least need of the care of the community services. In the past, the setting up of a community monitoring system has taxed many medical officers of health who have more or less successfully walked a tightrope between unnecessary interference and effective health monitoring of the aged.

More research is probably needed at the present time to find those elderly persons who are in need of special observation. It is, however, on the at risk aged person that the majority of the community services should be concentrated. It is generally agreed that the following can constitute the basis of an at risk group in the aged population.

(1) The recently bereaved.

(2) Those recently discharged from hospital.

(3) Those living alone: this group can be sub-divided into those who are effectively monitored by family and friends, and those who have no other social contact.

(4) Those with a medical and/or social history.

(5) The obese.

(6) Those who have had difficulties with walking, or with feet.

Other categories may be included, but the foregoing would seem to those who are most at risk of handicapping and permanent disability.

The setting up of an effective monitoring system would involve much more co-operation between the various services responsible for the aged than has hitherto been found in most areas. It is extremely difficult at times to define the aged population, and sometimes even more difficult to get the information which would lead one to place an aged person in the at risk categories mentioned above. However, the community physician has an undoubted part to play in this system of monitoring, not only as a means of secondary and tertiary prevention but also as a means of finding out the changing balance in the aged in their demands for hospital and other health service care. So far there has been little published work on the morbidity patterns in the aged population. The relationship between the morbidity patterns of disease in the aged and the demands for health service care is obviously of great importance for the manager in the health services, and the community physician can provide much valuable information.

Monitoring in the Intermediate Aged Group

Epidemiological studies of the patterns of morbidity between the time of leaving school and the onset of retirement would be of major interest to the health services. This is the group of the population with a continuously changing pattern of morbidity which, nevertheless, makes heavy demands upon the acute resources of the health services. It is in this group where the apparent and actual needs of the health services need to be most closely monitored. The demand for treatment is obviously a subtle interplay of actual demand with the needs which the patient and his medical practitioners have come to expect from the services. It would be difficult to lay down stringent guide lines about the type of case that can be managed within the community and those that need hospital care, but it is obvious that a great deal more stress will be laid, in future years, on the care of the patient within the community. The hospital services, as such, may well find that they are needed mostly for the most acute episodes of an illness which demand specialized and intensive treatment. The Oxford Regional Hospital Board's plan for community hospitals serving the District General Hospital is one in which this kind of assessment of hospital and community care could most readily be carried out. Until we know the effects of different types of health service care and management on the progress of a disease, our whole therapeutic approach is likely to be based on intuitive experience which may or may not represent the optimum in care for the patient.

SCREENING AND THE COMMUNITY

Screening type methods may be used both as a means of finding the actual needs of the community in relationship to health care and as a diagnostic procedure at an early stage of the disease. The idea of multiphasic screening at the present time is not likely to be advanced within the health services. However, the second use of screening is becoming more prominent as research evidence shows the value of screening methods in the detection of disease at a stage when it is amenable to treatment. There is some evidence to show that certain serious conditions may be arrested and the traditional mortality data improved in certain areas of screening. The community physician has a particular interest in this field as, in order to keep effective checks on screening methods, a community record must be set up so that the effect of early intervention may be properly evaluated. The use of community records in this setting is particularly relevant at the present time. As detailed questions about the confidentiality of such records are bound to be raised, it is essential to know by whose hands the records should be finally controlled. The community physician is in a special position to ensure that records are properly collated, and are available to the relevant health service personnel for the use for which they are intended. He has had a long experience, as a Medical Officer of Health, of handling confidential information which has been presented to him in the interests of the community, and he is uniquely placed to balance the needs of the community with the necessity of preserving the private nature of the information.

The Community Physician as Administrator

It will remain to be seen how far long experience in administration is to be utilized in the Area Health Boards of the future. It is likely that at the transitional phase many Medical Officers of Health will, in fact, become the medical administrators of the Area Health Boards. However, the future may show that the stage of the community physician is an essential part of the training of the medical health services manager. It is to be hoped that a training in community health will be an essential part of every senior manager in the health services. Without the expertise and insight the community physician can bring to the health services, much of health services management and administration must of necessity be rather limited at present. The Medical Officer of Health has had long experience of balancing what is ideal and what is practical in the community with the limited resources that have been placed upon him in the setting in which he works. Many will rejoice that, as community physicians, the new emphasis on community care will bring a change of emphasis in the health services which may be financially beneficial to the provision of community facilities.

5—The Administrative and Managerial Structure for Nursing

Patricia Morton

Introduction

The pattern of nursing administration was little affected by the event of the N.H.S. in 1948. Although the introduction of a nationalized service brought about major changes in the organization of the hospitals and defined the nursing services to be administered by the local health authority, the traditional structure of the nursing profession remained substantially unaltered. In the long term it became evident that an imbalanced nursing service was emerging, and there was a need to revise the framework of nursing administration to define more clearly the status of senior nursing staff and accord them the right of official representation at meetings of governing bodies to present the professional concept of nursing policy. This is particularly important in the light of proposed changes for a unified health service in which the nursing services have a vital part to play.

The nursing task is twofold. First, it is primarily centred on ministering to the individual in need of care and assistance because of adverse health circumstances. By its action it seeks to promote maximum physical, mental and emotional well-being and to prevent, as far as possible, the occurrence of secondary manifestations. Secondly, nursing lends clinical and therapeutic support to medical care and undertakes a paramedical function.

The demand for technically competent nurses to keep pace with the advances in medical science in the treatment of patients in hospital, providing short-term care in acute illness, has, perhaps, taken precedence over providing the quality of care in long-term incapacity. The status within the profession of the different branches of nursing has possibly led to a maldistribution of administrative nursing expertise. A policy for the reorganization of nursing to meet the concepts of total nursing care was difficult to formulate without means of expression through official channels. This has been a limiting factor in achieving a true partnership with medical and lay administrators, but the profession itself has also kept the basis of nursing firmly rooted in the hospital system. Collaboration with professional colleagues in the interest of continuity of nursing care has developed slowly compared with the demonstrated need of individual patients and the resources already available in the community.

It is felt that the resolution of three major issues may restore the balance of the nursing service and enable the quality of care to be maintained and improved. (1) One is the availability of supporting staff to carry out non-nursing tasks at present undertaken to a greater or lesser extent at all nursing levels. (2) The second is for the improvement in status of the nursing students, and their release from providing service needs in order that their educational and training needs can be adequately met. These two issues are probably interwoven in that it may be that the nursing students carry out proportionately more of the non-nursing tasks than qualified nurses, thus accelerating the demand for them to provide service. (3) By decentralizing nursing administration, each grade of staff can carry out managerial functions at the appropriate level. A redistribution of nursing tasks, based on job analysis, will determine the range of managerial activity accorded to each level.

In the *Report of the Committee on Senior Nursing Staff Structure* (Ministry of Health, 1966) the opening paragraph points out that the lack of representation at committee level in the N.H.S. had restricted the right of the nursing profession to be heard on matters relating to nursing policy. The following two extracts from this report may clarify the emerging position. 'We see the nursing function in hospitals as caring for patients and carrying out treatment under the direction of doctors and in co-operation with other professional and technical staff. The primary function of the nurse administration then is the ordering and co-ordinating of nursing jobs, and the people who do them, and these constitute her *sphere of authority.*' 'In the ordering of all things which go towards the well-being of the patients nurses have a duty to make their requirements known and a right to be heard. This constitutes their *field of influence.*'

The impact of the Salmon Report, to give it its short title, has been profound and it will certainly provide a basis for the coherence of nursing in hospital and in the community. It has been said that what is a new thing for one generation becomes the commonplace of the next. The present generation of nurses has been presented with an outstanding list of revolutionary ideas on the internal structure of their profession.

Management has been defined as the creation and maintenance of an internal environment in an enterprise where individuals working together in groups can perform efficiently and effectively towards the attainment of group goals. Management is the body of organized knowledge which underlies the art of managing. The goal of nursing is the attainment of the highest possible standards of care; this is the prime objective of nursing care, and the decisions for the formulation of overall policy rest with the senior nursing officers. In the precise words of the Salmon Report. 'In top management nurses have policy forming tasks of proposing the objectives and limitations of nursing in achieving the purpose of the hospital.'

At this point it is worth considering the wider implications of a nursing policy, not only for achieving the purpose of the hospital but also the possible aims of nursing within a unified health service which would provide an administrative framework for the achievement of integrated health care. The organizational changes proposed in the Green Paper *The Future Structure of the National Health Service* (1970) refer to the new responsibilities which will be created for nursing. 'The area health authority's chief nursing officer will be concerned with both hospital and community nursing and midwifery services.' Essentially, the hospital is concerned with the care of the sick where home care and treatment is neither feasible nor possible. In the community, nursing is concerned with health teaching, the prevention of ill health and with care and after-care. Although there are differences in the nature and scope of work undertaken by nurses in these two spheres, the continuity of care relies very much on a common core of nursing policy to link the hospital and community service effectively. To provide for this the Working Party on Management Structure in the Local Authority Nursing Services (Department of Health and Social Security, 1969), under the chairmanship of E.L. Mayston, had in its terms of references, 'to consider the extent to which the principles of the Salmon Report on senior nursing staff structure in the hospital service are applicable to the local authority nursing services and what changes in the structure of senior posts and changes in the definitions of posts may be required'. The aim of the proposals of this report was to facilitate a smooth transition to a more integrated nursing administration, in the light of foreseeable changes, in the structure of the N.H.S. Full co-ordination under one authority, with integration of services at local level, will succeed if communications within the service are efficient.

The keynote of the Salmon Committee recommendations, the principles of which are echoed by the report of the Mayston working party, is perhaps 'communication'. This is essential for the gathering of information and knowledge to plan co-ordinated care and for the understanding of professional responsibility. As part of the policy the use of conferences is recommended through which all grades of staff, by representation, can contribute information and advice for the making of decisions. These decisions should be made at the requisite management levels by either informal or formal meetings. A real exchange of ideas, the opportunity to participate in decision making within one's sphere of authority, gives greater job satisfaction. Lateral communication systems have not hitherto been a common feature and this, in the view of Salmon, has been a limiting factor in effective communication between nurses themselves and with other members of the team. An understanding of the sphere of authority in relation to subordinates and supervisors and the means of co-operating with those who provide other than nursing service are important parts of professional training. Solving problems of communication is perhaps the most difficult task of administrators, and it calls for the appreciation of social skills in human relationships as well as clear lines of control. In the interests of the continuity of patient care and the full implementation of health care, the channels of communication need to link effectively with the health and social services in the community.

The Future Pattern of Nursing Administration

If nursing policy is to be decided by the nurse administrators of the future, the revised structure should improve the channels of communication to provide the information essential for decision making and facilitate its implementation. The three levels of management are first, middle and top and at each level there are grades appropriate to the functions and sphere of authority relative to the needs of the service. At the first level, in hospitals, the grades of staff nurse and charge nurse have an executive function and carry out the work programme of a section. They are responsible for direct nursing care and the organization of the nursing team. Programming the policy and working out procedures for its implementation are the tasks of the two grades at middle management: the nursing officer of a unit which may consist of up to six sections, and the senior nursing officer of an area are comprising two or more units. They accept responsibility at consultant level and order and co-ordinate other nursing staff within the area. The formulation of nursing policy, and responsibility for its implementation, is the task of top management — the principal nursing officer at divisional level, and the chief nursing officer at group level.

Nurses in top management posts are the advisers to the governing body in all matters related to nursing.

With modifications, these three levels of management are appropriate for the structure of nursing outside the hospital environment where a separate nursing service meets the needs of the community. The services provided by health authorities are home nursing, health visiting and domiciliary midwifery. Co-ordination of staff undertaking these specialist functions at executive level is recommended at middle management level. The grades within each management level are not analogous with those of hospital nursing staff. At field level, nursing staff work on a more independent basis, taking decisions in respect of their direct professional service to individuals and families and working in close liaison with workers in other disciplines. Most of the field workers have undertaken an additional course of education and training which includes the management and organization of their working area. The content of first-line management is acting as consultant and adviser to a group of field staff, promoting new ideas and often undertaking some field work which may be of a specialized nature. Many of the functions equate with the lower grade of middle management. As organizational changes take place and services become more integrated, clearer lines of first-line and middle management will emerge. The major activities of middle management are for the systematic programming of policy decisions and the co-ordination of the services to meet the growing concept of the team approach to meet the health needs in the community.

Although traditional aspects of functional management may be retained at middle management, the trend towards the appointment of nursing officers to control and co-ordinate the three main branches of community nursing service is likely to continue and emerge as the most efficient pattern for the future.

Again, in the community there may be need for only one grade at top management to provide a single avenue of communication on policy and to direct home nursing, health visiting and domiciliary midwifery.

Overall control of a comprehensive service is the possible ideal for the future, linking all nursing specialties within the N.H.S. under one director of nursing services at each local level, to achieve its primary objective of policy which is a high quality of nursing care.

Within such a framework for the nursing services as a whole, a new look could be taken at the preparation of nursing students for entry to the nursing profession. Administration is a process through which the nurse educationalist can obtain the essential practical instruction and experience for students to be prepared in accordance with professional requirements. At basic level the health services are still responsible, with the hospital schools of nursing, for the education and training of most of the entrants to nursing. This present system raises conflict between educational needs of the student and the service demands of a hospital, and it has been often recommended that schools of nursing should be administered separately and that preventive and caring aspects should be included in the basic course.

Preparation for Management

For a fuller appreciation of the managerial responsibility in nursing, a systematic scheme of training is recommended. As the management potential should develop from within the profession, there will be a need for prescribed theoretical courses of preparation organized by educational establishments. Basic principles of management have been introduced at an elementary level into the syllabus by the General Nursing Council. The nursing student will gain an understanding of the skills of management, teaching and communication which are pertinent and relevant for performance in the first-level post accepted on qualification. This inclusion into the syllabus will enable the student to make a more critical appraisal of the needs of patients in general and the role of the nurse within the organization. Efficiency and confidence come with practice, and the newly qualified nurse has to assume responsibility gradually and accept guidance from experienced members of staff who always have a teaching relationship to fulfil as well as a supervisory role.

It is recommended that preparatory courses should be taken by all staff before promotion to a higher level or grade. *First-line management* courses consolidate areas of professional learning, reinforce the understanding of duties relating to the organizational area and give opportunity for the reappraisal of interpersonal relationships. Such courses, planned in local educational institutions, are of about four weeks' duration. The syllabus includes the study of the broader operational principles of management relating to organizations, and a more advanced study of the administration of the health services specific either to the hospital or to the community. Also included is a more detailed examination of functions entailed at first level, for example team management, teaching of practical skills, the art of communication, and staff appraisal.

Further courses of training appropriate to the level of management will prepare nurses for the functions they are required to undertake at each level. These functions are defined as professional, administrative and personnel; they will vary proportionately in accordance with the job specification for each grade of staff.

Middle management posts are more concerned with the organization of the nursing area which, in hospitals, is sub-divided into units each with an overall control of a number of sections. Nursing officers have responsibility for ordering and co-ordinating other nursing staff and programming the work. They act as consultants to those in charge of the sections and provide information essential for the formulation of overall policy. This expanding field of nursing management will, by creating a direct-line relationship, balance the organization of the service. It is perhaps the most vital of the recommendations which have been made for the structure of the profession because, by combining the use of clinical and management skills, it will allow for the maximum potential development of nursing expertise. Promotion prospects will become available for those who wish to remain in a specialized or clinical nursing post as well as for those who become teachers or administrators. These officers will give support to nursing staff and will undertake day-to-day responsibility for control of the clinical situation and promote professional knowledge in the interest of providing an expert nursing service. It is at this level that direct links could be established with the community nursing services for planning a programme in relation to the discharge of patients, and care and after-care with consultation and collaboration on specialized rehabilitative measures or supportive care needed by an individual.

Many posts in middle management grades will require an additional professional qualification, but such courses may not have included sufficient content of the theory of management needed for the job to complement their professional skills. Nurses entering this grade will require a more advanced course of preparation in management theory and its practical application, particularly to administrative and personnel functions undertaken at this level. A minimum of 12 weeks is recommended to cover the general principles of management and control, together with an introduction to the behavioural sciences. Emphasis is placed on the inclusion of the use of case studies and discussions on innovation in a changing environment.

The formation of policy and the organization of its implementation comprise the principal function of *top management* who are directly responsible to the governing body on all matters relating to nursing, both for service and nurse training requirements. The creation of posts within this sphere of authority, both at national and local level, will establish an authoritive source of advice on all matters pertaining to nursing. General administrative ability and experience in nursing, rather than specialized clinical expertise, are the requirements, for the level of management. For such posts the qualities needed are a mature personality, a developed critical sense and the ability to make sound judgements. If the profession is to obtain individuals of this calibre who will be the future leaders of an independent profession, the educational aspects of nursing need to be directed to the fostering of such potential and its retention.

Preparatory courses recommended at present are, if possible, shared with lay and medical health service administrative staff undertaking advanced courses and are organized mainly by university departments.

The impetus for the development of management potential of senior nursing staff will come through the National Nursing Staff Committee, a directive committee with the responsibility to advise on the provision of management courses, with concern for their location and content of the syllabus. Two other functions of this committee are to appoint a panel of assessors for the selection of persons appointed to top level posts and to promote opportunities for further study and research in the field of nurse management. It will inevitably be some time before actual courses fully reflect the theoretical and practical needs of the three lines of management. This is partly because there is still great scope for experiment as organized management training for nurses is of recent origin, and partly because many present staff are very experienced and the need is for transitionary courses. These members of staff have much to contribute to the orientation of future management courses particularly by the evaluations they make. The National Nursing Staff Committee consider that management expertise is in no way incompatible with the traditional role and that management training is a most important supplement to the professional skills of nursing.

The future

Nursing is not a static service but is constantly adjusting as changing patterns of disease affect the delivery of health care. This calls for the ability of nurses to undertake more responsibility for the control and planning of their professional field of work for which a greater understanding of management and administration is needed. Social, scientific and technical changes affect the interpretation of nursing, which cannot afford to remain too deeply rooted in tradition.

Bibliography and References

Baly, M. (1969). 'Changing Demands for Health Services: 1 and 2.' *Nurs. Times* **69**, (*Occ. Pap.* 21 and 22)

Biggart, J.H. (1968). 'The Challenge of Nurse Education.' *Int. Nurs. Rev.* **15**, 292

Christman, L. (1969). 'The Role of Nursing in Organizational Effectiveness.' *Int. Nurs. Rev.* **16**, 248

Department of Health and Social Security (1969). *Report of the Working Party on Management Structure in Local Authority Nursing Services.* London; H.M.S.O.

Koontz, H. and O'Donnell, C. (1968). *Principles of Management – An Analysis of Management Functions* (4th ed.). New York and Maidenhead; McGraw-Hill

Jacobs, D. (1970). 'The Future of Nursing, Professionalization, Profanation and Prophecy.' *Int. Nurs. Rev.* **17**, 16

Ministry of Health (1966). *Report of the Committee on Senior Nursing Staff Structure.* Scottish Home and Health Dept. Edinburgh; H.M.S.O.

National Council of Nurses of the United Kingdom (1968). *Administering the Local Authority Nursing Service*, London; Royal College of Nursing

– (1969). *The Future of Public Health Nursing in Relation to the Needs of the Community.* London; Royal College of Nursing

Peters, R.J. and Kinnaird, J. (Eds.) (1965). *Health Services Administration: A Source Book.* Edinburgh; Livingstone

6—Use of Management and Administrative Techniques in Nursing

B. Watkin

Outline of Nursing Management

The term management techniques is used in a variety of ways, and often the emphasis is on quantitative techniques. In this section the term will be used in the simple sense of techniques that are used in management in particular those which are, or ought to be, employed by the nurse manager. There will inevitably be some overlap with other more specialized contributions, but it is hoped that the nursing administrator may find this section a useful synopsis of the areas which are of chief interest to her (or, increasingly, him).

As far as hospitals are concerned, some guidance on the functions to be discharged by the nurse manager in the new nursing administrative structure is provided in the Salmon Report (Ministry of Health, 1966). Included in this Report are specimen job descriptions for a number of posts at top management, middle management and first-line management levels. Analysis of these yields the following principal areas of concern.

(1)   The manpower function.
(2)   The communications function.
(3)   The management decision and control function.

The emphasis naturally varies according to the level of management. At what the Salmon Committee is pleased to call 'top management level' (if what the chief nursing officer of a group does is top management, one wonders what levels of management are represented by the group secretary, the Hospital Management Committee, the Regional Hospital Board and the Department of Health and Social Security), the manpower function includes advising on nursing establishments and recruitment, as well as the selection and appointment of staff, induction, appraisal and staff development. At first-line level the manpower function is represented by induction, appraisal, supervision, the scheduling and co-ordination of activities, counselling and training.

As far as the communications function is concerned, all levels have in common the need to submit and receive reports, to engage in face-to-face interaction with subordinates and colleagues, and to participate in meetings. While the first-line manager has the greatest contact with patients and their relatives, middle and top management are progressively more involved in meetings and in tendering advice to committees. At top management level there is an important public relations function which involves the nurse manager in extensive contact with the outside world, public speaking being a necessary skill.

All levels take decisions, but the scope of these decisions is much wider at middle and top management levels than at first-line management level, where the ward sister or charge nurse is subject to fairly tight constraints, and where many of her decisions are choices between alternatives laid down by those above her in the hierarchy. Top management has a responsibility to devise and install systems of management information and control, while middle and first-line management have it in their power to determine whether such systems do or do not function effectively.

The Manpower Function

The health services are labour-intensive: wages and salaries account for more than 70 per cent of running costs of hospitals and the wages and salaries of nurses and midwives for about 27 per cent of total running costs. It has been predicted that by 1980 the dominating problem of the health services, will be not shortage of money but shortage of manpower in particular skilled manpower. The importance of the manpower function does not require any further emphasis, but it is worth remarking that nursing staff establishments and personnel policies cannot be considered in isolation from the rest of the health services manpower picture. The major costs of a Salmon-type reorganization of the senior nursing staff structure in a hospital group often fall under headings other than nursing. Policies that nurses shall not be used for duties that do not require their special skills may demand the employment of more domestic, technical and administrative staff. This is as true in the public health as in the hospital field. On the other hand, a willingness on the part of nursing staff to acquire new skills may avoid the need to create new grades of technical or paramedical staff, or may help to eke out scarce manpower resources in such departments as physiotherapy, occupational therapy or social work. Before such ideas are condemned out of hand as either dilution or mis-use of nursing skills, the possible advantages in terms of a more closely integrated patient care team should be pondered. Such considerations as these cannot be pursued here but they lead naturally to discussion of what kind and what number of staff are required.

HOW MANY NURSES?

Organizations need manpower to achieve their objectives. The types and numbers of staff they need are determined by the tasks that have to be carried out to achieve these objectives. The first stage of manpower planning is therefore clarification of the objectives of the organization. This requires thinking at the level of the total organization, and not merely a part of it. In this context the total organization is the Health Service (an increasingly integrated Health Service, it is to be hoped) and not merely the particular hospital, health centre or domiciliary nursing service in which the administrator happens to be working. Still less is it merely the nursing component of the service. At a senior level the nursing administrator is entitled to regard herself as a part-manager of the whole, rather than as merely the manager of a part; a departmental head responsible for only the nursing service. When faced with pressures that, at first sight, seem to indicate a need for more staff, she is bound to ask if this is work which should be done in the hospital, or would a better service to the patient result if it were done elsewhere, for example in the patient's home, or in welfare accommodation. If the answer is yes the matter should be raised in the appropriate quarter. Sometimes it is useful to ask how many of the tasks that feature in this work load which is causing problems need to be done at all. Could they be eliminated without an unacceptable fall in the level or quality of service, or would it, at present labour costs, be economical to eliminate them by the use of machinery and labour-saving devices?

The nursing administrator would be wise to seek the help of experts in operational research and work study to find the answers to such questions as these, but it is important that she should pause to ask the question, and not merely fall into the habit of asking for more and more when pressures build up. It is important that she should invite study of the work of nurses in clinical areas and contexts. The current pre-occupation of hospital boards' management services teams with laundries, domestic work and portering services is understandable, in view of the pressures being exerted by the Department of Health towards the introduction of incentive bonus schemes in these areas, but is regrettable, for it is in the clinical areas that the quality of the service is primarily determined and that most costs are either directly or indirectly incurred.

A good deal of work has been done in the search for optimum nursing establishments in hospitals, and the most useful reports are those by Goddard, for the Leeds Regional Hospital Board (1963), and the Work Study Department of the North-eastern Regional Hospital Board of Scotland (1969). Roberts (1963) produced for WHO a valuable review of the principles and techniques relevant to the staffing of public health, and out-patient nursing services.

The North-eastern Regional Hospital Board work study team produced a formula for the staffing of general hospital wards, which deserves to be put to the test of more widespread experiment and evaluation. The formula is

$$W = N[F(B + T) + A + D + M]$$

where W is the average weekly nursing work load in hours,

N is the average number of patients in ward,

F is the patient-dependency factor for ward specialty,

B is the time in hours per week required to maintain the standard of basic nursing care prescribed by the advisory panel for a totally helpless bedfast patient,

T is the time required for technical nursing of the ward specialty, expressed as a percentage of the time spent on basic nursing,

A is the time per patient per week for administrative duties,

D is the time per patient per week for domestic work,

M is the time per patient per week for miscellaneous duties.

The study appears to have established that basic nursing care, at an acceptable level (as judged by a professional panel), of a totally helpless bedfast male patient requires on average 12·5 hours per week, and of a female patient 14 hours per week. In addition, each specialty was found to have its characteristic dependency mix and its characteristic requirement for technical nursing. The portion of the formula F(B + T) can therefore be rendered for a male surgical ward as follows.

The patient dependency factor is given as 0·5 (if all patients in the ward were totally bedfast and helpless, the dependency factor would be 1·0), and the requirement for technical nursing is 67·5 per cent of the time required for basic nursing care. So this portion of the formula becomes 0·5 (12·5 + 8·4) = 10·45.

In hospitals training nurses for the register, the allowance for administrative duties is four hours per patient per week; for domestic duties the allowance (based on an assumption that the recommendations of an earlier report on domestic staffing have been implemented) is 1·25 hours. The allowance for miscellaneous duties, including personal time and so on, is estimated at 6·5 per cent of the total time spent on other duties. The formula for a 30-bed male surgical ward thus becomes

$$W = 30(10·45 + 4 + 1·25 + 1) = 501$$

This figure is then subject to (*a*) an adjustment for ward layout and (*b*) an adjustment for additional duties. The final figure for weekly work-load is divided by 42 to give the numbers of full-time staff required. In the example, assuming that no adjustments were required for layout or additional duties, this would be 501/42 = 11·9. This figure is, of course, for day-time staffing only. At night, the numbers of staff required to maintain observation and supervision of patients is likely to exceed the numbers needed to discharge the actual work-load therefore the formula is not applicable.

The various norms and allowances used in this formula have been carefully validated and checked, as far as the north-eastern region of Scotland is concerned, but as the authors themselves point out, 'The time allowed for administrative duties, domestic work and miscellaneous duties, represent current practices in hospitals in the north-eastern region and may not be in accordance with usage elsewhere. Before attempting to use the tables in Appendix E of this paper in any hospital outside the north-eastern region, it would therefore be necessary to check that all the figures used in the tables apply to that particular ward.... it would be necessary to carry out an activity sampling study combined with a detailed record of patient dependencies to establish this. If differences are found, new tables should be compiled using the appropriate figures.'

A more fundamental limitation is that the norms rest on unvalidated professional judgements of what is an acceptable level of patient care. In one instance, at least, the judgement of the advisory panel was in direct conflict with research findings. Norton, McLaren and Exton-Smith showed that for a helpless patient two-hourly attention to pressure areas is necessary, but the advisory panel thought four-hourly attention was sufficient. In most instances, however, there are no research findings against which the recommendations of the panel can be set, and there is an outstanding need for more clinical research in nursing in order that assessments of what care patients require, and how many staff are needed to provide that care, can be more firmly based.

JOB ANALYSIS

Appendix B to the Scottish report sets out duties appropriate to various grades of staff, and is again open to the criticism that it is based on subjective judgements and, indeed, incorporates some surprising inconsistencies. The ideal in such matters is to work systematically from the objectives of the organization, to the tasks that have to be done to achieve those objectives, and thence to the skills and knowledge required to perform these tasks. Industry has used the techniques of skills and knowledge analysis in the design of training programmes for both manual and non-manual workers for some years (Seymour, 1968), but as far as is known no attempt has been made in the United Kingdom to achieve as fundamental an approach as this in the design of a training course for one of the health professions.

On the other hand, the Salmon Report has popularized the use of job descriptions to clarify organizational structure and organizational relationships. It is doubtful whether they are yet being used effectively in the health services as a basis for the specification of the attributes and qualifications required in a job, or to indicate training needs. But job analysis – the process leading to the writing of a job description – has been stated (Roff and Watson, 1969) to have the following seven major uses.

Placement. – For this purpose it is necessary to have a description of the job, supplemented by a description of the kind of man or woman who could perform the job satisfactorily (personnel specification).

Training. – For this purpose the job description would emphasize the skills and knowledge required by the job.

Establishment of wage or salary scales. – For job evaluation information is needed which shows the relative importance, difficulty or unpleasantness of a range of jobs.

Safety. – For this purpose detailed information of hazards which may be encountered is required.

Job classification. – For this purpose it is necessary to have a description of the essential features of a job so that it is clear in which respect each job resembles other jobs and in which respects it differs.

Methods improvement. – This requires detailed information; breaking down tasks into smaller units to permit closer examination.

Organization planning. – Here considerable emphasis is placed on the purpose underlying the tasks that are performed – the objectives of the job – and the relation of these tasks to others.

Systematic job analysis is required in order that sensible decisions should be made on such matters as: does the hard-pressed ward sister require the help of a clerk, a housekeeper, a receptionist, an extra nurse, or merely improved central services? What is the right combination of nurses and technicians (and what sort of technicians) in the intensive therapy unit? To what extent can non-nurse administrators play a part in the administration of nursing services? What is the optimum mix of health visitors, home nurses (S.R.N. and S.E.N.), social workers, secretary/receptionists and aides to support a group general practice?

The technique of preparing a job description will vary according to the purpose for which it is intended to be used, and according to whether the job is one that is already in existence, or one that has not yet come into being. The starting point should always be to define the principal objectives of the job; what is the point of having a person in that post at all? The existing or prospective job content can then be analysed in the light of its relevance to the stated objectives.

The completed description should answer the following questions.

(1)   What are the objectives of the job?

(2)   What are the duties and responsibilities of the job and how do they relate to the stated objectives?

(3)   How does this job relate to other jobs in the organization?

(4)   How can success in the job be measured?

The duties and responsibilities of the job must be described in sufficient detail to enable at least an approximate assessment to be made of the skills and knowledge required to do the job. A more detailed account will be required if the purpose of drawing up the description is to design a training course. Any special features of the job, such as disagreeable working conditions, should be recorded. It should not be necessary to stress that job descriptions should be based, wherever possible, on direct observations. It is a recurrent finding that managers do not know exactly what their subordinates do with their time, even though they may think they do (in some cases subordinates are found to be undertaking tasks which the manager says, and believes, he does himself), and that identical job titles may conceal substantial differences in job content even within the same organization.

PERSONNEL SPECIFICATION, RECRUITMENT, AND SELECTION

From the job description is derived the personnel specification, which sets out the *minimum* requirements for the job in terms of qualifications, experience, aptitude and ability. A useful framework is the Seven Point Plan devised by the National Institute of Industrial Psychology (Rodger, 1951). The headings in the Seven Point Plan are as follows.

Physical make-up. — Covers health and physique, including appearance, bearing and speech.

Attainments. – Includes educational and occupational attainments.

General intelligence. – Ability to reason quickly and accurately; to learn quickly and to handle complex ideas.

Specialized aptitudes. – Includes manual dexterity, mechanical aptitude, verbal facility and artistic aptitudes.

Interests. – (*a*) Intellectual; (*b*) practical and constructional; (*c*) physically active; (*d*) social; (*e*) artistic.

Disposition. – Characteristics shown in the individual's relationships with other people and his work; his steadiness; his self-reliance; the extent to which he is acceptable to others and the extent to which he influences others.

Circumstances. – Includes financial and family background.

It is necessary to stress again that the qualities specified should be the minimum requirements to enable the job to be done satisfactorily; any qualities over and above this should be specified as desirable but not essential.

Some of the headings in the Seven Point Plan lend themselves more obviously to objective measurement than others, and for some jobs measurable aptitudes are more obviously important than others. A case in point is the numerous attempts that have been made to devise a battery of tests to assess suitability for nursing. Much of this literature was reviewed by Millott (1963), who concluded that the difficulty of devising useful tests was 'partly due to the lack of data about the defining characteristics of nurses in general, or of the successful–unsuccessful nurses in particular', and that studies of the characteristics of nurses showed that they were 'much like anyone else'. MacGuire (1966) has demonstrated that wastage during nurse training is associated with characteristics of the particular training school rather than with individual characteristics of the students. None of this is surprising since the range of jobs and the range of activities in nursing is extremely wide. It might be possible to define the characteristics which would make for success as a scrub nurse in the operating theatre, as a geriatric health visitor, or as a paediatric ward sister, but a list of desirable characteristics of the potential nurse is likely to be either too general to be of use, or based on a conventional stereotype which does not take into account the wide range of jobs available in the profession.

However, given that we are now discussing the filling of a particular vacancy for which a personnel specification has been prepared, the remaining stages in the selection process are: (*i*) notification of the vacancy; (*ii*) receipt and acknowledgement of completed application forms; (*iii*) preparation of short-list; (*iv*) the taking up of references; (*v*) interviewing the short-listed candidates and making the appointment. Vacancies should normally be notified both internally and by public advertisement. It is not common practice in the health services to send particulars of vacancies to people working for other employing authorities who have not enquired about the post, but who might be interested if it were brought to their notice. There is, however, nothing to debar this practice. For some grades in the health services references will be supplemented by the availability of staff annual reports. To discuss in detail here the requirements for acknowledging applications, taking up references and calling short-listed candidates for interview would merely duplicate much of what appears under the subsequent heading 'The Communications Function'. As is emphasized in that section, an organization will often be judged by the tone and appearance of the letters it sends out.

Cuming (1968a), whose brief guide to selection procedures in the hospital service was prompted by the mounting evidence that appointments are often badly handled, lists three purposes of the inteview.

(1)   For the employer to obtain all the information about the candidate necessary to decide his suitability for the post.

(2)   To give the candidate all relevant information about the post and the organization of which it is part.

(3)   The public relations function of leaving the candidate with the impression that he has been treated fairly.

Often the first purpose is emphasized and the other two, particularly the third, are forgotten. As Cuming remarks, the ultimate aim of any employing authority should be to send unsuccessful candidates away feeling genuinely sorry that they have not got the job because it seemed such a good place to come and work. As it is, many committees seem quite oblivious to the amount of goodwill they lose as the result of bad interviewing practices.

Participation of committee members, two or three senior officers, and perhaps one or more outside assessors, makes it difficult to achieve in interviews for senior posts the degree of relaxation and informality that is most conducive to the fulfilment of the purposes of the interview. Every effort should be made within the limits set by national policy to keep the numbers involved in the interview to a minimum. At lower levels, where there is more discretion and committee members are unlikely to be concerned, three should be the maximum. This should, of course, include the immediate superior to whom the candidate would work if appointed. The larger the interviewing panel the more important is detail preliminary briefing and planning of the interview.

INDUCTION

Just as the first few days of a baby's life are the most hazardous it will experience until it is well past middle age, so the first few weeks or months in a new job are the time when a worker is most likely to leave. Once the induction crisis, as this is known, is over, it is likely that he will settle down to give years of contented service, or at least that he will stay with the organization for an appropriate period given the particular post and the likelihood of further progression in his career. Labour turnover is not wholly a bad thing; if all workers stayed in the same jobs until retirement the organization would become dangerously static. There would be no opportunities to introduce new blood and new ideas from outside and the ability of the organization to adapt to change would be reduced. However, wastage due to the induction crisis is invariably undesirable, because the new worker leaves before he has had time to make a solid contribution, and all the costs — in terms of time and disruption as well as money — of notifying the vacancy and selecting a new worker have to be incurred again.

Fortunately this waste can more often than not be prevented by careful induction into the organization and into the job. Naturally, if selection has been poor and a worker has been appointed who does not have the right qualities for the job, wastage will occur anyway. It will also occur if there is a great discrepancy between what the new worker has been led to expect of the job and what the job in fact entails. That is one reason why it is important at interview to ensure that candidates understand what the job entails and have a realistic appreciation of the demands that will be made on them. But given appropriate selection, and given that the new worker has a reasonable understanding of what he can expect when he takes up his post, it is still necessary to ensure that premature disillusion does not set in and that the employee becomes part of the team in which he is to work as soon as possible.

Effective induction starts with the letter of appointment, which should be friendly and welcoming in tone, even if it has to include formal statements relating to salary, superannuation and leave entitlement. The letter may be accompanied by a brochure or leaflet specially compiled to give new employees basic information about the work and structure of the organization, conditions of service, amenities, layout of the buildings, social facilities and so on. Induction courses, ranging from half a day to a week or more, have long been used in industry and are becoming more common in the health services. Because in many grades people enter into employment in ones or twos at odd intervals, it may be necessary for the new employee to work from a few days to a fortnight before he can join a group large enough to justify an induction course. This is quite long enough for him to grow discontented and leave if his immediate superior assumes that the formal induction course will do all that is required.

Because it is so important that the new worker should be given time and attention by his immediate superior on his first day, so that special features about the job and the working situation can be explained to him, and so that a relationship can be established, it is worth considering the question of starting times and dates. If a Monday is a particularly busy day, or if the morning is a specially busy time for the head of the department, it is an advantage if the worker can be asked to start on the Tuesday morning, or at lunch time.

WASTAGE, TURNOVER AND ABSENCE

Samuel (1969) commented 'It is an irony of British management that while most firms can quote a figure of return on capital employed few make any calculations of the cost of wastage of their manpower resources'. One can go further: relatively few organizations keep effective records of wastage during training, staff turnover, or absence, and although hospitals, in particular, often express themselves as extremely concerned about wastage during nurse training, the loss of trained staff, and absenteeism or sickness rates among various grades of staff, it is usually extremely difficult to get facts, as distinct from impressions, and more often than not it is necessary to arrange for data to be specially collected that could more usefully be monitored on a routine basis as part of an overall system of management information.

Most organizations can produce a crude percentage figure for labour turnover calculated in the following way

$$\frac{\text{Number of leavers during year} \times 100}{\text{Average number of employees during year}}$$

It may be possible to produce such a figure for specific groups of staff, such as staff nurses, sisters, nursing auxiliaries, ward clerks and so on, but a percentage turnover figure calculated in this way has only a very limited usefulness because it does not give the kind of information that is required in order to assess what kind of labour turnover problems the organization has, and what kind of approach might be fruitful in dealing with it.

For example, does a turnover rate of 50 per cent in a labour force of 100 mean that 50 posts were vacated during the year, which might indicate that there is something wrong with the organization as a whole, or does it mean that there were 10 jobs which fell vacant five times during the year, no one staying in any of these posts for more than about two months? This is a quite different situation, and one in which attention must be directed at the particular department or type of job in which the high turnover is occurring. Again, it is useful to know how long the wasters stay with the organization before they leave. It is a common finding that a disproportionate amount of turnover occurs in the first few weeks of employment – the induction crisis – and this points either to faulty selection or inadequate induction. Wastage during training may follow a characteristic pattern of peaks and troughs that can be associated with particular events in the training course; such as first night-duty.

The crude labour turnover rate therefore needs to be supplemented by other measures including the labour turnover rate broken down for particular departments, jobs, and class of employee (that is, classified by age, sex, educational attainments and so on), the survival rate, and the length of service. The survival rate can be plotted on a graph or chart to show the percentage of employees joining who leave in each successive quarter, month or week of service. Length of service can be shown in the form of a chart setting out the percentage of staff with varying lengths of service. All these measures must be taken together to give a complete picture. For example, the percentage turnover rate might be high, the survival rate might reveal that most of the departures took place within the first few weeks of service, and the length of service analysis might show that in spite of the high percentage turnover the bulk of the labour force was relatively stable and the turnover was, therefore, occurring in only a small proportion of the jobs. The compilation and uses of these indices are clearly explained in a useful publication of the Hotel and Catering Economic Development Committee (1969). Samuel (1969) also refers to various measures of labour turnover.

The term absence from work can be neutral, used to encompass certificated sickness, uncertificated sickness, and absence from other causes. There is little point in trying to compile statistics that distinguish between sickness and other forms of absence. The dividing line is too uncertain. Does one accept a person's statement that he was sick, or even a doctor's certificate which may be based only on what the patient himself told the doctor? One may, of course, have to accept such a certificate or claim for pay and disciplinary purposes, but from the point of view of monitoring the morale of the work force it is better to treat all absence as one, although it is useful to break it down into short-term (up to three days) and long term (more than three days), and by sex, age, marital status (in the case of women), type of job, and department. The breakdown into short-term and long-term absence will be useful in establishing whether the dominant problem is one of odd days off, or whether a relatively small number of workers, suffering from more serious or chronic conditions are contributing disproportionately to the total days lost. Another useful measure is the annual inception rate, that is, the number of incidents of sickness or absence per employee per annum. This again can be broken down by category of staff and department.

The object of collecting this kind of information is to enable management to take appropriate remedial action when either turnover or absence rates appear to be unduly high. Appropriate action cannot be taken unless the nature of the problem is clearly understood. Often the help of a competent statistician will be needed in the design of a personnel records system to collect this information and to interpret its significance, but such advice is normally readily obtainable, either within the Health Service itself, or from the management studies department of a local university, polytechnic or college of further education.

MOTIVATION AND MORALE

Labour turnover and absence can both be regarded as forms of withdrawal from the work situation. In Revans' (1964) hospital studies the two were found to be associated and among student nurses 'coming events cast their shadows before them' – those who discontinued training spent more time off sick than those who did not. A less extreme form of withdrawal is low productivity. This is often difficult to measure in the health services, but there is no reason to believe that it does not occur.

The manager will be interested not only in techniques of measuring various manifestations of withdrawal from the work situation (or low morale), but in what he can do to improve the position. First, however, there is the question of the point at which the manager starts to feel concerned about turnover or absence. Not only is there probably an irreducible minimum in both cases but, as has already been pointed out, turnover at least is not wholly a bad thing. An organization or department with a crude turnover rate of 10–15 per cent or less per annum, and an average of fewer than 10 days lost per annum per employee, probably has little to worry about on these scores at least, although it is still possible that in this kind of very stable situation productivity may be low. Revans argued that hospitals where morale was low were those where communications were poor, but various social scientists have since refined this concept a little so that it is now appreciated that the communication of information and ideas is not in itself enough. The information and ideas conveyed must be seen to influence events. People need not only to be listened to, but to be allowed to have some influence on policies and decisions that affect them. The new Salmon structure gives ample opportunity for the development of participative patterns of management in the nursing service itself, although it could reasonably be argued that there are few decisions or policies which affect only the nursing service and that therefore participation needs to be rather more widely based than this at every level, from the ward or section upwards.

Another factor which has been prominent in research into student nurse wastage, in particular, is a clash between expectations and reality. MacGuire (1966) has written of the student nurse's need to see her training as a coherent, planned experience, and of her disillusion when this expectation has been disappointed. A Ministry of Health circular (H.M. (67) 58), drew heavily upon the researches of MacGuire and others to suggest a checklist of factors which might be contributing to the loss of student and pupil nurses during training. Students and pupils are in some ways a particularly vulnerable group, but many of the factors which contribute to student and pupil wastage may also be responsible for poor morale among trained and auxiliary nursing staff. If there still remains a gap between expectation and reality after all feasible improvements have been made in the working situation, induction programmes, which have already been discussed, have their part to play in closing the gap.

Again briefly touching on a vast subject, the present system of staff appraisal in the organization has important implications for morale. Where there is no formal system, staff will glean impressions of what their superiors think of their work from chance remarks or from the way their superiors act toward them. This is not very satisfactory; staff need to know where they stand with those who are important to them in the organization and, both from their own point of view and from that of the organization, they need to know their strengths and weaknesses. This kind of feedback can be provided by an open system of appraisal in which the counselling interview at regular intervals is a central feature. Some appraisal and reporting systems are closed, that is, the person appraised is not allowed to see the report that is made upon him and has no opportunity to discuss it. However, the best industrial and commercial systems, and the type which it is hoped will be introduced into the nursing service, allow the person appraised to see his report, to discuss it and, perhaps, record his comments. In this way, appraisal can make a positive contribution to the individual's performance and development, since he can see clearly what is required of him, what he is doing well, where he is falling short and what he needs to do to improve. The counselling interview is also the occasion when the manager can establish what help his subordinate requires in order to achieve better performance. This may range from the clearer delegation of authority to sending him on a course. A sound appraisal system will make a positive contribution to the individual's sense that he has a well-defined place in the organization and that his contribution to it is valued.

The Communications Function

BASIC PRINCIPLES

Effective communication is communication that is *understood, remembered,* and *produces the desired effect.* To achieve this clarity in the use of language is not enough. There must also be an understanding of the factors, emotional as well as cognitive, that may interfere with the ability to understand, retain or act upon the message that has been transmitted. The basic principles of effective communication are the same, whether the particular context is an instruction to a subordinate, the giving of clinical information to patients or their relatives, the drafting of a notice or a letter, the submission of a report to a committee, or the issue of a press release. The chief requirement for effective communication is the power of empathy; the ability to identify with the person for whom the communication is intended so that it can be framed in a way that he can understand, that he will regard as appropriate and acceptable, a way that will produce in him the desired response.

Barriers to effective communication

Empathy can only be achieved by conscientiously striving after it, clarity of expression only by endless practice and the study of good examples. Gowers (1966) remains the supreme teacher in this field. It is, however, helpful to be aware of the most common barriers to effective communication. The following list is based on an account by Parry (1968).

Limited capacity

There are limits to our capacity to absorb information; there are limits to our ability to attend while information is being imparted to us. These limits are not fixed, but variable. There are variations between people, and the same person will vary in capacity at different times and in different circumstances. The sustained lecture is seldom a very effective way of imparting information because lecturers tend to outrun the capacity of their audiences, both to attend to what they are saying and to retain what they hear. Active participation increases the amount retained and this is why the emphasis in education has shifted in recent years from straight lecturing to seminars and discussion groups.

Distraction

Distraction interferes with attention and thus with the effectiveness of communication. It can take many forms: physical distraction such as noise, discomfort, undue humidity or too high or low a temperature; preoccupation with other matters that have for the moment more importance or interest; a reaction of distaste or amusement to some aspect of the presentation or the person speaking, for example, a badly set out letter or unpleasant facial mannerisms.

Unstated assumptions

It is a common error to assume that the person with whom you are communicating already has certain information which, in fact, he does not possess. Nurses are often sent to fetch instruments that they have not been taught to identify. The charge of the Light Brigade was a disaster because Lord Raglan assumed that Lord Cardigan could see all that he could see from his own position on the heights above.

Incompatible views of the world

We perceive the world in the way we have been taught to perceive it and this social learning goes on, for the most part unconsciously, from birth. Thus ethnic origins, upbringing, social class, educational experience, professional training will all help to determine the things we see as important, the things that agitate us and the things that please us. This is why misunderstandings can easily arise between managers and workers, doctors and administrators, Englishmen and Americans. To be conscious of this problem is to be a long way towards overcoming it.

Unconscious mechanisms

Unconscious factors that can hinder effective communication range from deep-rooted attitudes about relations between the sexes (for example, when a woman manager gives an instruction to a male subordinate), to the disruptive effect of anxiety. The worried patient may hear only those things which tend to confirm or dispel his fear that he may have cancer; the nurse who is expecting a reprimand will have ears for little else.

Confused presentation

Confused presentation may take the form of a lack of clarity in the use of words, or it may be a case of poor design and production of a printed or typewritten communication. The appearance of a form, a letter, a notice or a brochure can assist or retard understanding of the content. This is notably the case when research workers want people to fill in questionnaires and have no means of compelling them to do so. A badly designed questionnaire will be thrown away because it is difficult to follow and complete, but a well-designed questionnaire is more likely to be returned with the required information.

How to communicate effectively

Many of the suggestions made to improve communications in organizations amount to changes designed to bring people into situations and relationships in which there exists the opportunity for effective communication. This, however, does not mean that effective communication will necessarily occur, and since organizational structure and design is outside the scope of this chapter the following brief discussion will concern itself exclusively with the factors the individual must bear in mind when attempting to communicate, whether the content of the message be information, instruction, opinion or argument.

The fundamental need to establish empathy implies that consideration must be given to the characteristics, situation, beliefs, attitudes and expectations of the person or group to be addressed. How much does this person know already about the matter, and how much background information will he need to be given? How readily will he listen to you? How difficult will it be for you to get his attention? What problems or anxieties has he that might affect his reaction to your message? Will his interests or his prejudices be affected by it?

The presentation of the message must be related to the person or group addressed. The choice of words is important. Not only must they be words that will be clearly understood, they must be words that will convey the right tone and implications. A letter will conjure up in the mind of the person who receives it a picture of the person who wrote it. What sort of picture do you want the recipient to have of you? Consider the difference between the following two examples.

'Thank you for your letter of the 13th August. Your complaint is being investigated and I will write to you again when I have more information.'

'I am so sorry you feel your wife was not treated with every consideration when she was in our hospital. I hope you will give me a few days to look into the matter and then I will write to you again.'

The first is official, defensive: the second personal, concerned. Similarly, when giving a talk the first essential is to establish rapport with the audience. When the audience is an unfamiliar one it may be difficult to plan the presentation in advance, and it may be necessary to feel your way towards the right level and right type of presentation by breaking away from the pattern of the formal talk and getting some interaction going right from the start. This demands considerable skill and cannot be done with a large audience, so the importance of getting as much information as you can about your audience before planning your presentation is underlined.

For example, you are going to give a careers talk to an audience of schoolgirls. What age are they? From what kind of school? Is this a school that usually sends a number of its pupils on to nursing, or does the headmistress discourage girls who show ability from applying for nurse training? What kind of questions do these girls normally ask careers lecturers? Are they interested in pay, or would a more vocational emphasis be the right approach? Are there among them a number who might be qualified and interested to consider the possibility of a university nursing course? Enough has been said to indicate that the essential skill of communication is an ability to tailor presentation to the needs of the particular group or individual person.

Finally, it is important to know how effective your communication has been. This means follow-up and the opportunity for feedback. Has your message been understood; have people been affected as you hoped; has the task been carried out as you intended? If not some further action, some further communication, may be required, and it may be necessary to modify your approach on future occasions.

THE SPOKEN WORD

Communication at the informal level

Most communication goes on between people encountering each other in twos and threes. Most of it is unplanned, a good deal is unconscious, but all the time one human being is with another he is communicating even though he is silent. He is communicating with his eyes, his gestures, the slight movements that indicate inattention or impatience, the way he stands, and the clothes he has chosen to wear. When he speaks he communicates not only by what he says and the words in which he chooses to express it, but by the tone of voice he adopts and by the movements of his eyes, his body and his hands as he speaks. Even on the telephone much more is communicated than a bare record of the conversation would indicate. Post Office telephone operators are, with good reason, taught to 'put a smile in your voice', and it is a salutary exercise to record a telephone conversation in which you have taken part and then play it back. A pause sounds much longer on the telephone than in ordinary conversation and may fill the person on the other end of the line with consternation. What is he thinking? Have I said something wrong? Have I been cut off?

A point that is often forgotten when making a telephone call is that most people, when they pick up the receiver, need a moment or two to orientate themselves to realize to whom they are speaking, and to turn their minds to the matter that is being raised. When the telephone rang they were probably engaged in something quite different, or deep in conversation on some other topic. So it is wise to speak relatively slowly and deliberately at first, identify yourself clearly, and give the other person that moment or two to grasp what you are talking about. You can then gradually increase the speed at which you are talking so as not to waste time. Once again, effective use of the telephone depends on putting yourself in the shoes of the other person.

When Ley and Spelman (1967) reviewed the literature on communications between doctors and patients and went on to conduct some experiments of their own, they drew some conclusions that can be applied in a much wider context. Their interest was to discover why it was that even when doctors tried to communicate with patients and tell them about their illnesses, the treatment they should have and the restrictions they should observe, patients so often failed to understand what was said to them or to abide by the doctor's instructions. Most of the barriers to communication described above were found to be operative in this context. More particularly, doctors often made wrong assumptions about patients' existing level of knowledge and therefore used terms that were either misunderstood or not understood. Patients and doctors often have different ideas about what is important. Many patients remembered what they had been told was wrong with them but forgot the instructions they had been given and a marked degree of anxiety interfered with understanding and retention. On the other hand, moderate anxiety, just enough to make the patient interested in what the doctor had to say, helped the patient to remember.

The following positive advice came out of these studies.

(1)   Make the patient write down what he is told. He will then have a record to consult.

(2)   When giving information to patients give the most important information first.

(3)   If advice or instructions are given, emphasize their importance.

In other contexts it will not always be possible to proceed in this way – staff will generally resent it if they are asked to write down what you tell them! But much the same purpose can be served by following up a conversation with a letter or note setting out what you understand to have been the conclusions reached and the action agreed although this degree of formality will only be appropriate when the matter is a fairly significant one.

It is also sound practice to break down the content of the communication into easily assimilable units, and to structure the conversation in such a way that you can be sure each unit has been understood before you pass on to the next. The most important points should be mentioned first and, if possible, repeated two or three times, preferably in slightly different words each time. If one way of putting the matter is not acceptable, another may be.

On the other hand, it is a mistake to be so intent on getting your message across that you do not listen to what is being said to you. It may be important! It may need to be taken into account, and it may modify what you had originally intended to do or say. At the very least, your evident willingness to listen will increase the chances that people will be willing to listen to you. To listen effectively is at least as important an art as to communicate effectively – as Nichols (1959) has shown. One way of checking that you are listening effectively is to reformulate what the speaker is saying and feed it back to him: 'As I understand you, what you are saying is...' or 'So what you would like is...'. He will soon correct you if you have got it wrong.

Committees and meetings

Frequent attendance at committee meetings is an occupational hazard of working in the health services. Senior nurses are sometimes members of hospital boards or committees, or they may attend as senior officers with the right to speak, either freely or when invited to do so. These meetings may be conducted in a relatively formal way with the rules of procedure observed, while at the other extreme a group of ward sisters who have come together spontaneously to 'thrash out' standard procedures for use on their wards may function quite effectively without any formal procedure at all, and without a designated chairman. There are numerous books on committee procedure and practice, but probably the most practical and readable, and one that does take fully into account the wide variations found in the ways in which committees conduct their business, is that by Anstey (1962). Perhaps the most useful formulation of the factors making for success at any meeting is McGregor's (1960) 'Characteristics of the Effective, Creative Group'.

(1) The atmosphere . . . tends to be informal, comfortable, relaxed . . . .

(2) There is a lot of discussion in which virtually everyone participates, but it remains pertinent to the task of the group.

(3) The task or objective of the group is well understood and accepted by the members.

(4) The members listen to each other! Every idea is given a hearing. People do not appear to be afraid of being foolish by putting forth a creative thought even if it seems fairly extreme.

(5) There is disagreement . . . disagreements are not suppressed or overridden by premature group action. The reasons are carefully examined, and the group seeks to resolve them rather than to dominate the dissenter.

(6) Most decisions are reached by a kind of consensus in which it is clear that everybody is in general agreement and willing to go along. . . formal voting is at a minimum; the group does not accept a simple majority as a proper basis for action.

(7) Criticism is frequent, frank and relatively comfortable. There is little evidence of personal attack, either openly or in a hidden fashion.

(8) People are free in expressing their feelings as well as their ideas, both on the problem and on the group's operation.

(9) When action is taken, clear assignments are made and accepted.

(10) The chairman of the group does not dominate it nor, on the contrary, does the group defer unduly to him. In fact the leadership shifts from time to time depending on the circumstances. . . there is little evidence of a struggle for power as the group operates. The issue is not who controls, but how to get the job done.

(11) The group is self-conscious about its own operation.

Perhaps this is a counsel of perfection, but the criteria set out by Anstey for the successful committee shows in practical terms what the individual committee member, or chairman, can do to set his sights on this goal.

Public speaking

Public speaking is an art that can only be acquired by practice, but it is one that the senior nurse must acquire if she is to discharge her responsibilities for the following.*

(1)   Participating in conferences relating to nursing.

(2)   Undertaking public relations work, both locally within the community and generally on behalf of the nursing profession.

(3)   Exercising leadership in the hospital group.

Concentration on the needs of the audience can help to overcome the self-consciousness of the beginner. What can you do to make the experience interesting and useful for them, however traumatic it may be for you? Content must be judged in the light of what you can discover about them and what you are trying to achieve, but the technique of public speaking in the relevant contexts depends on three fundamentals.

(1)   Familiarize yourself with your material.

(2)   Convey warmth and an interest in your audience as people.

(3)   Avoid monotony.

Familiarity with the material does not mean learning your speech by heart. It means knowing enough about your subject and how you wish to present it to be able to *ad lib* effectively if, for example, a previous speaker has made many of the points you intended to make and thus stolen your thunder, or an unexpected interruption throws you off your stroke. Always practise difficult words and names beforehand. For example, some people have difficulty with the letter 'r' in a word like primarily, and they may find it helps to pronounce it with the emphasis on the second syllable.

Some people naturally convey more warmth of personality than others, but if a speaker smiles at his audience they are more likely to smile back at him! An audience also appreciates a talk that appears to have been prepared for them, even though it may be basically the same talk that was given last week to a different audience. If you do your homework on your audience as conscientiously as you do on your subject, you should have no problems in modifying material and presentation to meet its needs.

Monotony can be avoided if you ensure that you can be heard. Remember that your voice will sound louder to you than to anyone else in the room: do not shout, but project your voice to the back of the room. Vary the pace and tone of your delivery; do not be afraid to speak slowly and deliberately at times and more quickly at others. Look at each part of your audience in turn, and control your mannerisms.

*(Salmon Report – job description: Chief Nursing Officer)

Restrained gestures are better than clutching your hands feverishly in front of you. Take care not to drop your voice at the end of your sentences so that you become inaudible. Practise the effective use of pauses, which have the same function of emphasizing your important points as white space has round a heading on the printed page.

THE WRITTEN AND PRINTED WORD

Almost everything that has been said so far applies also to correspondence, memoranda, reports, notices, publications for patients and their relatives, brochures and publicity material and house journals. These are only a few of the many forms of written and printed communication with which the senior nurse may need to concern herself.

Routine correspondence is often badly handled because care is not taken to predict the effect a particular form of words will have on the recipient. A reply to an enquiry about employment or training is an exercise in public relations; – even when there are no vacancies. An organization will often be judged by the tone and appearance of the letters it sends out.

Reports

Reports to committees are particularly important in a service where committee members may lack detailed knowledge but will take decisions on the basis of information supplied by officers. As the Farquharson–Lang Report (Scottish Home and Health Department, 1966a) observed:
'Too often officers are content to put forward (and boards to accept) either a letter raising a problem or an oral report, based perhaps on some earlier reference in the minutes. This probably means that members are not fully aware of all the factors which should be taken into consideration until they come to the meeting and their officers explain the situation; if all the information is not then available, consideration of the problem may have to be deferred until the following meeting. We recommend that boards should, in consultation with their officers, review the arrangements for the presentation of material to them to ensure that members have, in advance of meetings, a comprehensive statement of any matter on which they are being asked to give considered views.

A report needs to include the following elements: summary (this may appear at the beginning or at the end); introduction – what the report is about, why it was written; source of the information, including an account of any investigations carried out; findings; conclusions; recommendations. There may also be appendices setting out more detailed information or supporting data than it is appropriate to include in the body of the report. The report must include a clear statement of the terms of reference.

Write clearly and simply. Be careful to define key terms. Use headings to break up your text, but be clear whether you are using them as a logical framework or as attention-catchers (like newspaper headlines). Has the report persuasion as its objective? Then let the facts speak for themselves as far as possible. Separate facts from comment. Are you making recommendations? Check that they are soundly based on your findings, that they are practicable, and worth the money, effort and time involved. What savings or other advantages would accrue? Can you quantify these? Will your quantification stand up to rigorous examination? Have you examined the arguments *against* your conclusions or recommendations — is it worth refuting them in advance? Are you justified in coming to firm conclusions at all? Finally, if you use visual aids — charts, diagrams, tabulations — make sure that they are consistent with your text, and that they clarify rather than confuse.

Brochures and publicity material

Enough has been said on the content of written communication to limit discussion under this heading to matters of physical presentation. Visual layout and design are often considered secondary matters but, however inspired the content of a publication, it will not be read if the physical appearance repels. Good design, photography, artwork and printing are not cheap, and the cost of an effective job should be allowed for. The difference may be between throwing away £250 and spending £800 wisely. The King's Fund published, in 1965, a useful report *Brochures for Schools of Nursing,* and some further points in this connection were made by Watkin and Baynes (1966) in an article that is available as a reprint from the King's Fund. Much of what is said in this report is equally applicable to other types of printed material and will not be repeated here. However, most publications issued by hospitals have, as their main object, either *persuasion* (training school brochures, back-to-nursing campaign material) or *reassurance* (e.g. leaflets for patients). While both these objects require that certain information should be included, it is as well to pause to consider whether the total effect of the publication as written and designed is, in fact, persuasive or reassuring. As Watkin and Baynes pointed out:

'The provision of information obviously has an important part to play in persuading, attracting and motivating, but if we look at the production of a brochure as an exercise in persuasion rather than as the provision of information for its own sake, we are less likely to produce brochures that look like something from the Department of Inland Revenue, comprehensive, formal, and utterly forbidding.'

House journals

House journals are increasingly used in hospitals to open up channels of communication between management and staff as a whole, and to promote a feeling of identity with the hospital or group. Scrutiny of the 60-odd hospital house journals submitted for the King's Fund competition in 1969 gave rise to a strong impression that live hospitals tend to produce live journals. This is reasonable; even the best editor cannot produce an effective journal in an organization where management is dead from the neck up and the prevailing atmosphere is one of apathy. In many hospital journals there is a reluctance to discuss current management problems and policies, but this is hardly a criticism of the officers, many of them relatively junior in the hospital heirarchy, who edit the journals. They can hardly be expected to reform the service single-handed and to wrest from an unwilling management information that it does not wish to share with the staff.

This means, of course, that the successful house journal is not the individual creation of its editor. It is the creation of the organization that appoints a suitable editor, and gives him the freedom and scope, the support, resources and facilities that he needs to do a good job. If management truly understands the value of an effective house journal, it will be prepared to assign the resources of staff, time, and money to enable the job to be done properly.

PUBLIC RELATIONS

The standard definition of public relations – and it cannot be bettered – is that of the Institute of Public Relations...'The deliberate, planned and sustained effort to establish and maintain mutual understanding between an organization and its public.'

This definition makes it clear that the public relations function is two-way; it helps the public to have a better understanding of the hospital, and the hospital to have a better understanding of its public. This applies equally to relations with the press. These will only be fruitful if an effort is made to appreciate the needs and problems of the press. A journalist's prime task is to get news for his readers; he is not an advertising agent retained by the hospital to publicize its achievments and play down its shortcomings. What he considers to be news will not always be what the hospital would like to appear, but nonetheless the cultivation of friendly relationships, on a personal level, frankness when things go wrong, and willingness to draw to the attention of newspapers — particularly local ones — things that may interest them will, in the long run, pay worthwhile dividends.

In the wider sense, the best forms of public relations are a standard of care that will be reported by patients to their relatives and friends in glowing terms and a staff who are both satisfied and informed. Public relations techniques that will persuade a community, in the long term, that its hospital is first-rate and the staff devoted when this is not in fact the case, just do not exist.

The Management Decision and Control Function

A STRUCTURED APPROACH TO PROBLEM SOLVING

A manager's effectiveness turns on the decisions he makes when confronted with problems. The more scrupulous he is to adopt a scientific approach to the decisions he has to make, the more likely he is to make the right decisions. The scientific approach to problem solving may be set out in six stages.

(1) Define the problem.
(2) Analyse the nature of the problem.
(3) Identify alternative solutions.
(4) Choose the best solution.
(5) Implement the decision.
(6) Check that the solution works.

The first stage is perhaps the most important, for the other stages depend on how the problem is defined in the first place, whether dispassionately and objectively or in a superficial, subjective way that seizes upon the presenting symptom and does not trouble to identify the underlying problem that has given rise to it. Coupled with definition of the problem should be early recognition that there is a problem, and that a decision is called for. Decisions are often made not consciously, but by a process of creeping commitment. The manager responds to a series of situations in such a way that he ends up with only one possible course of action. He can avoid painting himself into a corner in this way if he makes the conscious effort to look at the situation at a sufficiently early stage. Care must be taken that the problem is correctly identified — it is a waste of time to find the right answer to the wrong question. Efforts to recruit more staff are futile if 75 per cent have left by the end of the first month. The problem is one not of recruitment, but of retention. Problems that are initially thought to be problems of shortage are often, on closer inspection, seen to be problems of maldistribution or ineffective utilization.

To analyse the nature of the problem it is necessary to collect all relevant information that is available. It is accepted that managers often have to make decisions on inadequate information and in circumstances and under pressures which do not permit the collection of all the data on which a fully informed decision could be made. Nonetheless, decisions are seldom, and then only by chance, better than the information on which they are based, and important decisions should not be taken without adequate information. The consequences of delaying a decision must be weighed against the likely costs of a wrong decision.

The stages of analysing the nature of the problem and identifying alternative solutions often merge. The danger here is that the range of solutions considered may be limited because the manager plumps for one that seems attractive as soon as it occurs to him, without sufficiently pursuing the possibility that there may be other and better, although perhaps less obvious, alternatives. It is worth examining even the most improbable solutions and at this stage the technique known as brainstorming (Cuming, 1968b) has much to offer. The solution chosen must be the one that best contributes to the achievement of the organization's objectives, and the more clearly these are defined the easier it will be to determine which is the best solution.

Objectives in health service organizations are commonly diffuse and ill-defined. 'To serve the community' or 'to get patients better' are phrases that beg more questions than they answer. While defining objectives at the level of the total organization is often extremely difficult it must be attempted, for these objectives are a necessary framework for departmental and unit objectives. These are frequently easier to define. A medical laboratory, for example, might define the service it wished to give in terms of same-day reporting on certain types of test, with the percentage of error falling below a certain figure, and unit costs within a stated range. The objectives of an out-patient department might include the requirement that 95 per cent of patients should be seen within 30 minutes of their appointment time. These are things that can be measured and success or failure can be clearly demonstrated. It is not always possible to express objectives in such clear terms, but it should not too readily be assumed that it cannot be done.

The identification of alternative solutions and choosing the best of these should ideally be shared by the people who will be affected by the decision. If participation occurs at these stages, the implementation stage will present few problems since those chiefly affected will already be committed to the chosen solution. The final stage consists of monitoring the effects of the decision to see whether, in practice, it does solve the problem it was intended to solve and does contribute to the achievement of objectives. This leads naturally to the discussion of management information and control.

MANAGEMENT INFORMATION AND CONTROL

As motor cars have become more complex and road conditions more congested, increasing instrumentation enables the driver to get the best out of his car and to complete his journey swiftly and safely. Like the driver, the manager needs information about how the machine he controls is behaving and about what is going on around him. He needs his equivalent of a revolution counter to see whether he is pushing his organization to the limit of its capacity. As a simple rear-view mirror is no longer enough for the driver, and he needs wing mirrors to cover his blind spots where traffic police may be lurking, or the foolish driver who may be trying to overtake him on the nearside, so the manager needs an increasing amount of information about the environment which impinges on his organization.

The driver uses the information he receives directly via his senses or indirectly through mirrors and instruments to adjust his speed and direction of travel, and he may need a further glance at his instruments to see if his action has had the desired effect. It is well known that it is difficult to judge speed on the motorway, and when approaching the roundabout marking the end of the motorway the wise motorist discards his subjective impressions and relies entirely upon his speedometer reading. In just the same way a manager may, through familiarity, misjudge the state of morale in his organization and an attitude survey may be required to shake his conviction that 'we're all one big happy family here'.

A manager in a service industry needs principally to monitor the *cost* and the *quality* of the service he is providing. However, he is wise if he also monitors certain *intermediate variables* which are likely to affect cost and quality, for example, labour turnover, resource utilization and staff attitudes. Financial control and costing is discussed in Chapter 11, and the need to maintain personnel records that provide information about staff turnover and absence is stressed earlier in this section. In the health field it is not possible to suggest a single or simple measure of the quality of service provided. A number of measures and techniques may have to be employed to give an adequate picture of how the organization is performing. Some approaches that have been tried, either routinely or experimentally, are listed below.

Accreditation

The term accreditation is derived from the scheme administered by the Joint Commission on Accreditation of Hospitals in the United States of America. The scheme is based on a manual setting out minimum acceptable standards, although attempts are now being made to shift the emphasis from minimum standards to the setting of objectives. Accreditation does not directly monitor the care provided, but is designed to ensure that the facilities and processes necessary to ensure high quality care are present and used. In the United Kingdom there is no such accreditation of hospitals, but the recognition of hospitals for training purposes by the General Nursing Council and other statutory or professional bodies is a form of accreditation.

Medical audit

In the United States of America medical audit is usually carried out by a committee or committees of the medical staff. The emphasis is on review by colleagues of individual cases. The audit is based on agreed standards, for example, tests that ought to be carried out in all cases of particular conditions. All cases, or only a random sample, may be discussed. The system is seen as one that ensures high standards of care and provides continuing educational experience for the staff. The Brotherston Report (Scottish Home and Health Department, 1966b), suggested that a similar system might be set up in Scottish hospitals, although it preferred to call it patient care evaluation. If patient care evaluation became a recognized function of the divisional medical structure there would be a strong case for the involvement of nurses below the senior management level who are now in some hospitals invited to attend divisional meetings. It is difficult to see how patient care can be adequately evaluated without taking into account those aspects of care for which the nurse is responsible.

Utilization review

Utilization review again derives from the United States of America, and is carried out mainly by the medical staff themselves. The utilization committee reviews, for example, long-stay cases; certain short-stay cases (was the stay too short for safety?); unnecessary admissions; doubtful emergency admissions; operations performed that were not indicated by the diagnosis on admission and so on. The object is to promote the most effective use of hospital facilities, but also to provide an educational experience for the staff concerned. Once more, participation by nursing administrative staff is indicated should this kind of function be undertaken by the divisional medical structure recommended in the Cogwheel Report (Ministry of Health, 1967).

Hospital activity analysis

Hospital activity analysis is a system based on an American model for analysing information about patients treated in general hospitals. It is hoped that it will soon be operative in all N.H.S. general hospitals. At present, information on each patient discharged is copied onto a special form, coded and electronically processed. The object is to feed back to the hospitals information about their patterns of work that can be used for management purposes, and to review clinical and management policies.

Patient welfare measures

Measures of patient welfare were developed in the course of the 'Nurse Utilisation Project' (1960). They were designed to make it possible to quantify the relationship between nursing activity and patient welfare. The measures included days in hospital; days of fever; number of post-operative days; narcotics, analgesics and sedatives required; mobility; mental attitude; physical independence; skin condition; patient opinion; physician's evaluation of patient's progress.

The nursing administrator needs not only to monitor the quality of care received by patients, but also the work-load which her staff have to carry. The most useful measure here is *nursing dependency*, as described in a publication of the Operational Research Unit, Oxford Regional Hospital Board (1967). A technique and *pro forma* for the *patient satisfaction survey* has been evolved by the King's Fund (Raphael, 1969), and is suitable and available for routine use as a means of monitoring patients' subjective experience of hospital care.

Management can only be effective if it is based on sound information, and this applies as much to nursing administration as to any other form of management. If the collection of the necessary data appears to impose an additional burden on an already overworked staff, it should be considered at least possible that the better planning and ordering of priorities, which is possible when objective measurement replaces impressions, will in the long run increase the effectiveness of the service to the patient and make it feasible to achieve a reasonably satisfactory relationship between staffing levels and work-load.

Bibliography and References

Anstey, E. (1962). *Committees: How They Work and How to Work Them.* London; Allen and Unwin

Cuming, M.W. (1968a). *Reducing the Odds.* London; King Edward's Hospital Fund for London

— (1968b). *The Theory and Practice of Personnel Management.* London; Heinemann

Gowers, E. (1966). *The Complete Plain Words.* Harmondsworth; Penguin

Hotel and Catering EDC (1969). *Staff Turnover.* London; H.M.S.O.

Leeds Regional Hospital Board (1963). *Work Measurement as a Basis for Calculating Nursing Establishments.* Harrogate; The Board

Ley, P. and Spelman, M.S. (1967). *Communicating with the Patient.* London; Staples

McGregor, D. (1960). *The Human Side of Enterprise.* New York; McGraw-Hill

MacGuire, J. (1966). *From Student to Nurse – Training and Qualification.* Oxford Area Nurse Training Committee

Millott, H.L. (1963). *Selection of Student Nurses.* Melbourne; Royal Australian Nursing Federation

Ministry of Health (1966). *Report of the Committee on Senior Nursing Staff Structure* (Salmon Report). London: H.M.S.O.

— (1967). *First Report of the Joint Working Party on the Organisation of Medical Work in Hospitals.* London; H.M.S.O.

Nichols, R.G. (1959). 'Listening, What Price Inefficiency?' *Office Executive* **34**, 10

Norton, D., McLaren, R. and Exton-Smith, A.N. (1962). *An Investigation of Geriatric Nursing Problems in Hospital.* London: National Corporation for the Care of Old People

Nurse Utilisation Project (1960). *An Investigation of the Relation between Nursing Activity and Patient Welfare.* Ames; Iowa State University Press

Oxford Regional Hospital Board, Operational Research Unit (1967). *Measurement of Nursing Care.* Oxford; The Board

Parry, J. (1968). 'Comunication Barriers'. *New Society* **11**, 671

Raphael, W. (1969). *Patients and Their Hospitals.* London; King Edward's Hospital Fund for London

Revans, R.W. (1964). *Standards for Morale.* London; Oxford University Press

Roberts, D.E. (1963). *Staffing of Public Health and Out-patient Nursing Services: Methods of Study.* Public Health Paper No. 21. Geneva; WHO

Rodger, A. (1951). 'The Seven Point Plan.' London; National Institute of Industrial Psychiology

Roff, H.E. and Watson, T.E. (1969). *Job Analysis.* London; Institute of Personnel Management

Samuel (1969) *Labour Turnover? Towards a Solution.* Institute of Personnel Management

Scottish Home and Health Department (1966a). *Administrative Practice of Hospital Boards in Scotland.* Edinburgh; H.M.S.O.

– (1966b). *Organisation of Medical Work in the Hospital Service in Scotland.* Edinburgh; H.M.S.O.

– (1969). *Nursing Workload per Patient as a Basis for Staffing.* Edinburgh; H.M.S.O.

Seymour, W.D. (1968). *Skills Analysis Training.* London; Pitman

Watkin, B. and Baynes, K. (1966). 'Nursing School Brochures.' *Br. Hosp. J. Soc. Serv. Rev.* **76**, 399 and 453

7–The Quantitative Foundations of Health Services Management

H.P. Ferrer

Introduction

The use of quantitative techniques in health services management cannot be considered in isolation from other sections of this book. These techniques involve the ability to select and maintain correct records, the use of epidemiological methods in community needs, and the application of these techniques in operations research. The relationship of quantitative techniques in decision making cannot be discussed adequately in this section. It is evident that there has been an increasing use made of these methods in recent years, and that measurement in management cannot be relegated to a second-class position but form an essential part of the techniques that a manager in the health services uses, both in his day-to-day decision making, and in the forward planning of the services.

Qualitative decisions have to be given a much more formal basis in the consideration of their value for management. We may say, for example, that a certain entrance to an out-patient clinic is better to use than another, but quantitative data may or may not have been used in coming to this decision. We have used many qualitative judgements.

97

For example, the entrance may look better and give a better image to the out-patients. However, in starting to measure the consequences of the use of this entrance for the patients and staff, it may be found that it is not in fact the best way in for the patients, and the use of this entrance is inefficient for the staff. It is then necessary to define the objectives involved; and if the conclusion is that the image of the out-patients is more important than the efficient use of patient and staff time, we shall go back to the original qualitative judgement. However, it may subsequently be necessary to justify these decisions. Is the better image justified in terms of cost and convenience to staff and patients, or will the image eventually be tarnished anyway as more and more frustrations arise in the inefficient use of staff and patient time? If we have gone about our decision making in consultation with the patients and staff, how have we used quantitative techniques in the measurement of opinion?

Quantitative measurements may not give a ready and easy means of decision making, but it will help to define more sharply the basis upon which we are trying to base our decision. The subtle interplay of readily available data, with our own subjective and often qualitative judgement, is outside the scope of this section. However, many persons brought up in the tradition of experience being the best guide in management may not find it easy to accept the challenge that quantitative methods present. It is also true that the misuse of such methods has cast a certain shadow over these techniques in many people's minds. Many managers in the health services, particularly medical personnel and nursing staff, may have had a training in life sciences which has not included use of quantitative techniques, and they may find it difficult to adapt to this particular method of thought.

Undoubtedly, quantitative methods should ideally form part of the almost unconscious approach to management by the modern health services manager. As such, it does not form a ready-to-use diagnostic tool which is applied in certain circumstances and not in others, but is rather a deeper method of training which is available at all times. It should be remembered that quantitative techniques may use any mathematical method, and often the simpler methods may be more appropriate to the problem in hand. However, by his training, the manager will be able to present his data in a readily available form and will know how to seek expert advice if he finds that the problem cannot be solved by the techniques that he has available himself. The major part of this section will deal mainly with the collection of data, an introduction to available techniques and some of the more useful methods which may be used to solve problems.

INTRODUCTION

The collection and handling of data

The collection of statistics can be divided into two main groups.

(1) A special survey, with the express intention of gathering material which can be subsequently processed.

(2) Material collected during the routine day-to-day administration which is accessible for statistical analysis.

In (1) it has to be decided whether the cost of a special survey is justified from the results obtained and, in (2) there has to be a meaningful use of the statistics to the personnel whose job it is to fill in the various forms, or to provide the information in other ways.

Observer observed

It seems inevitable that every observer of phenomena should be biased in a particular way, or that his observations may be subject to errors. Errors that can be classified occur between individuals, or *inter*-observer variation, and those that occur within the same individual observing different phenomena, or even the same phenomena, at different times. This we call *intra*-observer variation. It is important in the collecting of data to minimize these variations and, although it is not possible to eliminate them completely, at least they should be available for assessment. Assessment shows not only how accurate individual observers are but also, be feeding back the information to the original observers, can provide a training which enables them to standardize their techniques and to look critically at their methods.

Quality control and observers

It is obvious that from time to time the results obtained by different observers, or change in the circumstances which give a certain result, will affect the data that may be collected from a particular source. For example, if we are monitoring the bed occupancy rate throughout a large number of hospitals over a period of time, each hospital will not only vary in the average number of days that its patients will occupy beds, but also variations will occur within each specialty catered for in the hospital. It is possible to obtain some idea of this variation, and to get an early warning of, and changes in, variation, by some simple method such as the cumulative sum technique. The cumulative sum technique is a method of quality control which has been applied in industry for many years. The implications of this technique for use within the health services have still to be explored, but it is obvious that it provides a ready means of quality control that enables the monitoring of data to be kept up to date, and also to observe variations and trends in that data. Some of the implications of the cumulative sum technique may be recognized from Table 7.1. and *Figure 7.1.* If the number of days that the average patient occupies a bed changes

TABLE 7.1

Cumulative Sum Technique Applied to Bed Occupancy
Mean number of days per patient for 1969 = 4·5

1970	x (days/patient)	y (4·5 − x)	$y_1 + y_2 + y_x$
January	6·8	−2·3	−2·3
February	7·2	−2·7	−5·0
March	3·5	+1·0	−4·0
April	4·2	+0·3	−3·7
May	3·6	+0·9	−2·8
June	4·9	−0·4	−3·2
July	5·9	−1·4	−4·6
August	6·7	−2·2	−6·8
September	7·3	−2·8	−9·6
October	7·5	−3·0	−12·6

the technique will highlight this and will show immediately whether the change coincided with change in personnel, in season, or whether there is some other explanation. It may thus be possible to find the reason so that the needs of the department concerned can be accommodated to those of others in the hospital. It may be found, for example, that there is an increased patient occupancy in the department during particular times of the year, and that this demand can be anticipated in future years if the same pattern is followed.

Changes in personnel can also be observed by this method. If it is found that compared with sister A, sister B has a lower rate of bed occupancy, then it may be worthwhile investigating whether this has any serious implications for the rest of the hospital. Obviously this kind of continuous monitoring − a form of quality control within the health services − must be handled with some degree of tact. The whole field of observer variation and quality control of observers is likely to cause difficulties if the data is not presented constructively to the personnel involved.

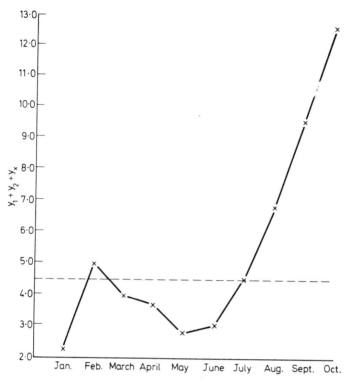

Figure 7.1. Graph drawn from figures in Table 7.1. (opposite)
  (1)   *The variations in occupancy due to season etc. are cancelled*
out by equal numbers appearing above and below previous mean (4·5)
  (2)   *During July and August some other factor has entered which has*
increased bed occupancy. This factor may be changes in policy, staff etc.,
which can be investigated

Methods of Collection of Data for Special Purposes

THE PERSONAL INTERVIEW

This method of collecting data is most difficult because of the expense involved in terms of staff time, and also because of the dangers of bias being introduced by the observer or interviewer himself. A certain degree of skill is needed by the interviewer and, in addition, certain qualities of character — neutrality, accuracy and amiability. Also,

101

the time chosen for an interview could be rather important and may bias subsequent collection of the data. The interview obtained from a doctor during a busy afternoon is likely to be more difficult than that obtained when the doctor is less rushed and in a more reflective mood. Obviously an interviewer has to have the kind of approach that is not going to give rise to a feeling of resentment in the person interviewed when in a field in which he may regard himself as an expert. Special skills are needed for the technique known as depth interviewing, and the task of finding personnel who are trained in this area is not an easy one. However, depth interviewing may be the only way in which it is possible to find reasons and the hidden factors that lead people to answer questions in a particular way.

THE QUESTIONNAIRE

Questionnaires are used widely in the collection of data. It is, of course, a much less costly method than using special staff for interviewing. However, unless a questionnaire is particularly well designed certain errors may be introduced. In particular, the questions asked may not convey the same meaning to the person questioned as that which the designer of the questionnaire intended. Although it is free from the personal bias which might be introduced by an interviewer, there is the danger of the other kinds of bias being introduced. Many people will not reply to a questionnaire or will reply haphazardly and inaccurately particularly if it is regarded as yet one more intrusion into their particular field of work. The questionnaire should be simple, as short as possible, and should not contain emotive phrases which are likely to cause reaction on a particular problem which may be bothering personnel or patients at a particular time.

Preferably, the answers should be of easy access and be capable of being ringed or answered in as simple a way as possible. It is important to avoid answers which could be biased and lead to misunderstanding. One example is the misuse of units. If a patient is asked, 'How long did you have to wait before receiving your appointment to the out-patient department?', then it is necessary to specify whether the answer is required in days, weeks, months, or years. Questions which rely on memory can cause some difficulty. One example is the notorious problem which many patients have of remembering their illnesses. Although most patients can remember major events, they cannot remember fairly trivial illnesses they may have suffered in the past five years. When the questionnaire asks, 'When did you last see your doctor?', there may be considerable difficulty for some patients who may not have seen their doctor for some years, with the results that they tend to round off their answers, whereas those who have seen their doctors fairly frequently in the recent past may give a more accurate answer.

Although it may be instructive in some cases to find detailed replies to questions such as, 'What would you most like to see in the hospital out-patient department?', this kind of question can cause a lot of difficulties if it involves the person writing something of an essay about the facilities of the out-patient department. Such essays could be useful, and with proper means of sampling it is possible to get some consensus of opinion which could be used later in a questionnaire that could be applied to larger numbers of people. If a few selected people are asked the above question about facilities in the out-patient department, the answers could be analysed and applied. For example, the facilities most people would like to see may be as follows.

(1) More comfortable chairs.
(2) Warmer conditions.
(3) Canteen facilities.
(4) Shorter waiting time.
(5) More accurate or easily heard patient call-system.

It is then possible to include these particular items in a subsequent questionnaire which could be supplied to larger numbers of people using a phrase such as, 'Which of the following would you most like to see in your out-patient department? Please number in order of preference'. It is possible to leave a blank for other facilities so as to obtain reactions of a different kind which may not have been included in the original heading.

Questions of a technical nature should be avoided as far as possible, because many people who lack the expertise that the question implies will take a middle course rather than betray their ignorance. Questions which involve the use of futuristic or even clairvoyant qualities in the person being questioned should also be avoided. A phrase such as 'Will you require more, less, or about the same theatre time next year, or in five years' time as you have at present?', requires a guess which even a consultant surgeon may find difficult to make. It would be more relevant to ask the question, 'Is your theatre time at present too much, too little, or just about right?', and to probe the reason for the answer given in subsequent questions, rather than ask for predictions which may involve many kinds of personal bias and prejudice of which the person being questioned may not be aware. The use of questions involving calculations on behalf of the person being questioned are also difficult. It may be valid to ask a relatively sophisticated health services manager questions which involve the use of calculations, but be much more difficult to ask a patient who may be attending an out-patient department 'How much do you spend each month on smoking?'. Asking for this kind of calculation can introduce inaccuracies which may not be easy to check when the questionnaire is analysed.

Pilot Surveys

Any large survey should be validated, preferably before being launched, by means of a pilot survey. The cost of a pilot survey will be more than amply repaid by possible waste that could occur if a large-scale survey was launched without adequate preparation. No matter how carefully a survey or questionnaire has been designed, the actual use of this method of obtaining information cannot be fully understood without adequate investigation under field conditions. It is, perhaps, at the stage of the pilot survey when most of the problems which subsequently may be met are highlighted. Perhaps in the future reorganization of the health services each area Health Board may have some kind of statistical unit which specializes in carrying out this kind of pilot investigation. The pilot survey is essentially a small-scale replica of the actual survey which it is hoped to carry out in the future. Its size is important, and although the pilot survey should be carried out on as representative a sample as possible, major faults will be highlighted in a way which no other method could bring about. Situations and questions which may appear perfectly clear to somebody in an office may look very different to personnel involved in the field, or to the patients from whom information is sought. The only sure answer is to check all surveys and questionnaires by means of a pilot study, and to be prepared, if necessary, to conduct several pilot studies as the original ideas are analysed and improved upon.

METHODS OF SAMPLING

Information can be obtained in several ways. First and foremost it is necessary to define what kind of information is required. Secondly, from whom or for what is this information required? This last is not always easy to define. One may decide to ask a group of hospital porters their opinion on a new trolley, or information may be required about prescribing habits from general practitioners. In the first case, one must define which of the hospital porters to ask about the new trolley: there would be no point in asking porters who have had little or no experience of it. In the second case, it is necessary to define which general practitioners to question. Should all the G.P.s in a certain area be questioned? If only a few of the G.P.s are to be questioned, it is necessary to ensure there is a sufficient number of urban, rural, and mixed practices.

The group chosen for study is called a universe or population. This still applies if the items in that universe are inanimate or abstract. It is seldom possible to ask every member of such a universe or population for the required information, and even if the full facilities for this were available there are some advantages in using a sampling method. The basic concept behind sampling is that once the desired population has been defined, whatever method is subsequently used, every member of that population must be given an equal opportunity of appearing in the subsequent sample. Ideally, every sample should be an exact miniature of the population or universe itself and should contain all the normal distributions and abnormalities which one might expect to find in the larger universe. However, this is seldom possible, and one can never be absolutely certain that the sample will be the exact copy in miniature that is required. We have also to decide how much confidence can be placed in the estimate of the sample and, generally, this can be done by specifying certain limits within which the true answer can lie. If one calculated from a sample, that the arithmetical mean number of prescriptions written each day by a G.P. in urban practices was 28 compared with arithmetical mean 17 in rural practices, it would be necessary to define the limits of reliability that could be placed on these figures because the calculations are based on a sample. These methods will be discussed later.

TAKING SAMPLES

It is seldom possible to obtain a sample which is completely free from bias. Many subtle factors come into play, such as the measurement of non-response, as it is seldom that every person asked a particular question, or subject examined from the original sample, will be available. Although it is desirable to get as many persons or objects as possible required for the sample under scrutiny, it is a very good sample indeed that contains over 80 per cent of the total population.

Random numbers

Probably the best method of drawing random samples is to use random sampling numbers. Various tables containing these numbers have been published. In practice, it has been found that these tables have no obvious bias. To obtain a random sample of 1,000 G.P.s throughout England and Wales take from a list of all the G.P.s in the country 1,000 names using a list of random numbers. Several random sampling number lists, however, do not contain sufficient number for the size of population being selected. In this case it is necessary to run several of the numbers together, reading them off in groups of, for example, six or more digits, which would cover 1,000,000 of the available population.

The non-response rate from the sample has to be studied carefully, particularly when using the interviewer method. If a certain person is not available the interviewer may turn to the next available person, and this may unconsciously add a certain bias to the sample. It is important therefore when instructing interviewers to be very exact as to where alternatives are to be drawn from, particularly if one is using a random method of selection.

Arbitrary numbers

Another method of drawing a sample is to select an arbitrary number, such as 15, and then to draw every fifteenth member of the population or universe. This method is particularly useful in dealing with hospital or G.P. records. The importance of the original number is that all the cards should be covered several times during the selection process, so that once the entire universe or population has been sampled one can return to the beginning of that population and continue to take out every fifteenth member. Occasionally this method introduces some difficulties particularly hidden bias. For example, to ask every tenth household in an area about the amount of illness within that household may unconsciously have introduced an error by doing so, in that these houses may not be typical of the population as a whole. Every tenth household, for example, may be of a different social class from the others, or it may be a recurring error in that every fifteenth household is definitely not of the same type as the rest in that area, so that approximately every fifth time round a bias would be introduced into the sample which would not have come about had random numbers been used. This kind of variation or fluctuation according to a definite pattern may be quite unknown at the time the original sample was drawn.

Averages

In the survey of the number of prescriptions that G.P.s write, it has been shown that it is possible to describe the characteristics of two groups of G.P.s (those in urban and those in rural practices), in that one prescribes, on the average, a larger number of prescriptions each day than the other. It is necessary to define what is meant by the average, as this is a very much overworked, over-used and somewhat misunderstood term. The total number of prescriptions from a group of urban practices is divided by the number of G.P.s selected for the sample. This gives the arithmetic mean, and it is the best-known type of average. In common parlance, this is known as the average. It is important to realize, however, that it only describes one particular attribute of the group, that is, rural compared with urban general practitioner. It does not give any idea of the distribution of the numbers or prescriptions. If these were plotted on a graph the *range of distribution* would be shown, but the average falls only at one point of this curve.

Grouped data

The arithmetic mean does not apply in the same way to grouped data. The following examples show methods of calculating the average number of prescriptions per G.P. in (1) single-handed practices, and (2) group practices.

(1)   The number of prescriptions per practice in seven single-handed urban practices are shown in line (*a*) below. The assumed arithmetic mean number of prescriptions per G.P. is 50, and the deviation of each practice from this is given in line (*b*).

(*a*)	55	72	10	35	60	55	75
(*b*)	+5	+22	−40	−15	+10	+5	+25

Add   64 − 55 = 9
Divide by total G.P.s   9/7 = 1·27
Add assumed mean   50 + 1·27 = 51·27 prescriptions per G.P.

(2)   The simple arithmetic mean does not apply when the items are arranged in class intervals and are numerous. It would be incorrect to divide the total number of prescriptions by the total number of G.P.s.
The assumed arithmetic mean number of prescriptions per G.P. is 15.

Prescriptions per practice	G.P.s per practice	Deviation from assumed mean
60	4	+45
75	5	+60
80	6	+65
65	3	+50
10	2	− 5

Add   220 − 5   = 215
Divide by total G.P.s   215/20   = 10·7
Add assumed mean   15 + 10·7 = 25·7
                                          prescriptions per G.P.

Disadvantages

The disadvantages of using arithmetic mean are that a few items of a very high or very low value may upset the average and therefore make it unrepresentative of the whole distribution. A few G.P.s in the urban areas who write a very large number of prescriptions may make the arithmetic mean of 28 prescriptions in a representative day quite untypical of the prescribing habits of most urban practitioners. Similarly, in the rural practices a few G.P.s writing only one or two prescriptions in the day of this example may make this also untypical of the prescribing habits of most rural G.P.s. This kind of situation is sometimes exploited where it is desired to bias the particular average for special purposes. If one takes the number of prescriptions written in an urban practice as being five times the average for urban practices as a whole, it may cause concern to think that the G.P. in question is over-prescribing. However, although this may highlight a particular G.P., and may cause some questions, it is by no means certain that he is abusing his prescribing habits or that his habits for that particular type of G.P. are unusual. However, the use of the arithmetic mean *is* sometimes abused, and it is necessary to use other types of averages.

The arithmetic mean, however, does have one particular *advantage* in that it is a figure which can be used in subsequent calculations. It is a very widely understood average, but it is important to remember that there is no real value which corresponds to the arithmetic mean. To say that an urban G.P. writes 27·26 prescriptions in the day under review obviously is absurd as no G.P. can write the 0·26 of a prescription.

THE MODE

The mode is the most fashionable value in a series, and for those expert in questions of fashion it is easy to remember as *a la mode*. If one groups each G.P. in a survey with the number of prescriptions written on a particular day the mode, or the most common number of prescriptions written, is different from the arithmetic mean just described. It may be found that the modal value of numbers of prescriptions written is 20 per day. If a curve was plotted of the number of prescriptions against the number of doctors, the modal value would be found at the highest point of that curve.

A particular advantage of the mode is that it is not made unrepresentative by an extreme value as is the arithmetic mean. The mode is also a real value and represents the majority of cases. Thus, in the example, the few G.P.s who write a large number of prescriptions in a particular day make the arithmetic mean seem rather high. On the other hand, the modal value gives a much more easily understood example; namely, what most G.P.s commonly do with respect to the number of prescriptions that they write each day.

As a value, however, it does lack exactness. If the distribution of numbers of prescriptions had two peaks when plotted on a graph, in other words a bimodal distribution, this becomes much less useful as a means of conveying the necessary information.

THE MEDIAN

With ungrouped data, or data grouped in a single unit, the median value may be found by writing down the numbers in ascending or descending order. Thus, if the number of prescriptions written by each G.P. on the day of the survey were written in order, from the least to the highest number of prescriptions, the number exactly in the middle of the series is the *median value.* This is easy to pick out when it is the middle item of an odd series of numbers. When it is in the middle of an even series then it is necessary to take the two middle items and find the arithmetic mean of them.

The median is much less used than the previous two methods of calculating averages. It is useful, however, in situations where it is desired to divide a distribution exactly in half. These are used in score situations; for example, intelligence testing.

The median can be subject to some abuse. For example, if the median value of the number of prescriptions was calculated, it could be claimed that half the G.P.s wrote above average number of prescriptions. This use of the median can be misinterpreted. The median is not distorted by extremely high or low values, but if there are large numbers of erratic and irregular numbers above and below it, the median value may be the only one of its kind in the particular series of numbers.

The other averages sometimes used are the *geometric mean,* and the *harmonic mean.* Both of these are of less importance than those previously described.

Briefly, the geometric mean is used in cases where we wish to measure changes in the rate of growth where the size of one quantity depends directly on the size of a previous quantity. For example, in studying the maternity patterns in a particular community not only does that community's birth rate depend on the population which precedes the point of time being measured but also depends on the number of married couples in the previous period.

The harmonic mean is used in the averaging of rates, for example, in calculating the number of patients per hour that went into an out-patient department, a more exact measure of the rate would be obtained using the harmonic mean than would be obtained just by adding the rates and dividing by the number of rates. Calculation of the harmonic mean involves taking the arithmetic mean of the reciprocals of the individual rates, then converting this back as a reciprocal. There is one difficulty, however, if the number of patients is constant, then the correct average to use is the harmonic mean, that is, if the length of time varies. On the other hand, if dealing with rates per hour, the correct average would be the arithmetic mean.

Dispersion

So far, one measurable quantity which any range of a sample might have has been discussed. The mode, median and mean give some idea of one of the attributes of the sampled universe. It also gives a figure which may be used in subsequent calculations. It is obvious, however, that there are other attributes of the universe which are not described by these averages. If the number of people who consult the doctor is plotted against the frequency of consultations, it is found that the curve approximates to what is called the *normal curve* (*Figure 7.2*). This has one centre point, and is therefore unimodal. It is also completely symmetrical. It bears out the generally understood and intuitive conclusion that most people are centred around the average, but there are extreme values both on the high and the low end of the variables which are shown in this so-called normal distribution curve. It is particularly useful in biological data, for example, height, weight, and intelligence of population. It also enables one to describe any typical distributions which may be higher or lower, narrower, or broader than this surve, but having nevertheless, the same general shape as the normal curve.

However, the normal distribution, may be skewed either negatively or positively. Examples of skewed curves are given in *Figure 7.2*. Again, the mode would be at the highest point of the curve whereas the median would be half-way along the length of the curve, and the mean probably somewhere lower or higher than that value. J-shaped curves may also follow positive or negative distributions. The U-shaped curve (*Figure 7.2*), on the other hand, is found when describing frequency of deaths in the very old and the very young.

Standard deviation and skewness

In the normal curve approximately 68 per cent of the population will be found on either side of the curve between the vertical lines

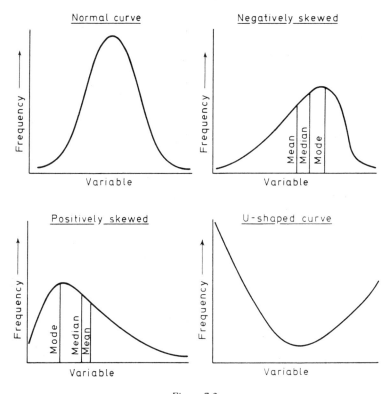

Figure 7.2.

shown (*Figure 7.3*). This is said to be one standard deviation on each side of the mean of this curve. If about 13·5 per cent is added to each of this distribution, then four standard deviations are included in this area, while adding 2·5 per cent at each end includes the total population in the distribution (69 + 2(13·5) + 2(2·5) = 100). It can be seen that approximately 95 per cent of the universe will lie within four standard deviations of the total. This measure gives a picture on which to work when discussing the universe in question. It is necessary to know only the mean, the standard deviation and the number of items to judge the approximate shape of the curve which will include the population or universe under discussion.

Although detailed methods of calculating standard deviation are not included here, it is sufficient to say that, first of all, the arithmetic mean of the sample of any universe is taken, and each deviation of every item in the sample is compared with this arithmetic mean and the final calculation is based on the arithmetic mean of these deviations. Even slightly skewed distributions may be described by means of the standard deviation.

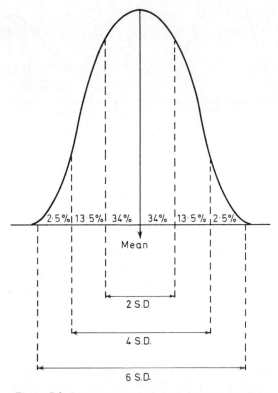

Figure 7.3. Proportions or standard deviations (S.D.). in normal distribution curve

Coefficient of Variation

The coefficient of variation is useful to compare two dispersions, as long as the units of measurement are identical. The coefficient of variation is

$$\frac{\text{standard deviation} \times 100}{\text{arithmetic mean}}$$

If the cost of prescriptions per week of a group of urban practices is compared with rural general practices, it may be found that in rural practices the mean cost is £40, and the standard deviation is £14. On the other hand, it may be found that in urban practices the mean cost is £45, with a standard deviation of £15. Rural practices would give a coefficient of variation of 35 per cent on these figures, whereas urban practices would give a coefficient of 33·33 per cent. From this it can be concluded that urban general practices may have a higher mean cost and, although the standard deviation might suggest that the cost was more spread out than in rural general practices, in fact, the dispersion of cost in rural general practices is higher than in the urban practices. This means that there is more variation in cost in rural practices than in urban general practices in the examples given.

Error Significance

If, in a survey of hospital occupancy, it is found that in over 1,000 beds every fifth patient is over the age of 65, one might expect that the same proportion of patients aged over 65 would occur in a sample of other hospital beds. However, the number may be one in four, and the age of every fourth patient in another hospital group may, in fact, be over 65. One has to ask whether or not this occurred by chance. Assuming that the sampling techniques are good, some other factor may be occurring which makes the proportion of persons over the age of 65 higher in one hospital group than in another. This difference between the two hospital groups is then said to be *significant*.

There is still the possibility that this difference could have occurred by change, but if the chances of this are so small the difference in age structure means something. It is, however, important to state at this stage that, in finding a significant result, one is not necessarily confirming or denying a particular hypothesis.

There is a danger of a result of this kind being used in the wrong way. There may be a significant difference in age structure between the two hospital groups for any one of the following reasons.

(1)   There is a difference in age structure in the populations in which they serve.

(2)   There is a geriatric unit in one hospital group which is not present in the other.

(3)   The consultants responsible for one hospital group tend to avoid taking aged persons.

(4)   The aged persons in the group with the least number of persons over 65 occupying hospital beds may be wealthier, and may prefer to go into private accommodation or private nursing homes.

The cause of the significance may have to be proved by other methods, but tests for significance are often undertaken in order to prove or disprove an original hypothesis. As can be seen from the above, it could be proved that if this result is significant any of reasons (1) to (4) may, in fact, be causing the differences, or it may be due to some other reason which has not yet been identified.

(*a*)   All the above causes may be acting in varying degrees, in which case the cause of this significant difference is said to be *multifactorial* in origin.

(*b*)   All the above causes, plus some other unknown and, as yet, unidentified cause, may be acting.

(*c*)   Some other unidentified and unknown cause may be acting alone. All that the tests for significance tell us is that the result is significant. There is a difference. It may give cause for hope that the original hypothesis is correct, but it certainly does not prove it.

Probability

The probability of getting patients over the age of 65 in the hospital groups being investigated can now be discussed. The probability (P) of an event is usually expressed as a decimal. If an unbiased coin is tossed a number of times one would expect the probability of getting a head to be one in two or, 0·5 as a decimal. In other words, P is equal to 0·5. If the probability of the events is one in 10, then P is equal to 0·1. Obviously, as the event becomes more and more rare, this probability becomes smaller. The probability of zero represents an absolute impossibility. Absolute certainty, on the other hand, is represented by the figure one.

PROBABILITY, POPULATIONS AND PATIENTS

If, in a particular population or universe, the number of males is exactly equal to the number of females, one would expect, on drawing a large sample, to obtain a result which gave a probability of getting a female of 1 in 2, or 0·5. If a sample of 50 persons were taken from this population or universe it would give 25 males and 25 females. In practice, however, one would get a variety of results from each sample of 50 persons, using random sampling numbers, ranging from 15—35 for this kind of population. The graph, or frequency polygon, in *Figure 7.4* shows the shape of curve when plotting the number of samples against the number of females obtained per sample. In strict statistical nomenclature, the obtaining of a female is counted as a success, whereas obtaining a male would be counted as a failure, that is, assuming that the original intention was to find the females in the population. It will be

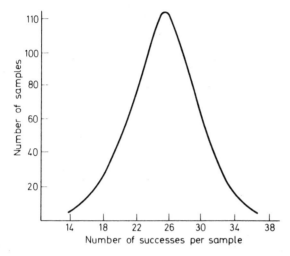

Figure 7.4. Frequency polygon, showing distribution of samples of 50, where $p = 0.5$, $q = 0.5$. Total sample of 1,000

noticed that this frequency polygon is very similar to the normal distribution curve previously described. If successes of obtaining a female is shown by the letter p, and the failure of obtaining a male by the letter q, then it follows that $p + q = 1$. It can be seen that from the frequency polygon the successes in samples of 50, when p is equal to 0·5 centre around the 25 mark. If the sample size is n, and the probabilities of obtaining female or male (or success and failure) are p and q respectively, then the arithmetic mean is equal to $n \times p$. The standard deviation would equal the square root of $n \times p \times q$. It will be remembered that 95 per cent of the total area of the normal curve is within ± twice the standard deviation on either side of the arithmetic mean of the population sample. In other words, 95 per cent of the samples will lie within the range of ± 2 standard deviations from the arithmetic mean. The chances of a sample falling outside this limit is 5 in 100, or 5 per cent. It can then be said that if a sample falls outside ± twice the standard deviation — it has only a 5 per cent chance of so doing – this is called the *5 per cent level of significance.* Looking back, again, at the normal curve ± 3 times the standard deviation includes practically the whole of the distribution of the population (actually 99·73 per cent). The chances of getting a sample outside the arithmetic mean ± 3 times the standard deviation is very small – about 1 in 1,000.

In drawing samples from a population with an equal number of males and females, the following observations can be made.

(1)   The arithmetic mean is equal to the number in the sample times the probability of obtaining a female.

(2)   In this particular case the arithmetic mean is equal to 50 × 0·5, or 25.

(3)   Standard deviation is equal to the square root of $n \times p \times q$ which, in this example, is the square root of 50 × 0·5 × 0·5, which equals the square root of 12·5, or approximately 3·5.

(4)   In drawing samples from this population, one can therefore say that 95 per cent of samples will lie within the range of the arithmetic mean, ± twice the standard deviation; that is, 25 ± 1 × 3·5, or 25 ± 7.

(5)   For every sample drawn it can be said that only in 5 per cent of the time will the result be outside the limits stated, namely 25 ± 7.

(6)   It is also known that from this distribution, the range of the arithmetic mean ± three times the standard deviation includes nearly the whole of the population, or 99·73 per cent.

(7)   In this example then, the chances of getting a sample with more than 36 females in it is only about 1 in 1,000 (the arithmetic mean ± three times the standard deviation is 25 ± 3 × 3·5, which equals 36).

(8)   If any sample of more than 36 females is obtained, it is to be rejected as it is so unlikely.

(9)   If such a sample does occur, one can assume that in some way it is no longer being taken from the original population which has an equal number of males and females.

In other words, there has been a change in the ratio of males to females. Such an example may occur if, for example, the number of hospital beds in an area was taken where we knew that the numbers of males and females in the general population were equal. If, in drawing the sample or in observing the hospital population, it is found that this sample of 50 contains more than 36 females, some other factor will have entered and for some reason, as yet undefined, the hospital population contains more females than would be expected from the proportions in the general population.

By using factorial numbers, it is also possible to predict the probability of obtaining a certain number of females in the sample.

These methods can be of great use in discussing trends, case loads, and requirements in the health services. It is not too much to say that they have highly significant application.

Correlations and Associations

Two sets of data may be correlated by plotting their values upon a graph (*Figure 7.5*). If the two sets of data follow each other closely, there may be said to be a *correlation* between them. Very often it is found that there is a correlation between the ambient temperature and the demand for hospital beds when these are plotted against each other. In this case, as the ambient temperature goes down, the demand for hospital beds increases. This is said to be a *negative correlation.* However, when the demand for beds goes up with rising temperature, as may happen in certain tropical countries, this is said to be a *positive correlation.* Although the relationship between these two variables may be represented by a straight line, very often other factors may make individual values lie outside the plotted line. By means of scatter diagrams of this particular type it can be shown that there is a correlation between two values, though the measurement of correlation by numerical means is a more complicated process.

It is important, however, at this stage to state that there should be some reason for thinking there may be a correlation between two values, otherwise it may be possible to get false correlations. This technique has been subject to a great deal of abuse in the past. Two factors may be found to be correlated which, in fact can be shown to have no real relationship. The same problems apply to correlation as apply to significance. It is easy to draw false conclusions from insufficient or imperfectly understood data and to say that there is a correlation or association between two values and then to go on from that to say that one thing is the cause of another. Correlation does not necessarily mean cause and effect. It is possible at times, to have quite lunatic correlations which bear no relationship to commonsense or to reality. Bearing this in mind, the results we obtain should be looked at critically. For example, it may be discovered that there is a correlation between the number of women in the community who have blonde hair, and the number of births in the community; it may be unwise on this data to draw the conclusion that blonde women are more fecund than those with other hair colours. There may, of course, be many other factors entering into the birth rates of a community whether it contained blonde women or not.

117

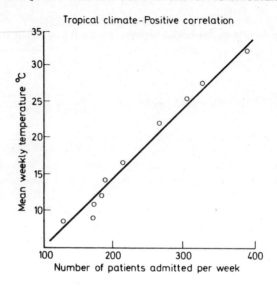

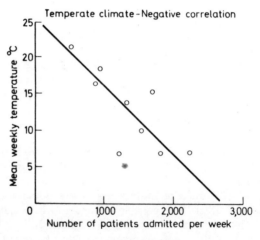

Figure 7.5.

Regression lines

In general, it can be seen that there are two such lines which can be used to give an estimate of the other variable. If there is a high degree of correlation between two factors the closer will be the estimate to the values that are found. If the angle between the two lines is very

118

small the correlation increases and, in fact, in the case of the perfect correlation this angle is zero, that is, the two lines virtually coincide. Where, however, the two lines are wide apart there is no correlation. One line will be parallel to the X axis, and the other to the Y axis.

By using regression lines it is possible to predict one variable from a known value of the other. In the former example in which hospital admissions vary according to the ambient temperature, it could be predicted that a certain ambient temperature would produce a certain load on hospital admissions in a particular area (*Figure 7.6*). If the ambient temperature for that particular area is known it could be

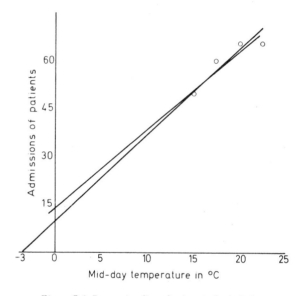

Figure 7.6. Regression lines for hospital admissions

predicted how many hospital admissions may be expected at any particular time. This is useful for forward planning, and for balancing routine admission with those expected in emergency situations. This technique is known as *interpolation*. Also, it is possible, by extending a regression line, to predict unusual situations. This is particularly useful when referring to temperatures or admissions which may not have been met before. It assumes, of course, a linear relationship. It is possible, also, to predict that for every unitary change in temperature there is a different number of hospital admissions. This is known as the *regression coefficient*. For example, it may be found that for every one degree drop in the ambient temperature, the number of hospital admissions in a particular area may have increased by 30.

The correlation coefficient

If the slopes of two lines for hospital admissions are represented by B_1 and B_2, the coefficient of correlation r is given by

$$\sqrt{B_1 \times B_2}$$

If the correlation is positive, r would be $+ 1$, and if the correlation is negative, r would be $- 1$. In the case of hospital admissions and ambient temperature, one would expect the value to be somewhere in the region of $- 1$. The value of zero indicates that there is no correlation. Values of unity or zero are very rare in practice. It is usually found that typical figures lie between 0·6 to 0·9. Small samples where the value of r lies below 0·5 could have arisen by chance, and it is not regarded as significant. The value of r is usually given in tables which show the size of sample needed for a given level of confidence.

Another method may be used when it is not possible to assign numerical values to a variable. In other words, when measuring qualities of dependability, trustworthiness and accuracy, one may rank the group of individuals to that particular quality. It may then be necessary to find out whether that particular quality, as assessed by some test which has been applied, is measurable in an actual work situation. First, the test is applied to a group of employees by assigning them to rank order, such as rank of reliability. Secondly, some other method of assessing the reliability must be found, such as the observed performance by their superiors. The two rankings are then compared to see if there is any correlation. If there is a correlation, the original test could be useful for predicting reliability in a work situation.

Test of Significance

The most commonly used test is the chi-squared test which can be used on samples of varying sizes. In the previous discussion about significance it was assumed that the sample was a large one. The chi-squared test can be applied to much smaller samples. Again, by means of this test, it is desired to find out if the differences between two samples could be due to sampling fluctuations, or if the differences are too large to be explained by such variations, and if they are real or significant.

The basis of the chi-squared test is that actual or observed phenomena are being compared, and the expected phenomena are in two or more samples. The result is then looked up in relevant tables, and the value of P (probability) obtained would indicate whether or not the result was significant; chi-squared should really be zero. If, however, the value of P is small, then the divergence from zero is unlikely to be due to sampling fluctuation. A value of P as small as 0·05, or less, is always significant. A very large value of P that approaches 1 means that there is little chance of obtaining a smaller value for chi-squared. This means that any significance in the results is unlikely, and even by taking larger samples the result would not be changed.

Quality Control

Quality control in the health services represents different problems from those encountered in industry. In most cases we are not monitoring an end-product, although there may be a place for discussing the use of quality control in monitoring the benefits brought to patients. The main purpose of quality control, in relation to the health services, is in the monitoring of needs both in the community and in the hospital, getting an early warning about possible changes in those needs, and about trends and changes in the resources that will be available within the health services.

It is interesting to speculate that few measures have been taken on the ultimate quality of life that comes to a sick person who may be regarded as cured. However, as many of the criteria for this may be based on subjective considerations, they are outside the scope of this work. In this sense, the patient could be regarded as an end-product of the industry of the health services, and the quality regarding their final benefit is something which has yet to be developed within the health services. Unfortunately, there is a tendency on the part of hospital services to regard a successful discharge of patients as tantamount to a cure. Whether the quality of life that patients lead has been improved, or maintained, compared with the state they were in at the beginning of their hospital stay, is still open to speculation. Ultimately, this depends very much on the subjective assessments of the patients themselves, as it is difficult for an observer to lay down what is the quality of life for another person. One must assume, however, that most patients will leave the hospital, in the words of Florence Nightingale, 'no worse than when they arrived in the hospital'. In this sense, such patients could be regarded as a success.

However, the second type of quality control in the health services is essentially related to the various changes and needs that go on within the service itself. One of the greatest difficulties that a hospital may have is adjusting its bed situation and admission rates to the real needs of the community, without creating an apparent need where none existed before. An example of this may be found in the specialty whose demands have changed considerably, reverting to the admission of minor cases with which it would not have dealt in previous years. The medical situation is one of great difficulty, as it is arguable that some of these minor cases could possibly have been dealt with better in the community; and in the overall planning of the hospital services the ever important question of *real* community need has to be considered. It is dangerously easy to create an artificial need in order to justify some particular type of expenditure which may have been created in the recent past for a situation which no longer exists. Industry has become more aware of these problems in recent years, and has an advantage which the hospitals do not necessarily have, namely, that profits will decline if a real need is not met. It is true that an industry can create an artificial need by use of pressure and advertising techniques, but how long this will survive depends very much on the relationship of this need to the real needs of the consumer of the product. The health services can be classed, loosely, as a service industry cushioned from more direct economic challenges. An artificial need could be created, albeit unconsciously, which could be perpetuated for many years.

Quality control in the health services, however, is concerned with changes and trends within the services, and the essential decision making which comes from deciding whether these trends and changes represent a need which will have to be met immediately or in some future planning programme.

PRESENTATION OF DATA

One of the principal difficulties, having obtained information, is to present it in a way which is immediately accessible for use by the manager. Too often, valuable data may be lost by not presenting it in a way in which trends and patterns may be comprehended immediately. On the other hand, it may sometimes be possible that exaggerated diagrams can lead to more difficulties by showing small variations as gross changes from the original pattern. This is an ever present difficulty which is sometimes exploited ruthlessly in a similar way to the misuse of averages discussed earlier. *Figure 7.7* gives examples of the use to which the results of the analyses may be put in order to present more comprehensively information to the interpreter.

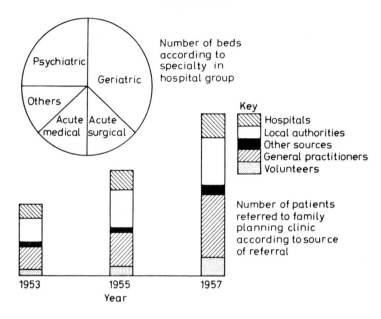

Figure 7.7. Two methods of presenting data diagrammatically. In the second example the method of presentation reveals that, although there has been an overall increase in the number of patients referred, the proportion referred from G.P.s has increased much more

Bibliography

Battersby, A. (1967). *Mathematics in Management.* Harmondsworth; Penguin (A good introduction to applications of methods and to operations research.)

Goldstein, A. (1964). *Biostatistics for Biological Sciences and Medicine.* London; Collier-Macmillan (A useful introduction for more advanced students involved in the medical sciences.)

Gregory, D. and Ward, H. (1968). *Statistics for Business Studies.* Maidenhead; McGraw-Hill (A useful introduction to the applications of statistical methods in business.)

I.C.I. (1964). *Cumulative Sum Techniques.* I.C.I. Monograph N.3. London (A very comprehensive account of this method of quality control in industry.)

Moroney, M.J. (1964). *Facts from Figures.* Harmondsworth; Pelican (A more meaty book than *Use and Abuse of Statistics,* which requires more concentration but which is well worth the effort.)

Reichmann, W.J. (1961). *Use and Abuse of Statistics.* Harmondsworth; Pelican (A good and easy-to-read introduction to the basics of statistics.)

8–Monitoring of Community Needs

Alwyn Smith

Introduction

The practice of medicine has long since ceased to be an essentially entrepreneurial activity by individual physicians and surgeons contracting with individual clients. During the centuries while medical practice was relatively ineffective such arrangements were tolerable. However, during the past one hundred years the development of effective practice has resulted in the practice of medicine advancing from the position of an activity marginal to public health to being one of its central resources.

The effective practice of public health is, of course, older than the effective practice of clinical medicine. The development and manipulation of public resources in the public health interest had been established by the early part of the nineteenth century, and during the remainder of that century it became increasingly possible to secure sustained improvements in population health. An important contribution was made to this successful development by the elaborate systems that were evolved for providing the authorities with a continuous flow of information about the health needs of the public and the extent to which they were successfully being met. Mortality statistics were well established by the middle of the nineteenth century, and since then a variety of procedures have been evolved for providing information on the prevalence and incidence of a wide variety of disabilities.

The branch of medical science under which these developments have been effected (i.e., that concerned with studying the distribution of sickness and health in human communities, together with the causes and consequences of their evolving patterns) has borne, at various stages of its development the names 'medical statistics', 'epidemiology', and, more recently, 'social medicine'. This chapter aims to provide an overall and necessarily brief survey of the objectives and characteristic methods of this science. In so short a review the coverage is necessarily selective and the approach employed has been determined by the desirability of reflecting current thinking and current advances.

Applications

EVALUATION OF POPULATION HEALTH STATUS

There is no country whose resources are so great or so small that it does not need to appraise carefully the health problems that exist so as to be able to direct available health and medical care resources with maximum effect. Although the means by which such direction is accomplished varies widely with the different circumstances and traditions of different countries, there is universal need for the most precise possible understanding of the health problems to be tackled.

The development of statistical reporting of the occurrence of illness within populations owes its origin to the pioneer work of John Graunt, a London shop-keeper whose work, 'Natural Political Reflections on the London Bills of Mortality', was first published in 1662. It was natural that early developments were substantially within the field of mortality statistics, since public concern for the state of community health was largely with diseases that usually culminate in death. Towards the middle of the nineteenth century an increasing capacity to understand and control epidemics of communicable disease led to the development of obligatory reporting of cases of such diseases. More recently other diseases have been made subject to statutory reporting (for example, in England and Wales, congenital malformations are now reportable although not obligatorily). Thus, monitoring of community health has traditionally been established on the idea of a complete reporting, from the population, of all cases of disease within certain restricted categories of severity and kind. Although such data are limited in their scope, they have revealed sufficiently the possibilities of health monitoring to provoke an intensive development of improved reporting and sampling procedures. The applications of such data are worth preliminary consideration since they, to some extent, specify the kind of health that is needed at present in the foreseeable future.

Description of current health status

Perhaps the simplest application of a monitoring system is the provision of an up-to-date account of the health status of the population. It is difficult to see how even the most elementary health administration can function without a knowledge of the health status of the population which the services are designed to serve. In the absence of such data, administration can accomplish little more than a resolution of the *conflicting pressures* exerted by the various different professional groups involved and the usually rather selective pressure groups within the Health Service clientele.

Detection of changes in health

The provision of early warning of the imminence of disease outbreaks involves two types of problems. It is desirable to be able to detect outbreaks of certain specified diseases for which procedures are available that might permit the outbreak to be averted or contained. Selected infectious diseases are usually made notifiable for such reasons. The second type of problem, exemplified by the outbreak of thalidomide-induced limb malformations, concerns the need to detect at an early stage new hazards which may arise from our continually changing environment. Since we cannot pre-select the diseases which may become important in this way there is a need for continual scrutiny of up-to-date information on disease occurrence. Suitable statistical detection procedures have been developed but appropriate data on morbidity are not yet widely available.

DETERMINANTS OF POPULATION HEALTH

Where detailed planning and administration of health services are important, it is necessary to investigate population health in more detail. An understanding of the determinants of the levels and patterns of disease occurrence in a community requires detailed numerical data on disease frequency in various specificable population groups and in identifiable circumstances of place and time. Such data may be applied to three distinct types of enquiry: (1) investigation of the causes of disease occurrence in individuals; (2) identification of the social and environmental influences that determine the characteristic disease experience of communities; and (3) study of the circumstances that determine the persistence and effect of diseases that have arisen.

Disease causation in individuals

Investigation of the mechanisms of disease induction and identification of pathogenic agents are traditional applications of epidemiological enquiry. The case for using nationally available morbidity statistics in such research rests mainly on the fact that many urgent aetiological problems require the use of data on a scale that is difficult to achieve by other means. Since governments are thus uniquely in a position to collect and analyse suitable data, they naturally incur the responsibility of doing so. Such responsibilities have traditionally been accepted by governmental health statistical agencies for many years. Examples of the kinds of enquiries that may be based on suitable morbidity statistics include the following. (1) Investigation of the influence of occupational or other general environmental hazards on the genesis of disease. (2) The increasingly important investigation of the pathogenic effects of procedures used in medical diagnosis and treatment. (3) Research into the effects of social and economic factors in the pathogenesis of disease.

Factors influencing the incidence of disease

The causes of disease occurrence in populations are often different from the causes of disease in individuals. They include the factors that influence individual exposure to disease agents. For example, the level of occurrence of lung cancer in populations is determined by those factors which determine the frequency of the smoking habit. These include the price and availability of cigarettes, the relative efficiency of the contrary influences which seek to persuade people to smoke or not to smoke, and other general factors that determine the attitudes which influence choice of behaviour. Such influences can only be effectively studied on large-scale representative data from complete populations. In addition, the steps which may need to be taken to control the responsible factors are frequently steps that can only be taken by governmental agencies. Responsibility for such studies is therefore naturally assignable to governmental health statistics agencies.

Factors influencing the natural history of disease

The prevalence of disease depends on its incidence and its duration. The factors that determine prevalence therefore include all the casual factors of disease incidence and factors influencing disease duration. These latter are specially important in the study of chronic diseases.

Statistics of the prevalence of morbidity may, therefore, be used to investigate the influences which determine the course and duration of diseases and the severity of the associated disability. Since governmental agencies now generally accept an increasing responsibility for providing medical care, and since medical care is an important determinant of the course of disease, studies of the prevalence and duration of disease are important for the planning of services.

Another important application of the study of the natural history and course of disease lies in the identification of the presymptomatic features of disease which may permit their earlier recognition. Many chronic diseases that do not lend themselves easily to primary prevention may nevertheless to substantially modified in their course by adequately early intervention. Since the early detection techniques will almost certainly require organization at national or regional government levels, it is natural that the studies on which they may be based should be derived from morbidity statistics collected and analysed at a comparable level.

EVALUATION OF EFFECTS OF SERVICES

The acceptance by governments of an increasing responsibility for management of health and medical services involves the duty not only to plan as effectively as possible, but also to subject to continuous appraisal the effectiveness of health service developments. Such appraisal may either be by continuous scrutiny of routine morbidity statistics, or by special studies of specific health and medical care programmes. Both kinds of study are included under the heading of morbidity statistics, but the techniques required will differ according to whether appraisal is of the effect of preventive services on incidence, the effect of therapeutic services on prevalence and outcome, or the effect of the provision of medical care on the severity of the disability associated with disease.

Effect of preventive procedures on incidence of disease

Monitoring may permit a continuing evaluation of the broad effect of preventive techniques. For example, trends in the notification of death rates from tuberculosis, poliomyelitis or diphtheria may confirm the effect of preventive techniques in these diseases and point to groups in which prevention has been less effective than in others. In some diseases more elaborate statistical studies are needed to take account of the many factors involved in determining occurrence rates. It is particularly important to be able to identify groups in which special preventive activity may be required. For example, the uptake of poliomyelitis vaccination has been shown to vary considerably between groups characterized by different social and educational backgrounds, and the use of cervical cytological screening services is usually least complete among those identifiable as having a particularly high risk of cervical cancer.

Effect of therapeutic procedures on prevalence of disease

While incidence relates to the frequency of new cases of disease, prevalence describes the current number of cases at a particular time. It is thus of more application in the statistical study of chronic disease. Prevalence levels are partly determined by incidence levels and are therefore influenced by preventive techniques, but since prevalence is affected by disease duration it is also influenced by factors which affect disease duration. Important among these factors is medical treatment and rehabilitation, and their influence on chronic disease is often evaluated by means of prevalence studies.

Statistics of disease prevalence require a different kind of organization from those of incidence, since they involve the need to be informed of current totals of cases rather than totals arising within a period. Establishment of disease registers or special census surveys may often be required.

Statistics of survival (for example in cancer patients) also require a more complex organization. However, incidence, prevalence, and duration of disease are simply related arithmetically, and if two of these are known the third can be derived by calculation.

Effect of medical care on disease severity and disability

The influence of medical care on disease severity has been most extensively studied in cancer. Other diseases might even more usefully be studied, as the factors determining choice of treatment are usually less complex than in the case of cancer. A particularly important area for study in many countries is mental illness which usually accounts for a large proportion of hospital utilization, and in which disability and severity may usefully be measured in terms of total duration of hospitalization. Therapeutic changes may greatly change the needs for provision of hospital accommodation and thus influence the provision of special hospitals and other facilities.

Sources of Data

Monitoring data may either arise from basic recording carried out in health institutions in connection with the operation of health and medical services, or may be the product of special surveys. Data of the former type are usually collected for statistical purposes by systems of continuous reporting which include procedures for the notification of selected diseases, hospital in-patient returns, statistics on other medical care; social security statistics, and statistics from established registers of various diseases. Continuous reporting through such systems represents the main source of statistical data at present. Special surveys, which will be considered later, have been gaining in importance during the last decade.

CONTINUOUS REPORTING

Since a great deal of data became available as a result of existing medical and civil formalities it is natural that they have been used for monitoring purpose. They may be considered as falling into three categories. First data based on the medical certification of causes of death; secondly, data arising from the obligatory notification of selected lists of conditions and thirdly, obligatory reporting of the utilization of certain specified health service agencies.

Mortality data

The oldest established source of data on the health of populations arises from the usual need felt by most communities to signalize the social importance of death by the institution of obligatory reporting procedures and professional attribution of an adequate cause for each death. The Medical Certificate of Cause of Death has a number of important advantages, as well as disadvantages, as a source of information on the occurrence of disease. The advantages are: (1) the relative completeness of the data, in most developed countries at least, the uniqueness of the event in the life of each individual: (2) the lack of any variability in severity which might affect completeness of reporting: and (3) the seriousness of the event, which tends to discourage irresponsible reporting of data connected with it.

The disadvantages are that many important illnesses are rarely certified as causes of death, and even some diseases which substantially contribute to mortality do not figure importantly in mortality statistics, (prematurity in developed countries, and malnutrition in the world as a whole are major contributors to childhood mortality and yet do not figure importantly among the certified causes of death used in statistical tabulations). A difficulty of increasing importance in developed countries, where death is increasingly postponed until the older ages, is the arbitrariness involved in selecting one disease process from among several which may have been evident at the time of death.

Nevertheless, it has always been and continues to be the case that statistical data on mortality furnish very valuable information on important health problems. A recent example in this country has been the epidemic of childhood deaths from asthma associated with bronchodilator areosols. This epidemic was first detected as an increase in the frequency of deaths from asthma among children. The use of perinatal morality, as an index of the quality of available obstetric care, is presently well established.

If the utility of mortality data for monitoring purposes is to increase, a number of developments will be required.

It will be desirable to make more efficient use of the diagnostic data recorded in medical certificates of cause of death. The selection of a single underlying cause involves the rejection of potentially valuable information. For example, official statistics do not permit an answer to important questions about the numerical frequency of different ways of dying. For example, there is no way of abstracting from mortality statistics any indication of the frequency of fatal renal failure. Experiments are current in a number of countries designed to develop ways of exploiting more of the available information by cross-tabulation of the various diagnostic terms appearing on the certificate. A major difficulty in these developments is that two quite different types of diagnostic data appear on death certificates, apart from the underlying cause of death. The first type of data represent stages in the morbid process initiated by the underlying cause and culminating in the terminal condition. The second type of data includes diseases present at the time of death and which are often capable of having determined that the sequence initiated by the underlying cause in fact resulted in a fatal outcome rather than a recovery. The difficulty of systematically unravelling these different classes of information on a population scale has not so far been adequately solved.

Important potential improvement to be expected from the analysis of mortality data will flow from the linkage of such data with data recorded during the life of the deceased individual. At present such linkages are generally rudimentary. For example, in no country of the world are there any nationally based routine statistics on the association between infant mortality and birth weight. The reason for this is that weight is recorded — if at all — at the registration of birth not at the registration of death, and the routine linkage of the two sets of data which would be required for such statistical analyses have not yet been developed on a national scale. This question will be considered in more detail in a later discussion on record linkage.

Notification

The practice of preparing lists of conditions, which must be reported when cases of them are encountered by doctors or other health workers, is the oldest procedure for obtaining statistical data on non-fatal illness. However, in the case of the infectious diseases notification was not established for the purpose of providing comprehensive statistical data but for the purpose of providing an early warning of the imminence of epidemics. The lists of notifiable infectious diseases in the various countries of the world show very great variety, but this variety is not always a reflection of the actual needs of the different countries for different kinds of information. In general, the notification of communicable disease is characterized by its incompleteness.

In Britain the recent institution of voluntary notification of congenital malformations illustrates an important difficulty about the use of notification as a useful source of information. This difficulty is in knowing in advance which diseases it would be useful to make notifiable. In the case of the dangerous communicable diseases which are subject to sporadic epidemicity, it is reasonable to establish notification as an early warning device. However, it is difficult, or impossible, to specify in advance the kind of diseases which may become of epidemic significance because of the continually changing environment to which we are increasingly subject. It would have been useful for congenital malformations to have been notifiable *before* the thalidomide epidemic. After the epidemic, it is questionable whether it is more useful to require notification of congenital malformations than of any other condition since we cannot know in advance which, if any, conditions will next show a sudden increase in frequency in consequence of some environmental change. If the next important epidemic is of a relatively uncommon malignant neoplasm with a fairly long duration of survival, it may be many years before we identify the phenomenon; still less before we discover its causes. Indeed, it is perfectly possible that a number of epidemics of severity and magnitude comparable with the thalidomide induced epidemic have occurred and will continue to occur without our having detected them.

The use of lists of notifiable conditions must continue to be mainly in the context of conditions known to be likely to show sudden epidemicity, and for which an effective means of averting an epidemic is ready-to-hand.

Reports from medical care agencies

The most obvious example of statistical reporting from medical care agencies is in its increased usage on patients admitted to hospital. In most countries the first examples of such hospital in-patient statistics were in connection with mental illness. Here, the reasons for instituting reporting were not so much concerned with monitoring of morbidity but with safe-guarding civil liberties. However, the successful exploitation of the available data in the epidemiological study of mental illness led to an interest in establishing comparable reporting systems in other types of hospitals.

In general, hospital morbidity statistics are based on reports submitted at the discharge of individual patients, and contain data on the sources of admission, disposal on discharge, utilization of significant hospital facilities, and some diagnostic data. It is this latter type of information that presents the most difficulty. Few systems of hospital morbidity statistics have succeeded in enrolling the hospital medical staff as principal recorders of the data. Diagnostic data have usually, therefore, to be abstracted from case notes by clerical staff. Since very many more diagnostic terms may appear in a patient's case record than can strictly be applied to the patient's actual illness, selection of the most appropriate term is not always very easy.

Attempts at a solution of this problem have usually been based on methods of encouraging medical staff to record systematically diagnostic data for each patient. The most hopeful line of development is to base statistical returns on the documents used for diagnostic indexing since even though they are rarely concerned with medical statistics, most doctors have occasional need to use a diagnostic index and may more easily be persuaded to treat the necessary recording adequately seriously.

Data from agencies other than hospitals are even more difficult to obtain. Although most doctors would accept the need to make records of presenting symptoms, signs, diagnoses and treatments, few doctors are prepared to make such records in a form lending itself to statistical reporting. However, in recent years a most remarkable exception to this general rule has been the development by the Royal College of General Practitioners of a series of systems whereby general practitioners can conveniently record the morbidity encountered in their practice. The systems have been used in a variety of studies sponsored both by the Royal College itself and by individual general practitioners. An additional result of the development of these systems has been that many general practitioners have been keen to collaborate in quite extensive studies of the morbidity encountered in general practice among a variety of patients of particular interest in the context of both health services research and general epidemiology.

A particularly interesting form of statistically accessible medical record is embodied in registration systems whereby cases of particular diseases, or groups of diseases, are made the subject of a register, primarily for the purpose of facilitating follow-up patient care and the evaluation of therapy, but also adaptable for statistical studies. Cancer registration is the most well developed example of systems of this kind. It was orginally designed principally as an instrument for the promotion of better long-term care but was adapted for statistical studies of survival and now forms the basis of general epidemiological studies of malignant disease. Other chronic conditions lend themselves to a similar approach, for example, diabetes, chronic bronchitis, and a number of mental illnesses. The use of registers in co-ordinating the long-term care of psychiatric patients, by many different agencies, has now developed in several centres to the point where these registers may be used to study the epidemiology of psychiatric illness as well as the efficacy of new patterns of patient care.

SPECIAL SYSTEMS

Surveys of sickness

Most continuously reported morbidity statistics relate less to morbidity than to use of medical care, since morbidity is not included in such statistics unless the patient seeks medical care from a reporting agency. This presents difficulties of interpretation, since it is well established that the probability that an illness is brought to medical care is dependent on many factors apart from its severity. Differences are demonstrable for different illnesses, for persons of different age and sex, and of different social and educational background. Since the probability may be subject to secular change, apparent changes in morbidity rates may reflect no more than changes in public attitudes to medical care; a situation that is well established as underlying much of recent apparent changes in morbidity from mental illness.

The difficulty is widespread among countries at very different stages of development although the diseases that are influenced may differ widely. Accordingly, countries of widely differing levels of development have made use of population surveys of morbidity.

General morbidity surveys

General surveys seek to define the extent of the total sickness load on a community. They may elicit information on morbidity either by interrogation or by physical examination. They may be either current, retrospective or prospective in method and individual surveys may combine two or all three of these methods. They involve examination of all members of a population or of a suitable sample, during a reasonably defined period and are therefore generally concerned with estimating the prevalence of disease.

The first problem in a general morbidity survey, once it has been decided what persons shall be included, is that of formulating workable definitions of morbidity. Many diseases do not represent simple qualitative departures from normal health but involve simply the exhibition of more or less extreme values for some quantity that is continuously distributed in the population. Obvious examples include hypertension, sub-nutrition and mental retardation but such diseases as bronchitis or neurosis may be equally difficult to define. Actual operational definitions will depend not only on the purposes of the survey, but also on the health investigational techniques employed. Data derived from interviews will permit a quite different set of definitions from data obtained by clinical or laboratory examination. It is, nevertheless, important to define morbidity for the purposes of the survey in as exact terms as possible.

Another difficult problem is the diagnostic classification of morbidity. Most existing classifications, including the International Classification of Diseases, are based on the assumption that the terms to be classified will be diagnostic terms as employed by physicians. Where morbidity is defined in terms of direct verbal reporting by the patients, classification may be difficult.

Surveys may be continuous, periodic or occasional, depending on the countries' resources and needs for data. Continuous and occasional surveys are at present undertaken in several countries and both have their advantages and disadvantages. Continuous surveys may make more economic use of the large investment in organization, training and experience that surveys involve, but they should permit some flexibility in the direction of emphasis on the population groups involved if they are not to generate more data than are required. Occasional surveys may be more closely tailored to current needs and may actually cost less.

Surveys based on actual clinical and laboratory examination are expensive of financial and trained manpower resources and may be difficult to organize. Usually the scope of the examination will need to be limited. For example, surveys of biochemical health, based on laboratory examination of blood or urine, have been developed in Sweden. Choice of a range of key investigations will eventually be based on accumulated experience. The health examination survey in the United States of America is relatively unrestricted in its investigational scope but is concentrated on special population groups of particular interest. It involves extensive clinical, biochemical and serological investigations which are performed by mobile teams. In many countries, investigations are limited to simple clinical examination and may be effectively carried out with modest resources, particularly if the examination is selective in its scope.

Interview surveys are usually directed towards the ascertainment of current or immediately past data on morbidity. Experience in many countries suggests that such surveys may yield valuable data if due regard is paid to the need for careful development of interview techniques and for validation studies. For example, comparison of morbidity reported for periods successively more remote from the interviews date permits estimation of the influence of defective recollection. Comparison of the frequency of morbidity reported to have been treated with data derived from actual treatment agencies is also valuable where possible. In fact, comparison between levels of morbidity reported at interview and levels reported as treated, is directly relevant to the problem of evaluating the importance of self-selection for medical care.

Recently, techniques have been devised for prospective enquiry into morbidity. These may involve the use of diaries for the recording of day-to-day illnesses. The diaries are distributed, together with instructions for their maintenance and collected after a suitable interval. If interviewers are available to supervise the recording at appropriate intervals the data may be very informative. Several countries have experimented with such methods on a sample basis.

Surveys of special diseases

Surveys of particular diseases have the considerable advantage over surveys of general morbidity that the establishment of definitive criteria of disease is usually very much simpler. Several diseases have been studied in this way to the point where the criteria are very widely established as diagnostic, or as adequately diagnostic, in population surveys. For example, establishment of malaria prevalence has long been based on simple survey methods. More recently, such diseases as chronic bronchitis have been studied by questionnaire methods aimed at supplying definitive symptomatic data and the symptomatic criteria have come to be widely accepted as defining the disease condition.

Such surveys also have the advantage that they are usually cheaper and easier to organize. This makes them possible in countries of relatively limited resources and on a large scale. The widespread use of such methods for measuring the prevalence of tropical infectious diseases (malaria, hookworm, trachoma, etc.) demonstrates their practicability and relative economy.

An advantage which surveys of particular diseases have over general surveys is the higher level of diagnostic ascertainment that is achieved when the examinations are more specifically directed. This may lead to some countries preferring a series of special surveys to a single general survey if the sampling system can be so devised as to avoid individuals being continually subjected to investigation.

Hospital censuses

Hospital censuses are valuable when continuous reporting procedures do not exist, or where they do not permit estimates of residence rates or numbers of residents. This is sometimes the case when data are not available for both admissions and discharges, or when the interval between admission and discharge may be very long as, for example, in the case of some mental hospital patients. Once a census has been carried out, establishment of admission and discharge statistics may permit a register to be maintained of patients in hospital so that current statements may subsequently be easily prepared.

Surveys on existing records

Surveys may be made from existing medical records where suitably complete records are available. Such surveys have several advantages. Since medical records are derived from medical sources the diagnostic data will usually be more specific than those derived from interview surveys, although possibly less so than data from examination surveys. Such surveys may be developed, eventually, into regular statistical reporting systems. Disadvantages include the likelihood of incompleteness of medical records — often in respect of important items which may involve exclusion of subjects from the survey. Such incompleteness cannot be assumed to be unrelated to items under study. Generally, medical records other than those from hospitals are inadequately maintained for survey purposes. Finally, since the data are not generally recorded with statistical purposes in mind they may not be suitable.

Nevertheless, it seems important that statistical use should be made wherever possible of the very large amount of clinical data that is placed on record in the day-to-day practice of medicine. If record systems can be improved and re-designed with such application in mind, record-based surveys would be particularly economical and informative. For such purposes records should contain a basic minimum of items which are common to all records and have common definitions.

Redesign of medical records systems is generally being undertaken in connection with the introduction of computer-based systems. Appropriate consideration of possible statistical applications should permit their organization in such a way that record surveys could be undertaken by means of suitable computer programmes for the retrieval and analysis of recorded data. National Health Statistics Offices in several countries have been studying the problems involved in such automated record and statistical systems. The simplest approach is by means of computer-based indexes to records libraries in which the form of each index entry is designed as a case-summary suitable as a unit for statistical analysis.

Sampling

Although it is often feasible to collect continuously reported statistical data from the whole of the population, in surveys, it is usually more practicable to restrict the observations to a suitably selected sample. Such samples may be taken from many different sources. Samples are often the only practicable means of collecting the required data: they are usually cheaper, quicker to carry out and analyse, and susceptible to more careful control of observational quality. There is often little point in sampling, however, where total population data are already available, where it is important to have reliable data on certain very small population groups, or where the required accuracy would involve relatively large samples.

The principal difficulty confronting the investigator who wishes to examine a representative sample of the population is usually the absence of a sampling frame, that is, a suitable list of the population from which a sample can be drawn. Extensive use has been made, in Britain, of the electoral register as a sampling frame and, for many purposes, it can be extremely useful. However, it is not a complete enumeration even of the adult population, still less of the whole population, and the way in which it is kept does not guarantee that it is up-to-date. A few countries have successfully used census enumeration data as a sampling frame. But in other countries such data are restricted in use by undertaking that census data are wholly secret. In some countries population registers are kept and are maintained reasonably up-to-date by a statutory obligation on people who change their residence to notify the appropriate authorities. Where the population register is up-to-date and kept in a suitable form it may make a very useful sampling frame.

In most countries a frame has to be devised to meet the particular needs of a projected sample, and the effort involved in constructing a frame is sometimes so great as to make it pointless to restrict one's final data to a sample.

Ideally, the procedure for drawing samples should be based on the principle of random selection; that is, all persons in the sampling frame should have equal probability of appearing in the sample and the selection of sample individuals should be made by a process governed only by chance. However, it is often perfectly acceptable to draw a sample by means other than a strictly random method. For example, in England and Wales the ten per cent sample of all patients discharged from general hospitals, which formed the basis of the Hospital In-patient Enquiry, was drawn by reference to selected terminal digits of the recorded day of birth.

Two-stage sampling has proved to be very valuable in a number of studies. Particularly when this has been based on the electoral register it has been very convenient. The technique involves a first stage sample of electoral districts in which each district has a probability of inclusion proportional to its population. In the second stage, a similar number of individuals are drawn from each district register. This method has the virtue that it makes it possible to concentrate resources, which may well be scarce, and to collect one's data with the maximum of speed and economy.

An admirable discussion of the principles of sampling as they relate to public health work is contained in a World Health Organization Technical Report Series (No. 336) entitled 'Sampling Methods in Morbidity Surveys and Public Health Investigations'. The writer knows of no other discussion of the subject which deals so comprehensively with all the problems in so short a space.

Analysis of Data

DATA HANDLING

The problems of data handling for population health monitoring are generally those common to all kinds of statistical processing. Nevertheless, it seems worth making a number of points.

Clerical methods

Almost all data handling procedures involve an element of clerical handling, although its extent may be very limited when advanced mechanical or electronic data processing devices are used. Nevertheless, it is perfectly possible to produce good analyses using solely clerical methods; indeed, mortality statistics were developed to a high level of efficiency in many countries before any other methods were available.

The most important factors when data are to be handled clerically are: (1) simplicity in the format of the reporting documents; and (2) a good book-keeping procedure which permits a continuous check on the timely and complete receipt of the incoming data.

Simplicity of format involves a rigorous exclusion of non-essential items, and this in turn involves a careful prior appraisal of what items of information are required. It is also important that documents are so designed that information may easily be recorded by personnel whose direct interest in the statistics may not be great. It is particularly important that reporting documents can be completed at one time by one person; if any different recording personnel are required, delays occur. Attention should be given to what items are readily available in basic records.

The importance of a properly organized procedure for central receipt and surveillance of incoming data is difficult to exaggerate. If analysis and publication of statistics is to be timely, then all stages in data collection and handling must be promptly carried out. Since, inevitably, some peripheral reporting units will default, it must be possible to monitor the incoming data and to identify defaulting units promptly. It is also often necessary to identify, and return for completion, forms that are either incorrectly or incompletely filled in. Delay on the part of the central collecting agency will render such completion more difficult and has the psychological effect of reducing the sense of urgency necessary to timely return of the documents. It is often useful to have an agreed set of dates by which the various kinds of data must be sent to the central statistical agency.

If clerical methods are to be employed for data analysis. incoming data will need to be sorted and counted. The process is greatly simplified if individual patient returns are made on individual documents and if these are sufficiently substantial to survive handling. Sorting and counting may often proceed concurrently with receipt, and thus permit periodic analysis as well as prompt annual analysis. Such timely analysis is highly desirable.

Simple machines

Simple machines are here taken to include sorting and tabulating machines and desk calculating machines.

There is no doubt that a very comprehensive statistical service can be provided by these simple punched card machines. They have been the main means of data handling in most health statistical offices for many years, and will no doubt continue to be for many more years. Even a simple counter-sorter is capable of a large amount of statistical data handling. Their principal drawbacks are their generally limited arithmetical capabilities, which necessitate the use of calculating machines (or clerical calculation) for obtaining rates and percentages, and their lack of speed compared with electronic computers.

Electronic computers

These machines are generally replacing simpler sorters and tabulators in the health statistics offices of the larger and richer countries. Their principal advantages are their virtually unlimited arithmetical capabilities, their greater flexibility in analysis, and their considerably greater speed of operation once they have been provided with operating instructions (programs). Principal disadvantages are their capital cost, the cost of investing in highly trained personnel needed for programming, and the relative time required for programming. This latter disadvantage would generally diminish as a set of suitable programs because available, and is often unimportant when programming of new procedures is facilitated by advanced systems.

Computers will handle statistical data, will carry out analyses, including calculation, will print the resulting tables, and perform complex logical manoeuvres which facilitate data interpretation. There is no doubt that they will transform the speed, flexibility and power of statistical analysis in the health statistics offices of those countries that can afford them.

Choice of methods

Choice of data handling methods will most often be determined by available financial resources. There is no doubt that elaborate methods will improve speed, flexibility and power of analysis but often at very substantially greater cost. There is also no doubt that useful statistics may be produced using very simple and inexpensive methods, particularly if careful thought is applied to the design of the procedures and the choice of data to be collected and analysed. It is impossible to suggest a general compromise since the sizes of populations, their needs and their resources vary widely, but it is recommended that all population monitoring systems employ at least some simple machinery, preferably involving punched cards, that would be generally compatible with more elaborate machinery if this became available later.

ELEMENTS OF ANALYSIS

Although it is important to suit the specific analysis of statistical data to the purposes for which they have been collected, it is nevertheless generally useful to have a number of standardized definitions and procedures which facilitate international comparability and which have been found generally useful.

Statistical units

Since morbidity statistics reflect the occurrence of sickness in the population, it would be desirable to be able to define sickness with some precision. Unfortunately this is not possible because sickness is variable in severity and duration and is inevitably complicated by variation in individual tolerance of disability. Such variation is fairly simply related to age and perhaps to occupation but its relation to psychological and social characteristics is much more complex. It is usually necessary, in the context of morbidity statistics, to frame the definition of sickness in such a way as to accommodate the particular features of the statistical reporting system involved. Usually, sickness is defined for statistics reported from medical care agencies in terms of contacts with these agencies, and for surveys in terms of abnormal states detectable by the survey technique.

Morbidity may be measured in terms of the numbers of persons who are sick, the number of episodes of sickness, or the duration of sickness. It is possible, for example, for a person to fall sick more than once and to have more than one diagnosis during a period under review. It is often not possible in currently available morbidity statistics to examine such possibilities in detail.

The simplest unit in many morbidity statistics is the case of illness. This is particularly true for acute diseases with a clearly definable onset and resolution, such as many of the acute notifiable infectious diseases. It is also possible to use such a unit for certain chronic diseases not having an episodic course. A principal requirement for useful statistics of cases of chronic diseases is that no case should appear twice in the statistics, and this may be difficult to achieve without quite elaborate methods.

A spell of sickness is a useful statistical unit for many purposes but it must be recognized that data from many commonly used sources will permit the multiple inclusion of a case of disease if the disease has an episodic course. For example, sickness absence statistics or hospital in-patient admission statistics deal usually with spells of sickness and they may therefore include several spells of absence or hospitalization in the course of a single case of an episodic disease such as bronchitis.

In hospital statistics, units may be admissions, discharges, or residents. Studies of residents are particularly useful in hospitals for chronic illnesses, such as mental hospitals, and as a measure of bed occupancy at a point in time. Admission and discharge statistics are generally easier to collect however. For hospitals dealing with acute illness, admission statistics are useful as a simple index of the work of the hospital. For hospitals dealing with chronic illness they are invaluable as a guide to trends in hospitalization. For most purposes, however, discharge statistics are the most useful because they permit more definitive diagnostic data, they permit data on duration of stay and on facilities used, and they permit data not only on sources of referral for admission but also on disposal at discharge. It is often useful for hospitals dealing with chronic illness to collect statistics on admissions and discharges and it may be particularly useful if the discharge reports carry copies of the data recorded at admission.

Statistics of sickness absence or of claims for sickness benefit are useful in that the units may be easily defined. Statistics of other generally treated morbidity may pose particularly difficult problems in the choice of units. For example, statistics of morbidity treated outside the hospital, whether by general practitioners or by other agencies, have no very natural unit except that of a consulation. For patients who make relatively frequent use of such consultation, an episode of illness can sometimes only be indeterminately defined in terms of a temporal clustering of consultations. Nevertheless, a consultation is not always a good unit since it often imposes a heavy recording burden. It may become practicable if such statistics are collected by means of a sampling technique which involves only occasional reporting days for individual practitioners, or if the first consultation in an episode of illness is selected as the reporting unit.

Record linkage

For studies of the demands made on services, it is often satisfactory to use a unit of sickness that does not permit consideration of multiple episodes or kinds of sickness in the same person. For general medical purposes, however, it is usually desirable to use data in which the person is the unit and his sickness experience a characterizable attribute. This experience may be in terms either of spells of sickness or cases of sickness, since a person may fall ill several times from the same or different diseases. A new requirement is to be able to study associations between the diseases experienced by persons over long periods of time. For such statistics the unit will be a personal medical history rather than a sick person's, case or spell of sickness. Recently developed methods for linking records of separate sickness events in the lives of individuals will permit such studies to be carried out far more freely than has been the case hitherto. For many purposes the process may need to be carried further so that a family's medical history is the unit. For example, it is often useful to be able to consider the pregnant mother and her subsequent child as a unit. Suitable linkage methods are now available and although they are greatly facilitated if a computer is available, it is quite possible to organize a linked record system using simpler data handling methods.

The term record linkage has been used in two different although related ways which exemplify two different practical approaches to the problems of linkage of suitable data on a national scale. The first approach involves the creation of a file for each member of the population into which all reported data on the occurrence of disease, or other relevant phenomena, will be entered. Such files would usually need to be kept by means of electronic computers and the files stored on magnetic tape or some equivalent medium. There are many difficulties apart from those of cost, complexity, unique identification codes, and the present limitations of actual electronic computers. Perhaps the most important is the emotional reaction which proposals of this kind have evoked from the general public. Computerized medical record files have been seen as yet another example of the capacity of electronic data processing equipment to facilitate the invasion of individual privacy. In the particular context of medical records, it has been claimed that the confidentiality of medical records must be maintained unless communication is made to another doctor and in the patient's direct interest. This raises a generally difficult question of the right of access of population doctors to data on the populations that represent their patients. If we are to develop monitoring systems which permit effective appraisal of health status and health services, and efficient monitoring of the imminence of potentially disastrous outbreaks, we shall need to redefine the ethical issues of medical confidentiality so as to permit the population doctor to have access to the necessary data on individual medical experience.

Another approach to medical record linkage, which to some extent circumvents these difficulties, is the identification of individual data so as to permit *ad hoc* linkages to be carried out when these are required. Such an approach can be effected with more modest data processing resources than are required for a fully linked system. However, in either system it will be necessary to develop highly specific identification devices for individual records and to develop linking methods which are not frustrated by the inevitable inconsistencies that will occur in identifying information. Such methods are being developed in several centres and are, from time to time, reported in the medical press.

Statistical methods

This is not the place for a long discussion of relevant statistical methods. Indeed, such a discussion might justifiably occupy a volume of its own. It may, however, be useful to consider some fields of innovation.

One particularly interesting development concerns the adaptation of statistical methods developed in the context of industrial quality control. An example has been the use of such methods for the analysis of data accruing from the system of notification of congenital malformations. The method employed has been that of cumulative sums in which the number of cases occurring in short intervals of time are substracted from a constant factor chosen so that in the absence of any disturbance of trend the accumulated sum of the negative and positive differences remains broadly constant. If there is a change in the basic trend this sum will cease to remain constant and a graphical plot of the accumulated sum at the end of each time period will exhibit a marked change of direction.

The method naturally lends itself to computer-based analysis of data and it is easy to arrange that the attention of the responsible authorities is drawn to any marked change in the frequency of a condition. Such changes may then be further investigated and the appropriate action taken.

Incidence and prevalence rates

It would scarcely have seemed worthwhile in a volume such as this to deal with such elementary questions as incidence and prevalence rates, except that in a number of recent discussions it has become evident that the distinction between these two measures of the morbidity load afflicting a community is not always clearly drawn. Incidence rates are fractions which express the frequency of incidents per unit population during a specified period of time. The incidents expressed in an incidence rate may be onsets of illness, terminations of illness (e.g. deaths), admissions to or discharges from hospital, or changes from one state to another. For example, the change of state from being negative to a cervical cytological examination to being positive to such an examination is an incident, and the rate expressing the frequency of such changes, during a period of time, is an incidence rate.

Prevalence rates should perhaps strictly be called prevalence ratios, since they are fractions which express the proportion of a population characterizable by a given state at a point either in secular time or in the life of individuals. For example, it might be argued that the proportion of new-born individuals affected by a congenital malformation is a prevalence rate. More familiar examples include hospital residence rates and prevalence rates for chronic illnesses determined by examining a population for the presence or absence of a disease state.

There will be an arithmetical relationship between a prevalence rate for any particular state and its incidence rate which defines either the entry into or exit from that state. The two rates are related by the average duration of the state. It is thus possible to calculate average duration if we know the prevalence of a condition and the incidence rate of its onset or termination. Indeed, if we know any two of these three factors we can determine the third. Thus, if the incidence rate for new cases of a condition is 6 per 100,000 population per year and the average duration of the disease is 1 month or 0·08 year, then the average point prevalence rate over the year is 0·5 per 100,000 population. This relationship is often useful when one of the quantities is unknown and the other two are known. For example, if we know the number of new cancer registrations per year and the total number on the cancer register at a given time, we can calculate average duration of survival. However, it is important to note that the relationship may be disturbed if any of the three elements is subject to secular change.

For many diseases it is not possible to determine the point of onset and it is not possible, therefore, directly to calculate the incidence of new cases. It may, however, be possible to infer it from changes in the prevalence over a defined period of time.

It is, nevertheless, important to remember that changes in the prevalence of a condition may be due either to changes in the incidence of its onset or to changes in its average duration. This is just as true whether the changes be secular or differences between the prevalence rates for categorizably different sections of the population. Thus, an association between prevalence and age may be due either to an association of incidence with age, or an association of duration with age. This may be particularly important in interpreting data on the age-specific prevalence rate for a positive result in a screening test.

Conclusions

No system for monitoring community needs will be effective however sophisticated its data collection and data analysis procedures if the results are not available to those capable of responding to the identified needs of the population. It has been a serious limitation of the health statistical services of many countries that they are located outside the agency responsible for the management of health services, and have come to regard their principal function as the compilation of annual volumes having a largly historical interest.

The reasons for this state of affairs have been various. In some countries the growth of a central statistics unit has preceded the development of central responsibility for health services and in such cases the health statistics agency has often been a branch not of the health administrative agency but of the general statistical office. In other cases, the separation has arisen predominantly because of the lack of interest in adequate numerical data on the part of those charged with responsibility for administering the health services. Such lack of interest may have arisen from lack of any suitable educational preparation for such administrative responsibilities — as has regrettably frequently been the case in this country — or it may have arisen because the monitoring agency has for a long time been relatively ineffective and administrators have perforce become used to muddling through.

The need which is now evident for a more efficient deployment of health service resources in relation to a more clearly identified ascertainment of the needs and priorities can only be met by health administrators who have been suitably educated in the necessary epidemiological skills. Such an education cannot be obtained from a single section in a wide ranging volume. Unfortunately no one book deals adequately with the problem. The bibliography attached to this section calls for selective reading and, ideally, the training of health administrators should include a substantial course in epidemiology. Until such courses are widely included in the education of health administrators, effective monitoring of community need is unlikely to be generally developed.

Bibliography

Hill, A.B. (1966). *Principles of Medical Statistics* (8th Revised Edition). London; The Lancet

MacMahan, B. and Pugh, T.F. (1970). *Epidemiology: Principles and Methods.* Boston; Little Brown and Co.; London; Churchill

Morris, J.N. (1967). *Uses of Epidemiology.* Edinburgh; Livingstone

Smith, A. (1968). *The Science of Social Medicine.* London; Staples

Witts, L.J. (Ed.) (1964). *Medical Surveys and Clinical Trials.* London; Oxford University Press

9–Operational Research in the Health Service

Anthony Hindle

Introduction

The definition of operational research is given on the front of every edition of the *Operational Research Quarterly* – the journal of the Operational Research Society, and it reads: 'Operational Research is the attack of modern science on complex problems in the direction and management of large systems of men, machines, materials and money in industry, business, government and defence. The distinctive approach is to develop a scientific model, incorporating measurements of factors, such as chance and risk, with which to compare the outcomes of alternative decisions, strategies or controls. The purpose is to help management determine its policy and actions scientifically'. The discipline of operational research is now firmly established in military, industrial and academic contexts in all the developed countries of the world.

In Britain the Operational Research Society started as a club in 1947 and has now close on 3,000 members. The majority of these members are employed in industry in a wide diversity of companies. It is recognized that operational research pays dividends. Most of the remainder are in the defence area or in academic institutions. Government based operational research is, as yet, at an embryo stage. However, a very rapid expansion is envisaged in this area of application over the next few years.

A certain amount of operational research activity has found its way into the health services and is the subject of this section.

Scientific Decision Making

It is clear from the definition of operational research, that it is very much concerned with decision making. In particular it is concerned with improving the quality of decision by subjecting the decision problem to rigorous and objective scientific analysis. Before we can fully appreciate the implications of this approach it is necessary to describe the general nature of decision making. Consider, as an illustration, the following decision situation.

A patient enters a doctor's surgery complaining of a spot on the end of his nose. The doctor immediately decides that this is a symptom of one of three possible diseases d_0, d_1 or d_2.

d_0 — a psychosomatic disorder. Both the patient and the doctor are imagining the spot on the end of the patient's nose. Or, more realistically, the patient is demonstrating a symptom of diseases d_1 and d_2 but, in fact, is suffering from neither.

d_1 — a common and non-serious and non-costly disease. It is easily the most likely cause of the patient's symptoms. It can be successfully treated by applying treatment t_1. If not treated in this way the patient will recover but only after a period of discomfort and time away from employment.

d_2 — a relatively rare and quite serious disorder. It requires a fairly expensive treatment t_2 which will cure it very quickly indeed. It will also respond, to some extent, to treatment t_1, although the patient will take a long time to recover. If untreated the disease can be very persistent although the patient normally shakes it off eventually.

The doctor has available to him a test or examination (E), which will detect, with considerable reliability, the presence or absence of disease d_2. The test is, however, expensive.

The society in which the doctor resides is cost conscious for the treatment of relatively trivial disorders such as diseases d_0, d_1 and d_2. It would like the doctor to minimize the total cost of treating the patient. It identifies the following costs.

(1) The cost, in lost productivity, of disease d_1; untreated.

(2) The cost, in lost productivity, of disease d_1; treated by treatment t_1.

(3)   The cost, in lost productivity, of disease d_1; treated by treatment t_2. A similar cost table can be produced for diseases d_0 and d_2. Other costs are as follows.

(4)   The cost of treatment t_1.

(5)   The cost of treatment t_2.

(6)   The cost of examination E.

It is assumed, for simplicity, that the doctor has to carry out his diagnosis, examination and treatment on this one occasion only, i.e., he cannot review the case at a later date.

What should doctor do?

The decision problem described above is one which we will attempt to solve later in this chapter. However, for the moment let us note that it contains two features common to all decision problems.

(1)   An *assessment* of the consequences of taking (or failing to take) various possible actions. For example, the doctor needs to know the consequences of deciding not to treat the patient who has the particular symptom in question.

(2)   A *valuation* of the various consequences in order that the 'best' action might be identified.

For example, the doctor needs to know the value to be attached to 'lost productivity'. Further than this, it is necessary that all the consequences of each action be measured in the same units, for example, in monetary units.

It should be noted that in this problem as in most real life problems the doctor's values are, to some extent, imposed upon him. This is clear from the statement: 'Society . . . . . would like the doctor to minimize the total cost of treating the patient'. In other words there is some purpose or objective to be attained by the taking of a decision, by the making of a choice.

Thus decisions are taken in order that objectives might be attained. This requires the assessment of the consequences of alternative choices and the valuation of these consequences in relation to the objective sought. Already we have posed questions which will normally prove very difficult to answer.

What is, or should be the objective to be sought?

What possible actions are available?

What are the consequences of these actions?

How can these consequences be measured on a common scale?

How can the best solution be deduced?

In order to help in the answering of questions like these operational research indulges in three primary types of activity.

Model building

Model building refers to the attempt to write down, often in mathematical form, an explanation of the reasons why certain consequences will follow from certain actions. A simple verbal model of part of the doctor's problem described above might be as follows.

If the doctor administers the test (E) to the patient with a spot on the end of his nose then there will be a positive reaction if, and only if, the patient has disease d_2.

A well known mathematical model is represented by the following equation.

$$PV = K$$

where P is pressure,
V is volume,
K is a constant.

This, of course, is Boyle's Law which states that pressure multiplied by volume, with reference to certain sorts of physical entities, remains constant. If you take an action to increase volume the consequence will be a proportional fall in pressure.

Model solution

A model or set of models is useless unless it can be manipulated to give answers to the questions in which the decision maker is interested. Let us say we have a model of the following form.

$$E = ax^2 + bx + c \quad (Figure\ 9.1)$$

where E is the measure of performance (e.g., total treatment cost in example),

x is the variable under the decision makers control (e.g., number of injections of penicillin),

a, b, c are constants.

In other words, we know precisely how performance depends on our decision with respect to x. However, the decision maker's interest is in knowing what value of x to choose in order to minimize (or maximize) the performance measure (E). It is necessary to be able to solve the model. In this particular case all that is required is an application of elementary calculus. However, very often, models are sufficiently complex to allow only partial solution.

Derivation of 'measures of effectiveness'

Very often, as in our doctor's problem, one of the most significant difficulties is that of deriving a single measure for all the diverse consequences of an action. For example, there are treatment costs directly related to the price of the drugs and so on; costs associated with loss of productivity; costs associated with obtaining information; the value of the doctor's time and so on. In order to obtain a single variable to maximize, all these diverse costs must be assessed and made commensurable. This is seldom completely attainable.

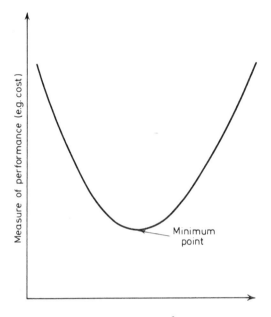

Figure 9.1. Graph of $E = ax^2 + bx + c$

In addition to these primary activities there are other aspects to a total operational research investigation such as data collection, data processing, systems design, systems implementation and so on. However these are activities common to all management services functions, whereas the characteristic feature of operational research is its direct attack on decision problems using scientific modelling and associated measures of effectiveness.

Model Building

What are the consequences of a particular course of action likely to be? What will happen if we build a new operating theatre? How will the nurses react to a new organizational structure? These questions require predictions to be made by the policy makers. The way operational research can help is by building a scientific model of the situation under consideration from which predictions and forecasts can be drawn.

In this chapter we will attempt to build several models which have proved particularly relevant in the study of health services — queueing models, simulation models, statistical forecasting models, and econometric models.

It is not intended, of course, to give a complete coverage, but merely to illustrate the concepts and principles involved in model development.

QUEUEING MODELS

Let us say that the provider of a service has a problem: the customers' waiting time for service is regarded as being too long on the average. Although, if a customer is lucky, he may arrive to find the service point unoccupied, he may find himself faced with a long queue. The service manager considers that long waiting times cost him money: either because he is responsible for the loss of money incurred by the customers when waiting or because he feels the 'expected' waiting time inhibits custom. His problem is whether to provide another service point which will also lead to costs due to extra wages. Although there are many facets to a problem of this type one aspect of it is to predict the customer waiting times resulting from the provision of an extra service point. In order to do this we require a mathematical model of the situation. Such a model is available to us.

If customers arrive at random at a service point and the time taken to provide them with service is variable but has a certain average value then the equation giving the expected waiting time is as follows.

$$\text{Expected waiting time} = \frac{\text{arrival rate}}{\text{service rate} \times (\text{service rate} - \text{arrival rate})}$$

Another measure which is of interest is the chance of not having to wait at all: this is given by the following equation.

$$\text{Chance of immediate service} = 1 - \frac{\text{arrival rate}}{\text{service rate}}$$

In a situation where more than one service point is provided a customer arriving at random has a choice: if one service point is occupied he can go to the other. The waiting time equation for a situation where there are two service points is as follows.

Expected waiting time $= \mu \times (\lambda/\mu)^2 /(2\mu - \lambda)^2 \times P_0$
where λ is arrival rate,

μ is service rate. P_0 is the chance of immediate service.

Using the equations above we are in a position to provide predictions for the service manager.

Clearly there are many situations in the health services where customers (patients) are expected to queue. In fact, could the problem of waiting time not be regarded as the main bone of contention between the hospital and its patients?

Consider the following problem. A doctor holds an out-patient clinic each week dealing only with new patients. The patients seen at this clinic will have previously put in requests for attendance via their family doctor. The hospital gives each patient an appointment date. They currently do this on an overflow basis in that the doctor will not see more than 10 patients in any one session. The requests are treated on a 'first come, first served' basis. However, the waiting time is, on average, five weeks which although satisfactory for some patients is much too long for others. For example, they may have been out of work in the interim period. The doctor would like to introduce a priority system by reducing the expected waiting time for urgent cases and increasing it for non-urgent. Let us build a model of this situation.

Suppose the demand of new patients occurs at random but is, on average, λ per time unit, i.e., we expect λ requests per week. Let μ be the maximum number of patients the consultant is prepared to see in any one session, 10 patients per week. Although the mathematics are somewhat complex if can be stated that

$$\tfrac{1}{2}(\mu - \lambda) \leqslant \text{expected waiting time} \leqslant \frac{(\mu - 1)}{2\lambda} + \tfrac{1}{2}(\mu - \lambda)$$

Now, if $\lambda \geqslant \mu$ then the waiting time will grow steadily to infinity. However consider the situation where λ is one patient per week less than μ (i.e. 9) then

$$\mu - \lambda = 1$$

Therefore from the equation outlined

$$\tfrac{1}{2} \leqslant \text{expected waiting time} \leqslant 1$$

In words, this means that if the maximum number of patients seen at a clinic is set slightly above the average demand (i.e. one patient per week more) then the expected waiting time should not be more than

155

the interval between clinic sessions. This is important because it means that the observed five weeks waiting time *cannot* have been caused by the random fluctuations of the request rate and must be due to other factors. However if demand is greater than 10 patients per week the waiting time will become, in theory, infinitely long. This being the case, the only sensible strategy for the doctor is to increase his clinic size.

A further possible reason for the doctor's problem, which ought to be investigated, is that the current five weeks wait is due simply to a backlog. Did the doctor take a holiday and allow a backlog to develop?

Our queueing model has helped us to pinpoint the real nature of the problem: given that the doctor is capable of meeting the out-patient demand then all patients could be seen quickly. If he is not capable of meeting this demand a priority system can only be a temporary solution because waiting times will grow indefinitely. In other words the maximum clinic size must be greater than the average demand. If long waits are due to backlogs then the doctor should work this off, since it is pointless to perpetuate what should be a temporary problem.

Can queueing theory also help with in-patient problems? Again we can give an affirmative answer. Consider the following problem. A hospital has 10 wards each with ten beds. Each ward accepts emergency admissions of a variable quantity. Although each of the wards can cope with the average number of emergencies the demand can often be much higher than this causing problems of availability.

If emergency demands occur at random then, subject to certain reasonable assumptions, the likelihood that a given number of patients (n) will be occupying beds in a ward is given by the following equation.

The likelihood of n patients being in the ward $= e^{-\lambda}(\lambda)^n/n!$

where λ is the average bed occupancy,
$\quad e = 2 \cdot 718$ (approx.)

Suppose for one of the wards average occupancy is eight beds, we can calculate from the above expression the likelihood that any given number of beds will be occupied. For example, below we have the calculation for 10 beds ($P(10)$).

$$P(10) = e^{-8} \ (8)^{10}/10! = 0 \cdot 1 \text{ (approx.)}$$

In other words, 10 beds will be occupied 10 per cent of the time. In fact it is possible to show that on 67 days of the year the ward will require more than 10 beds in order to cater for patient demand (given the average bed occupancy is 80 per cent). This will be the case for all 10 wards. However, let us now substitute the 10 separate wards for one large ward of 100 beds. Given that we still require an 80 per cent bed occupancy we can calculate the number of days on which more than 100 beds will be required. This turns out to be five days.

This is a clear indication of the advantages of a flexible, as opposed to a rigid, emergency admissions policy for a hospital. A hospital maintaining an independent ward system may appear to be underbedded (in our example each ward expects 67 days of 'underbedding' per year). However if the hospital is regarded as one large ward, for the same throughput of patients, the total hospital will be short of bed space on only five days of the year.

SIMULATION MODELS

Operational research increasingly makes use of the computer in order to produce a simulation of the real situation. In order to illustrate this approach a hypothetical hospital problem can be considered. A ward of 10 beds is faced with two types of demand: emergency admissions and waiting list admissions. The demand from emergencies is highly variable and results in the ward sister having to 'insure' against particularly heavy demands. She leaves beds empty which sometimes remain empty due to expected emergencies not turning up. If she fails to insure herself in this way she has to put up extra beds for unanticipated emergencies from time to time, causing some disorder on the ward. The ward sister considers that increasing the number of beds in the ward to 12 beds could considerably alleviate the problem.

The operational research problem is, in part, to predict the consequences of an increase in number of beds on the ward. How do we build a simulation model of this situation?

First, we construct a flow diagram of the system *Figure 9.2*. This shows patients flowing into the ward as emergencies and also from a waiting list via an entity called admission decision. Patients are also, of course, discharged from the ward after a certain length of stay.

Admission decision is a control device regulating the inflow of patients to the ward. We assume that emergencies must be admitted when they arrive at the ward but that patients can be taken off the waiting list at regular intervals. The number of patients selected in this way is dependent on the extent to which beds are available for them. In fact, in this simulation patients are admitted once per week and operated upon in a theatre session a day later.

The next step required is the collection of some data relating to the system. Clearly we need to know many facts before we can build a valid simulation model: we need to know about patients, resources, the interactions between patients and resources, and also about decisions.

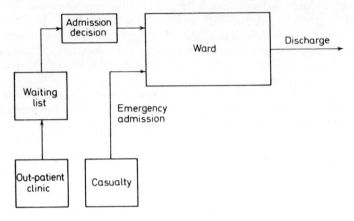

Figure 9.2. Simple flow diagram

The arrival pattern for emergency admissions, the number of days on which a given number of patients arrived unexpectedly on the ward is shown in Table 9.1. This information can be presented in the form

TABLE 9.1

Arrival Pattern for Emergency Admissions

Number of emergency admissions	Number of days during the year on which a given number of emergency admissions occurred
0	214
1	111
2	32
3	7
4	1
5	0
Total	365

of a histogram as in *Figure 9.3* representing the probability or likelihood of a particular number of patients arriving as emergencies on a given day.

Two further histograms, in this case illustrating patient lengths of stay, for emergencies and for waiting list cases, are shown in *Figure 9.4.*

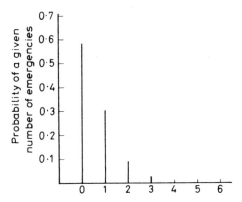

Figure 9.3. Histogram for emergency admissions

The decision to admit patients from the waiting list is made in accordance with simple rules of thumb. After detailed discussion with the ward sister and the medical staff the following decision rule emerges.

(1)   Patients are admitted on a first come, first served basis.

(2)   The number of patients admitted each week is given by the equation

$$N = e + d - \beta$$

where N is the number of patients to be admitted,

e is the number of currently empty beds (on the day the decision is taken),

d is the number of expected discharges (between the decision day and the admission day),

β is the insurance factor: the beds we need to allow for unexpected emergencies.

The ward sister and medical staff examine the waiting list every Thursday to decide on admissions for the following Monday. They count currently empty beds, forecast discharges and decide on an appropriate insurance against not having a bed for an emergency admission. This gives them a number of patients and the identity of the patients is decided simply on the basis of time on the waiting list. (N.B. No real hospital could work as simply as this example ward.)

We are now in a position to build an accurate simulation model of the system described above. First, we draw another flow diagram:

this time it is a logic diagram which will form the basis of a computer program which is a set of instructions for a digital computer. The flow diagram is illustrated in *Figure 10.5,* page 214 . The diamond shapes represent decisions to be answered by yes or no, and the boxes represent sub-routines.

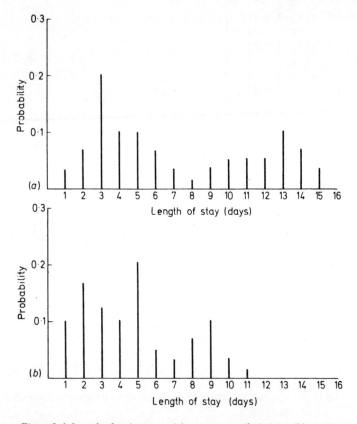

Figure 9.4. Length of patient stay: (a) *emergency admissions;* (b) *waiting list admissions*

The program instructs the computer to act as a ward having a certain number of beds and to admit and treat patients having certain characteristics. It instructs it to act on a day-by-day basis noting the events which happen on each day. The computer can be asked to go for years if required, and it is capable of generating ten years' data in a few seconds.

After moving to a particular day the first routine carries out daily modifications: it adjusts various counters in the computer which represent the current bed position in the ward. It then asks the question 'Is it decision day?': is it time to make a decision about the patients to admit to the ward next week? If so, it then estimates the likely bed availability and searches the waiting list in accordance with the decision rule equation. It next asks if there are any emergency admissions and, if not, whether it is admission day for waiting list cases. For either waiting list cases or emergencies a sub-routine called put-in-bed ensures that the patients are actually admitted: in the former case the waiting list is modified as a result of patients being taken off it. Do we want to continue? If so, we add more patients to the waiting list and go through another day. At some stage the computer is instructed to bring the simulation run to an end and so prints out statistics about the particular experiment and stops.

The output gives information about the day-by-day admission and discharge record and also the bed occupancy record.

Many experiments could be carried out with our simulation of the ward. We can vary two main factors.

(1) The number of beds available to the ward. (Remember that the sister considers an increase in bed complement to be the answer to her problem.)

(2) The insurance factor (β). (To what extent does she *need* to insure against the unexpected emergency.)

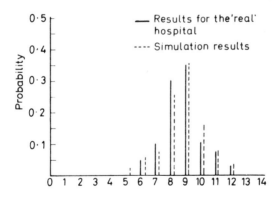

Figure 9.5. Bed occupancy results

However, the initial experiment should be to validate the model: the simulation is run with exactly the same bed complement as at present, namely 10 beds, and the same admission decision rule. The results of running the simulation in this form can be compared with the performance of the unit in practice. An example of this principle is shown in *Figure 9.5*. The two histograms illustrate the bed occupancy found in practice and in the simulated ward. They show the number of nights during a year on which a particular number of beds were occupied.

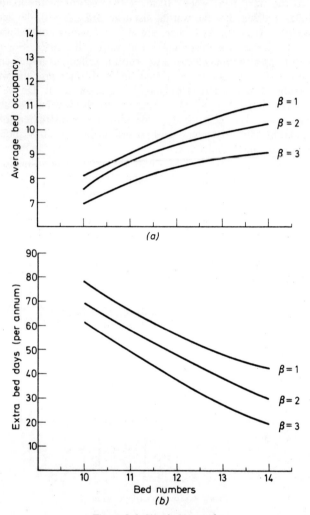

Figure 9.6. Simulation results

The histograms are similar but not identical. Is the agreement good enough?

In order to answer this question we would carry out a statistical test on the results known as the chi-squared test for goodness of fit.

This will tell us whether the observed differences between the real and simulated system are due to chance or to a fault in the model. Let us assume our model is valid.

The experiments which follow vary systematically the two key variables, bed numbers and insurance factor and give us results in terms of patient throughput, bed occupancy etc.

The two graphs in *Figure 9.6* show the types of result one might obtain from the simulation runs. *Figure 9.6a* shows for three values of β the way bed occupancy varies with bed numbers, and *Figure 9.6b* shows how the number of extra bed-days (beds having to be erected above the bed complement due to an unexpectedly heavy demand) varies with bed numbers; again for three values of β.

An example of a practical application of this simulation approach to hospital scheduling problems is given in Chapter 10.

SOME STATISTICAL MODELS

Among the most useful approaches in operational research and in other management services activities, especially in the health area, involve statistical modelling methods known as correlation and regression. Anyone familiar with the work on the relationship of smoking and lung cancer will realize the power of these techniques.

A group of school children are given an intelligence test and several years later the same children take their O level mathematics examination. The childrens' scores on the two tests are given in Table 9.2. The technique of correlation allows us to determine whether these scores are related. Let us plot a graph of these scores with intelligence on the x-axis and mathematical achievement on the y-axis. The result is in *Figure 9.7*. It is clear that there is a certain degree of relationship between the two variables but nevertheless the dots are somewhat scattered. A correlation coefficient is a measure of this lack of perfect relationship. The measure can vary between -1 and $+1$. These extremes imply that the dots fall on a straight line; in the first case on a line (a) and in the second case on a line (b). If there doesn't seem to be any pattern in the dots at all then the correlation will be close to zero. The correlation coefficient for the data of *Figure 9.7* is 0·8 approximately.

Table 9.3 gives some data obtained from hospitals in a particular hospital region. It gives information on lengths of patient stay and resource availability for eight hospitals. The hospitals are given a rank order on all the variables, i.e., the actual measurements are not given. However it is possible to calculate a statistic known as a 'rank order correlation coefficient'. The formula for this is as follows.

$$\text{Correlation} = 1 - \frac{6 \times \text{The sum of differences squared}}{(\text{number of hospitals})^3 - (\text{number of hospitals})}$$

where the sum of differences squared is equal to sum of differences in rank on variable A and variable B for all the hospitals with each difference squared.

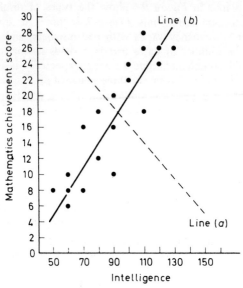

Figure 9.7. The relation between intelligence and mathematics scores

Let us work out an example which will make this clear. Consider length of patient stay for 'all emergency cases' and 'all waiting list cases' for the eight hospitals .
The ranks are as follows.

6	3	2	4	8	5	1	7
6	1	5	2	8	4	3	7

The differences between ranks are

0	2	3	2	0	1	2	0

The squares of differences equal

0	4	9	4	0	1	4	0

164

The sum of the differences squared is 22.
We can now calculate the correlation co-efficient from the formula

$$\text{Correlation} = 1 - 6 \times 22/(8)^3 - 8 = + 0.74$$

TABLE 9.2

Mathematics and Intelligence Test Results for 20 Children

Children	Mathematics score	Intelligence test score
1	12	80
2	18	80
3	28	110
4	26	110
5	8	50
6	8	60
7	16	70
8	20	100
9	18	110
10	26	130
11	10	90
12	8	70
13	26	120
14	20	90
15	22	100
16	6	60
17	10	60
18	24	100
19	24	120
20	16	90

The range of scores for the mathematics test is zero to 30 and for the intelligence test zero to 160.

This level of correlation hints at a relationship between the two variables which would suggest that in hospitals where length of stay for emergency admissions is long, so also is length of stay for waiting list cases.

Two words of caution are necessary at this stage. First, a correlation of this level could have occurred by chance selection of eight hospitals and might not reappear if another eight were selected. Secondly,

TABLE 9.3

Hospital Ranked by Length of Stay, Availability and Other Hospital Characteristics

Hospital	1	2	3	4	5	6	7	8
Length of stay (1 is short)								
All emergency cases	6	3	2	4	8	5	1	7
All waiting list cases	6	1	5	2	8	4	3	7
Medical emergency cases	3	5·5	2	4	5·5	7	1	8
Surgical emergency cases	7	1·5	1·5	4	8	5	3	6
Surgical waiting list cases	6·5	2	5	1	8	3	4	6·5
Bed occupancy (1 is high)								
Medical	6	5	1	8	7	2·5	4	2·5
Surgical	2	4	5	7	3	6	1	8
Proportion of emergencies (1 is low)	6	1	8	2	7	3	4	5
Mortality rate (1 is low)	7	3	2	4	8	6	1	5
Measures of resource availability (1 is high)								
Medical consultants	6	1	5	2	8	4	3	7
Junior physicians	7	5	4	2	6	3	1	8
Surgical consultants	6	4	7	5	2	1	3	8
Junior surgeons	6	7	3	4	8	1	2	5
Nurses	2	6	1	3	5	7	4	8
X-ray	3	6	7	4	8	1	2	5
Pathology	1	2	4	8	5	7	3	6

a correlation does not necessarily imply a cause and effect relationship — the correlation may be spurious. A good example of a correlation likely to be spurious is found in Table 9.3. This is the apparently perfect relationship between the availability of physicians and the length of stay of all waiting list cases. It is highly unlikely that this is cause and effect, in that waiting list cases are, in the main, seen by surgeons and not physicians.

Regression analysis is a more powerful method than the correlation approach. In order to understand regression it is necessary to refresh our memory on the nature of linear equations. Let us go back to *Figure 9.7*. This illustrates that mathematical achievement is related to, or depends on the student's intelligence. Expressed as an equation

$$y = f(X)$$

where y is the mathematics exam score,
    X is the intelligence test score,
    f means depends on, or is a function of.
Drawn through the dots is a best-fitting straight line (line (b)). We will return to the meaning of best-fitting in a moment. In the meantime, what is the equation for line (b)? The equation must tell us three things — that the line is straight; that the line has a certain slope and that it does not go through the origin. The equation will enable us to calculate the likely mathematics score given the individual's intelligence test results. The form of the equation is

$$y = ax + c$$

where a is a constant — slope of the line, x appearing without an exponent tells us the line is straight, c is a constant — the distance along the y-axis from the origin where the line intersects it.
The equation for the line in *Figure 9.7* is

$$y = 0.3x + (-10)$$

Thus, if an individual scored 80 on the intelligence test his expected score on mathematics should be calculated as follows.

$$y = 0.3(80) - 10 = 14$$

It can be seen from *Figure 9.7* that this is a reasonable result although this does not imply that people scoring 80 on x will necessarily score 14 on y: 14 is the *most likely* value. This is because the relationship between x and y is not perfect.
How did we draw line (b) in *Figure 9.7*? We use the least squares method. We take the distance from any line we might draw through the dots to every dot; square each distance and add up these squared distances. The best-fitting line is the one which has the lowest total for this sum of squared distances.

An example of the regression method in use for a health service problem concerns an aspect of the planning of an out-patient department. Let us say that we have a forecast of the number of patients who will attend a new out-patient department. How many nurses of various types will we require? There are, of course, many ways of answering a question of this sort. However, one way might be to examine the relationship between number of out-patient attendances and nurse staffing in existing hospitals. Fortunately data of this sort has been collected by the Department of Health and Social Security. The information can be plotted on a graph as illustrated in *Figure 9.8*. The relationship results in the following equation.

$$N = 9 \cdot 21 \times 10^{-5}x + 5 \cdot 67$$

where N is the number of nurses,

x is the arrival number of out-patient attendances.

In this example, as in the intelligence and mathematics illustration the dots are rather widely scattered, that is, the correlation between the

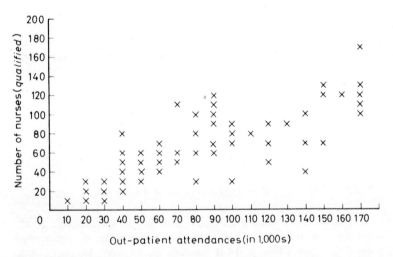

Figure 9.8. The relation between out-patient attendances and number of qualified nurses in 55 hospitals

variables is not very great. Thus reliable predictions of one variable from a knowledge of the other is not possible. Better results can be obtained using a multiple regression approach.

A given variable, mathematical achievement for example, may depend on more than one factor. It may depend not only on intelligence test scores but also on certain personality characteristics, for example, whether or not the person *is* an introvert or an extrovert. Let us assume that we have a measure of introversion—extroversion, and find that it is correlated with a mathematics score. We may be able to achieve a better prediction of an individual's mathematics score by using both the intelligence measure *and* the personality score than by using any one of these measures on its own. Thus the linear equation becomes

$$y = ax_1 + bx_2 + c$$

where y is the mathematics score,

$\quad$ x_1 is the intelligence score,

$\quad$ x_2 is the introversion—extroversion score,

$\quad$ a, b, c are constants.

Using this approach in relation to the nurse staffing problem it is possible to produce a reasonable multiple regression equation for the out-patient department, as follows.

$$y = 162x_1 + 84x_2 + 136x_3 + 154x_4 - 279x_5 + 127x_6 + 626x_7 - 17$$

where y is the number of out-patient attendances per week and $x_1 - x_7$ are the numbers of sisters, staff nurses, enrolled nurses, student nurses, pupil nurses, nursing auxiliaries and nursery nurses employed in the out-patient situation.

As a second example of the use of the regression method we can return to the study of eight hospitals in a particular region described above; the data for which are given in Table 9.3. Let us consider, first of all, a simplified model of hospital costs. Let us divide costs of treating patients into fixed costs and variable costs. Fixed costs are those which do not depend on the number of patients treated and variable costs are those which do. Thus the cost per bed per week (C_B) is given by the equation

$$C_B = (F + V(N))/B$$

where F is the fixed costs per week,

$\quad$ V is the cost per patient of variable costs,

$\quad$ N is the number of patients,

$\quad$ B is the number of beds.

Medical salaries can be regarded as a fixed cost whereas the cost of drugs varies with the number (and type) of patient. Consider what

169

happens to C_B if we appoint more doctors. First of all the fixed costs (F) increase. Also let us argue that employing more doctors allows us to treat more patients: thus N also increases. The cost C_B increases as a result of an increase in F and in $V(N)$. However, we can consider another cost, namely C_p or total cost per patient. This is given by the equation

$$C_p = (F^1 + V^1 (N))/N$$

where F^1 is the total fixed cost per annum,

V^1 is the cost per patient of variable costs,

N is the total number of patients treated per annum.

If we appoint more doctors and this results in more patients being treated then, under certain circumstances, C_p may decrease. Consider this example.

F^1 = £10,000 per annum,

V^1 = £5 per patient,

N = 1,000.

Therefore $C_p = (10,000 + 5(1,000))/1,000 = £15$ per patient.

Let us now increase our doctor cost by £500 and assume that this results in treating double the number of patients. Our accounts are now as follows.

F^1 = £15,000 per annum,

V^1 = £5 per patient,

N = 2,000

Therefore $C_p = (15,000 + 5(2,000))/2,000 = £12.50$ per patient.

This result is of considerable importance because total cost per patient is a much more sensible measure of the hospital's performance than is cost per bed per week. The reason for this is that minimizing cost per patient treated (effectively) implies an ability to treat the maximum number of patients within a given budget or, conversely, allows treatment of a given number of patients with the minimum budget. Where does the regression method fit into this picture? It is required in order to build a model relating resources to patient throughput, i.e., to replace our assumption that spending more on doctors will increase the number of patients treated by the hospital.

The number of patients treated depends on the number of beds (B), the percentage occupancy (P), and the average length of stay (L) as follows.

$$N = (365 \times B \times P))/L$$

where N is the number of patients treated per year.

By simple algebra one can substitute this result in the equation for C_p given previously. If we assume that for a given hospital $(365 \times B \times P)$ is a constant (K), then the equation for C_p becomes

$$C_p = (LF^1 + KV^1)/K$$

The only variable part of this equation is $L \times F^1$ illustrating the way cost per patient depends on the fixed costs and the length of patient stay. If increasing the fixed costs does not affect patient's length of stay cost per patient will increase. If, on the other hand, length of stay is reduced cost per patient may decrease. For example, consider these figures

$F^1 = £10,000$
$L = 10$ days
Then $F^1 \times L = £100,000$ days.

If by spending £2,000 it could be expected that length of stay could be reduced to eight days, total cost per patient would decrease.

$F^1 = £12,000$
$L = 8$ days
Then $F^1 \times L = £96,000$ days.

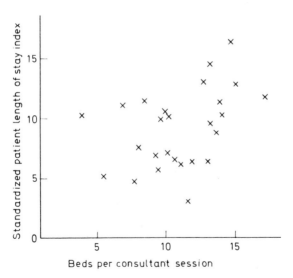

Figure 9.9. The relationship between length of patient stay and consultant availability

Do resources affect length of stay? The answer would seem to be affirmative. Consider *Figure 9.9*. This shows standardized length of stay plotted against the level of consultant staffing (measured in terms of beds per consultant session). Although the dots are again scattered there is a clear relationship for which we could derive an equation. We are now in a position to determine a level of consultant availability which will minimize cost per patient, that is, an optimal availability level. Rather than slip into the complex mathematics required, let us work through a hypothetical example which illustrates this point.

Let us consider that a hospital increases its medical cost per bed through five steps from 20 units to 60 units. This result is shown in Table 9.4 under the costs per bed (medical) column. This results in some increases in the other fixed costs labelled hotel costs. Also the

TABLE 9.4

Variable Costs

Costs per bed (F^1) Hotel Medical		Variable costs (V^1) per patient	Length of patient stay (days)	Total cost per case (C_p)
1	100 20	2·0	10	5·4
2	105 30	2·1	8	5·1
3	110 40	2·2	7	5·2
4	115 50	2·3	6	5·2
5	120 60	2·4	6	5·4

variable costs per patient may also increase slightly — perhaps due to receiving more attention from doctors. Average length of stay decreases, however, as established by the regression shown in *Figure 9.9*. Total cost per case has been calculated from the formula

$$C_p = (F^1 + V^1 (N))/N$$

where

$$N = \frac{365 \times \text{percentage occupancy} \times \text{number of beds}}{\text{average length of stay}}$$

The results hold for any number of beds.

It can be seen that cost per case decreases and then increases as medical cost per bed increases. In other words there is an optimal level, namely around the 30 units per bed mark.

Of course, in relation to a study of this type all the assumptions regarding statistical relationships need to be borne constantly in mind.

A statistical relationship may imply cause and effect and, at the very least, a detailed search should be made for an explanation of the phenomenon. Later in this chapter the detailed regression analysis derived from the information illustrated in *Figure 9.9* is presented.

Model Solution

In this section we will discuss some techniques which can be used to derive solutions from mathematical models. Initially we will cover methods which are particularly appropriate where the consequences of each possible action are known with confidence and our objective is clear. This is followed by a discourse on problem solution when many of the important factors are clouded by uncertainty: where cause and effect may be only hazily perceived.

MATHEMATICAL PROGRAMMING

Which action from a set of possible actions should we choose?

First, let us assume we know the consequences of each action with certainty. Let us further assume that we know what we want to achieve by the decision. Choice should be easy. But is it?

Consider the following problem.

You are in a position where you can buy three types of drug *A, B* and *C*.

The drugs are all intended for the treatment of the same type of disorder. However they are not all the same price and their clinical composition is not identical. In fact they contain three main elements *X, Y* and *Z* in various proportions. This data can be summarized as follows.

		Percentage		
Drug type	*X*	*Y*	*Z*	*Price per unit*
A	0·06	2·0	25	10
B	0·04	4·0	25	10
C	0·02	3·0	25	15

The doctor buying the drugs considers that the ideal drug should have between 0·02 and 0·03 per cent of *X* and between 2·0 and 3·25 per cent of *Y*: together with 25 per cent of *Z*. He has, therefore, been accustomed to buying drug *C* even though it is a little low on the proportion of *X* in the blend. However, the price of this drug is high.

OPERATIONAL RESEARCH IN THE HEALTH SERVICE

The trouble with drug A is that it is too strong on X and a little weak on Y. Drug B is strong on both X and Y. It is suggested to the doctor that he ought to purchase a blend of the drugs which will be remade to ideal specifications. He should attempt to achieve the purchased blend at minimum cost. What proportions of drugs A, B and C should he buy?

In this problem the objective has been precisely stated in quantitative terms and the consequences, in terms of chemical composition and price, of any action can be determined with certainty. It is clearly a mathematical problem and, in fact, can be solved using a technique known as linear programming. Linear programming and its variants are the most widely used (and useful) techniques of operational research.

Let us solve the drug purchasing problem using this method.

Consider that we have one unit weight of drugs blended from various amounts of drugs A, B and C. Clearly we can calculate the chemical composition of the blend and the price as follows.

Let x, y and z represent the amounts of drugs A, B and C, respectively, in the blend. Therefore the percentage of element X in the blend equals

0·6 × x (the amount of drug of type A), plus

0·4 × y (the amount of drug of type B), plus

0·2 × z (the amount of drug of type C).

That is

percentage of element $X = 0.06 x + 0.04y + 0.02z$

By a similar process

percentage of element $Y = 2x + 4y + 3z$

It should be noted that the percentage of element Z will always be 25.

The cost of this unit blended drug is easily calculated as follows.

$$\text{Cost (in units)} = 10x + 10y + 15z$$

Since the cost and chemical composition properties of any blend can be calculated one could experiment with different blends and note the results. With a simple problem like the above one would probably find the best answer. However if there were hundreds of equations to deal with the trial and error approach would break down.

Let us pursue the mathematics a little further. First, we need to represent in the form of an equation the statement 'the proportion of element X should be between 0·02 and 0·03 per cent'. From the proportions of X in the original drugs, it is clear that the proportion of this element cannot fall below 0·02 per cent. Therefore, we can state that the proportion of X should be less than, or equal to 0·03 per cent. This gives the following equation.

$$0.06x + 0.04y + 0.02z \leqslant 0.03$$

By similar arguments the equation for the statement 'the percentage of element Y must be between 2·0 and 3·25 per cent' is

$$2x + 4y + 3z \leqslant 3.25$$

A further equation is required

$$x + y + z = 1$$

This simply states that the units of quantity are proportions of one unit weight of blended drug.

Also for completeness we need to state that the proportions (x, y or z) cannot be negative they must be greater than or equal to zero. This is written as follows.

$$x \geqslant 0; \ y \geqslant 0; \ z \geqslant 0$$

The cost equation we have already written down previously.
The full set of required equation is

$$0.06x + 0.04y + 0.02z \leqslant 0.03 \text{ (for element } X) \qquad (1)$$
$$2x + 4y + 3z \leqslant 3.25 \text{ (for element } Y) \qquad (2)$$
$$x + y + z = 1 \text{ (total)} \qquad (3)$$
$$x \geqslant 0; y \geqslant 0; z \geqslant 0 \qquad (4)$$
$$C = 10x + 10y + 15z \text{ (cost)} \qquad (5)$$

The problem can be stated as follows.

Determine x, y and z such that they satisfy equations (1) to (4) and lead to the minimum cost as calculated from equation (5).

SOLUTION

There are several methods for the solution of the problem but we shall use a graphical method.

First, we can eliminate z by using equation (3)

$$x + y + z = 1$$

Therefore $z = 1 - x - y$

This gives for equation (1)

$$0{\cdot}06x + 0{\cdot}04y + 0{\cdot}02(1 - x - y) \leqslant 0{\cdot}03$$

that is $4x + 2y \leqslant 1$ \hfill (6)

For equation (2)

$$2x + 4y + 3(1 - x - y) \leqslant 3{\cdot}25$$

that is $4y - 4x \leqslant 1$ \hfill (7)

For equation (5)

$$C = 10x + 10y + 15(1 - x - y)$$
$$= 15 - 5x - 5y \tag{8}$$

We can now draw the graph shown in *Figure 9.10*. The limiting conditions, represented by equations (6) and (7) are illustrated by the graph lines.

The solution cannot be outside the shaded area and the cost decreases with increases in x and y. In fact, it can be seen from equation (8) that cost is equally affected by x and y increases.

Clearly the cost is minimized by taking x, y at point M. Thus $x = 0{\cdot}083$ $y = 0{\cdot}033$ $z = 0{\cdot}587$ (from equation (3)) and the minimum cost = $12{\cdot}935$ units per unit weight (from equation (8)).

Thus the doctor should be advised to purchase drugs in the following proportions.

Drug type	Proportion (percentage)
A	8·3
B	33·0
C	58·7

This will cost 13 units (per unit weight), as against 15 units with the present policy of buying just drug C. The blended drug when remade will be to ideal specifications.

The techniques of mathematical programming are designed for the solution of problems where a blending of elements is required. For example, they can be used to determine an optimal blend of resources for an organization: they can be used to suggest an optimal purchasing policy for raw material (say for a blast furnace) and so on. In the health services there have as yet been few successful applications, mainly because of the model building and measurement problems referred to earlier in the section. However, it is tempting to think that potential applications are widespread: determining optimal staffing ratios: allocation of nurses to wards: purchase of drugs and other raw materials: allocation of beds to consultants and so on.

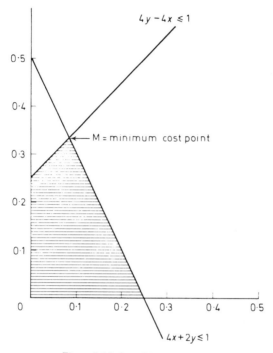

Figure 9.10. Drug blending solution

STATISTICAL DECISION ANALYSIS

It can be readily appreciated that the technique of linear programming has widespread applicability in situations where it is clear what is wanted and the consequences of an action can be predicted with certainty (or approximately so).

However in relation to many problems of decision the issues are clouded by uncertainty. One can never be sure, under English weather conditions, whether a cricket match, for example, will survive a forecast rain shower. One can rarely feel confident in predicting the result of a soccer match; a doctor can very often only detail a prognosis about a patient in terms of the likelihood of a variety of consequences. Statistical decision analysis attempts to deal with problems of this type.

Consider a simple game with a pack of cards. A gambler shuffles a pack of 52 playing cards and places three cards face downwards in front of you. He suggests that you pay him 2·5 p. if they are *not all red* and that he will pay you 25 p. if they are *all red cards*. He further suggests that the game should continue for one hundred plays, i.e. he will shuffle and deal one hundred times. Should you play this game? How much do you expect to win or lose?

This is a decision situation in which the only certain feature is the uncertainty of the outcome. Nevertheless mathematical techniques can again assist us. First, we need to know the likelihood or probability $P(R)$ that a card, selected from a pack of cards, is red. This is given by the following equation.

$$P(R) = \frac{\text{number of red cards}}{\text{total number of cards}} = \frac{26}{52} = 0.5$$

What is the probability that all three are red?

Here

$$P(\text{all red}) = \frac{\text{number of all red threesomes}}{\text{total number of possible threesomes}}$$

The following threesomes are possible

RRR	BRR
RRB	BRB
RBR	BBR
RBB	BBB

There are thus eight possible types of threesomes in terms of black and red cards and therefore, since only one of these sets is all red

$$P(\text{all red}) = \frac{1}{8} = 0.125$$

Clearly, by a similar argument, the probability that a set of three cards is not all red is given as follows.

$$P(\text{not all red}) = \frac{7}{8} = 0.875$$

What do these probabilities mean? They mean that if the gambler properly shuffles the pack between card selections and selects three cards, one in every eight selections on *average* will be all red cards. It does not mean that you will necessarily obtain one set of all red cards in *every* eight selections: only that this will be the long-term average.

We now need a way of deciding whether to play this particular game and we do this by calculating the *expected value* (*V*) of the game. This is given by the following equation.

$$V = \text{(probability of winning} \times \text{value of winning)} + \text{(probability of losing} \times \text{value of losing)}$$

therefore $V = (0.125 \times 25 \text{ p.}) + (0.875 \times (-2.5 \text{ p.}))$
$$= 0.94 \text{ p. per game.}$$

Thus by playing the game you will gain at the rate of 0.94 p. per game and you can expect to win approximately one pound sterling in one hundred plays. Again this does not mean you will necessarily win this amount, or even win at all, but that this is the *long-term* expected payoff.

What is the most you would be prepared to pay him for playing this game?

Statistical decision analysis forms the basis for the solution of the problem faced by the doctor treating spots on the ends of noses outlined earlier in this chapter. However before we proceed to solve that problem we need to introduce a further important concept. This is the idea of a *subjective probability*.

When we talked about the probability of three cards being all red we were talking about objective probabilities. If a pack of cards is shuffled properly and three cards selected and this process continued indefinitely then the proportion of all red threesomes will converge on 1 in 8. This is an objective fact. However, in asking the question, 'What proportion of patients having spots on the end of their nose have disease d_1?', we may have no more evidence than the experience of the doctor concerned. We may have to ask him to estimate this proportion or probability. If we then use this probability in further statistical analysis in exactly the same manner as an objective probability we become Bayesian statisticians. The term derives from the work of the Reverend Thomas Bayes whose paper in 1763, entitled An Essay Toward Solving a Problem in the Doctrine of Chance, suggested that probability judgements based on mere hunches could be used in the analysis of decision problems. In general, Bayesians are 'subjectivists' and are happy to introduce intuitive judgements and feelings into the formal analysis of the decision problem if relevant objective data cannot be found.

We can now attempt to solve the doctor's problem.

Data

Clearly it is necessary to have some probability statements in relation to the problem. These will probably have to be supplied by the doctor on the basis of his experience in treating patients with spots on the end of their nose. Also, of course, we will need the costs referred to earlier. Let us list the costs first of all. These are shown in Table 9.5.

TABLE 9.5

Relative Costs of Treatments for
Different Diseases

Disease	Treatment		
	t_0	t_1	t_2
d_0	5	20	40
d_1	70	20	50
d_2	150	100	20

The cost, in terms of treatment cost and loss of the patient's earnings of disease d_1 treated by treatment t_0, i.e., no treatment, is 70 units. If treatment t_1 is employed the total cost is reduced to 20 units.

The cost of disease d_2, if untreated, is 150 units. If it is treated by treatment t_2 this cost is reduced to 20 units.

Notice that even d_0 can be a costly disorder especially if the patient is treated as though he was suffering from diseases d_1 or d_2. This is due to the cost of the treatments and certain side-effects.

The cost of the examination (E) to detect the presence of disease d_2 is 15 units.

What probability assessments do we require?

First of all we need to know the likelihoods that a patient with a spot on the end of his nose has diseases d_0, d_1 or d_2. Maybe the medical literature will tell us this. However, it is more likely that the doctor, on the basis of his experience, will have to tell us. Hence, we must be Bayesians. Let us assume that the doctor states the following.

It is unlikely that the patient is suffering from a psychosomatic disorder. I would expect him to be suffering from either d_1 or d_2 of which the former is by far the most likely.

After further questioning he agrees to the following probabilities which, of course, add up to unity.

$d_0 = 0.1$ $\qquad\qquad\qquad$ $d_1 = 0.7$ $\qquad\qquad\qquad$ $d_2 = 0.2$

Secondly, by a similar process, it is necessary to obtain information about the examination (E). The examination is supposed to give a positive result if, and only if, the patient has disease d_2. But it may not be infallible. Let us assume that Table 9.6 represents the best available information about the test.

TABLE 9.6
Probability Assessments

Sign	d_0	d_1	d_2
Positive	zero	0·1	1·0
Negative	1·0	0·9	zero

Thus Table 9.6 indicates that the test works well: no-one with disease d_0 will give a positive sign, and everyone with d_2 will show positive. However, although 90 per cent of patients with d_1 give a negative result, 10 per cent give a positive sign. Thus the test is not quite infallible.

We now have all the basic data required to solve the doctor's problem. What should he do?

Should he treat the patient with treatment t_1 because disease d_1 is the most likely? Should he, on the other hand, offer treatment t_2 because disease d_2 is the most serious and costly? Should he test for d_2 using examination E, before deciding on treatment?

An answer based on Bayesian statistics is given below.

Analysis

The technique of analysis used is called decision tree analysis. The first choice that the doctor has to make is whether or not to use examination E. In a decision tree a choice between alternatives is represented in *Figure 9.11*.

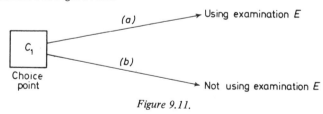

Figure 9.11.

At choice point C_1, a decision is made as to whether to go along branch (*a*) of the tree and use examination (E), or branch (*b*) and not use it.

Other choices are not under the doctor's control. For example, the patient may have either disease d_1, d_1 or d_2. This is not determined by the doctor. It can be referred to as a chance point as represented in *Figure 9.12.*

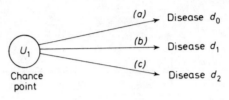

Figure 9.12.

At the chance point (U_1), represented by a circle, we might proceed (c). Which branch is chosen is not under anyone's control.

In general a decision tree looks like *Figure 9.13.*

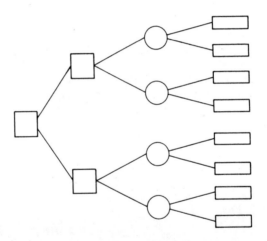

Figure 9.13. A decision tree

There is a sequence of choice points and chance points and at the ends of the decision tree, in the rectangles, are the consequences of following a particular path. In our example, the consequence will be in terms of a cost, that is, one of the costs indicated in Table 9.5.

Obviously the purpose of the decision tree is to provide the information to the decision maker as to the choices he ought to make at the various choice points.

182

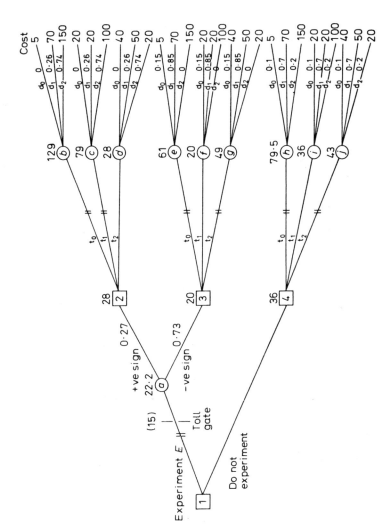

Figure 9.14. The decision tree for the doctor's problem

The decision tree for the doctors problem is shown in *Figure 9.14*. At the end of every branch there is a cost consequence — it is this cost we wish to minimize. There are four choice points, labelled 1 to 4 in the rectangles. Let us proceed through the tree.

Let us first of all examine the consequences of not carrying out the examination E at choice point 1. This leads us to choice point 4. At this point we decide on a treatment (t_0; t_1; t_2). Let us choose t_0. This leads to chance point (h) — the patient may be suffering from diseases d_0, d_1 or d_2 with likelihoods 10 per cent, 70 per cent and 20 per cent respectively. What is the expected cost of choosing t_0?

This is readily calculated as follows.

$$\text{Expected cost} = (0 \cdot 1) \times (5) + (0 \cdot 7) \times (70) + (0 \cdot 2) \times (150) = 79 \cdot 5$$

In other words this is calculated in exactly the same way as in our card game which we discussed earlier. This expected cost is written above chance point h in the diagram. The expected costs of the other choices is written above chance points i and j (36 and 43 units respectively). Obviously if we reached choice point 4 we would choose treatment t_1. Therefore branches t_0 and t_2 are blocked with ‖. However, the question remains, should we be at choice point 4 at all? Should we have gone down the other branch at choice point 1. Let us examine this possibility.

The first thing that happens along the experiment branch is that we have to pay 15 units to carry out the test (E) represented in the diagram by a toll gate.

We then reach the chance point a: the test may give a positive sign or a negative sign. What are the likelihoods or probabilities? These can be calculated as follows.

Imagine a thousand patients being given the test — they all have spots on their noses. What will be the result? First of all we expect that there will be 100 d_0s; 700 d_1s and 200 d_2s. All the d_0s will give negative signs: giving 100 negatives so far. Ninety per cent of the d_1s will give negative signs (630 negatives). Finally none of the d_2s will show negative. Therefore we expect 730 negatives and thus we get 270 positives. These probabilities are shown on the branches from chance point a.

Let us say we are now at choice point 2 and again in a position to choose treatment. Going along t_0 we reach chance point b. The disease may be d_0, d_1 or d_2. But having carried out test (E) and obtained a positive sign, the probabilities are now different to those associated with the diseases along the 'do not experiment' branch. In fact the probability of it being d_0 is zero in that d_0s always give a negative sign on test (E). The probability of d_1 can be readily calculated as follows.

Only 10 per cent of d_1 s show a positive sign on test (E) and d_1 s represent 70 per cent of the patient population. We want the probability that a patient is d_1 given that he gives a positive sign. The formula is

$$\frac{\text{probability of having disease } d_0 \text{ and giving a positive sign}}{\text{probability of giving a positive sign}}$$
$$= (0 \cdot 1) \times (0 \cdot 7)/0 \cdot 27 = 0 \cdot 26$$

The appropriate probabilities, calculated in the above manner, are shown over all the branches from chance points b to j. We can now calculate the expected costs at these points. For example at chance point d the expected cost of choosing treatment t_2 is

$$(\text{zero}) \times (40) + (0 \cdot 26) \ (50) + (0 \cdot 74) \ (20) = 28 \text{ units}$$

The expected costs at the chance points b to j have been written in and inappropriate choices at choice points 2 and 3 added to our knowledge about choice point 4. At choice point 2 we should choose treatment t_2 with an expected cost of 28 units. At choice point 3 we should choose treatment t_1 with an expected cost of 20 units.

We now need the expected cost at chance point a. This is clearly given by

$$(0 \cdot 27) \times (28) + (0 \cdot 73) \times (20) = 22 \text{ units (approx.)}$$

Our problem is now solved: the doctor should not carry out test (E) but should immediately offer treatment t_1. The expected cost is 36 units. The expected cost, if test (E) is carried out, is 15 units (the cost of the test) + 22 units (the expected treatment cost); giving *37 units* in all. Of course, if the cost of giving the test (E) could be reduced to 10 units then the doctor should always offer the test; offering treatment t_1 if a negative sign is the result.

Possibly the most valuable outcome of an analysis of this sort is that it gives a measure of the value of the test (E).

The cost of not giving the test minus the cost (excluding the direct cost of the test) of giving the test. In our case $36 - 22 = 14$ units.

How helpful is this approach? Clearly it is based on many assumptions and oversimplifies the doctors problem. Also he may feel that expected cost is not an appropriate criterion. He may feel that he would rather minimize his regret, i.e., reduce the risk of the more serious consequences. However the approach can provide guide-lines for doctors and throw light on the key problems of diagnosis and treatment in the health services.

Some Applications of Operational Research in the Health Service

Having discussed the nature of operational research and the techniques which can be used to solve certain health service problems it is appropriate to discuss some actual applications. However, before doing so it is important to recognize that the N.H.S. compares in size to an industrial giant but the proportion of its resources devoted to the analysis of its planning and management problems has been very small indeed compared with its industrial counterpart. Most of the work which has been carried out relates to the hospitals' service and I will describe some analysis carried out at Lancaster in this problem area.

The tone for operational research applications at the hospital level was set by Normal Bailey when he highlighted the problems of patients waiting for service. There can be very little doubt that waiting is a major bone of contention between the hospital and its patients. Bailey investigated appointments systems for out-patient clinics and developed a simulation of this process. An example of the sort of result obtained is shown in *Figure 9.15*.

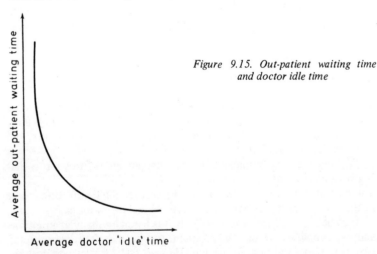

Figure 9.15. Out-patient waiting time and doctor idle time

It shows a relationship between average patient waiting time in a clinic and the expected doctor 'idle' time, i.e., the time spent by doctors waiting for patients. Very often it is the trade-off between these two variables which is the issue. It is still possible unfortunately, to find doctors who place a very high value indeed on their time in relation to patient waiting time even to the extent of having every patient present at the commencement of a clinic session.

Bailey also looked at the in-patient problem: the problem of patients requiring treatment in hospital beds and developed a queueing model of the process by drawing the analogy between a fixed number of telephone channels and a fixed number of beds, both faced with random demands.

His work raised many of the important questions. For example why do patients have to wait weeks to see a specialist and months to be admitted in many hospitals? The answer is very often neither simple nor obvious.

It is simply that demand is greater than that with which the hospital can cope; in which case we would expect waiting lists to be increasing in length steadily. Alternatively is it due to a variable service rate and random arrivals leading to long, but stable, waiting lists? Or could it be due to the failure to work off backlogs of work caused by holiday periods and so on?

Despite the importance that must be attached to these questions many hospitals have yet to come to terms with them.

At the Infirmary we have attempted to produce a simulation model of the hospital's patient treatment system. The hospital is conceived as a hierarchy of three levels as illustrated in *Figure 10.2* (page 205).

The total hospital comprises specialties such as general medicine, general surgery, gynaecology, ear, nose and throat surgery and so on, and these specialties in turn comprise consultant medical specialists, surgeons and physicians, together with their supporting staff. The key element or sub-system is regarded as the individual consultant specialist, or, more impersonally, the individual treatment unit.

The other resources of a hospital provide the back-up service to this element in the treatment of patients (e.g., nurses, radiography, pathology, beds and so on).

The aim has been to build a suite of simulation models appropriate to decision making at these three levels.

Consider, as an example, a surgeon having ten beds and three hours operating time per week. His unit deals with 'cold', i.e. non-urgent, waiting list cases. The consultant admits patients, operates, and then discharges them. The control problem is mainly one of selection of patients so that the resources at the disposal of the surgeon, particularly operating theatre time and beds, are used to their best effect. The particular consultant in question had difficulty controlling operating theatre duration and also felt that his bed and operating theatre time were out of balance.

A model was built of the process capable of acting in two modes – either 'on line' to the consultant to carry out experiments with the selection decision, or with automatic rules replacing the human decision maker. In practice, one of the critical problems involved is that of determining the extent to which patient demands on the facilities can be estimated prior to their admission. In some specialties statistical methods have proved feasible whereas in others it is difficult to devise them due to the variety and complexity of patients treated. In such situations we have attempted to model the doctors' own estimating abilities (and, of course, to use learning processes to try and improve them).

The results of a typical estimation experiment with the surgeon trying to estimate the operation duration per patient in advance of admission are shown in *Figure 9.16*.

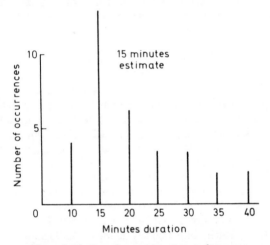

Figure 9.16. Consultant estimation performance

This is a histogram of operation duration estimated to take 15 minutes. Perfect control of operating session duration is clearly impossible for this consultant without a considerable improvement in his estimating ability. However, the simulation can examine the relationship between estimating ability and operating theatre control measures and particular consultant–patient–resource systems placed at appropriate points on the graph. This is illustrated in *Figure 9.17*.

Here it is seen that improvement in estimation leads to improved control. Although this is obvious enough the estimation parameter for the consultant tells us what we can expect of him and also what insurance factor to build into the resources provided for his use. It also helps in the monitoring of his improvement or lack of it.

Having modelled the patient selection–admission–operation–system it is possible to study the consequences on resource use of changes in, for example, the timetabling of various events such as: operating theatre schedules; patient admission days; clinic sessions; ward rounds and so on. Also, clearly, it is possible to examine the consequences of changes in the resource allocations and resource levels provided for the treatment of patients of various types.

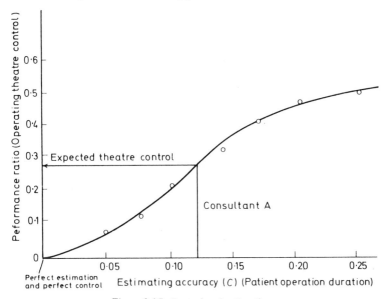

Figure 9.17. Control and estimation

The problem of the surgeon with ten beds and one three-hour operation session per week can be used to illustrate the resource balance question.

Having modelled the process and improved the effectiveness of patient selection procedures, simulation experiments can be carried out in which the number of beds (or operating theatre time) available to the specialist are systematically varied (*Figure 9.18*). Three performance criteria are used.

(1)   Bed occupancy (average number of beds occupied).

(2)   Throughput of cases (number of patients treated per annum).

(3)   Operating theatre utilization (the percentage of sessions taking 3 hours ± 10 minutes).

189

It should be noted that for this experiment the decision rule for patient admission was attempting to fill all the available beds.

It can be seen that theatre utilization reaches an optimal point. In fact this is the region of 14–15 beds, which defines a particular optimal balance point for the unit. This balance point is of course different from that which would have emerged without a study of the estimation and control problems of the unit: different in the direction of a higher ratio of beds to theatre time.

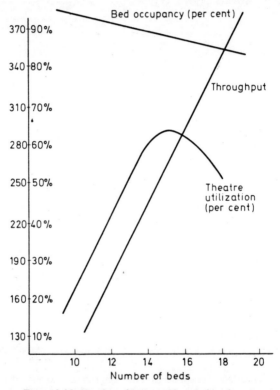

Figure 9.18. Number of beds and hospital performance

The most complex simulation so far built and used represents the joint activities of three surgical specialties as follows.

Ear, nose and throat surgery with two consultants.

Ophthalmology with two consultants.

Dental surgery with a single consultant.

The primary physical resources involved comprised: a general theatre; a minor operations theatre; and a male and female ward (40 beds).

190

The problem tackled involved devising the best feasible general theatre schedule and deciding on the way the minor operations theatre should be used.

One of the more general problems looked at using these models has been the length of patient stay question. Following discussion with doctors on length of stay problems, it is possible to modify the input in terms of treatment policy, and determine the consequences for resource utilization, timetabling and so on.

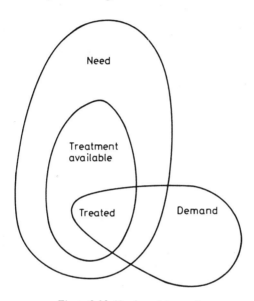

Figure 9.19. Needs and demands

In addition to analysis of the efficiency of use of hospital resources research has been carried out on problems of correct levels of provision of these facilities.

There are two basic questions to be considered.

What should be the total level of hospital resources in relation to a population?

How should different types of resource be combined in order to get the best value for money?

It is part of the folklore of hospitals that resources are inadequate, but it has proved more difficult to quantify convincingly the extent of the inadequacy. Two main approaches to this problem have been used, those based on need and those based on demand. The distinction between these is illustrated in *Figure 9.19.*

Out of a population which may be considered as the whole area of the figure some, those represented by the large circle, are not completely healthy. They *need* medical care. For some of these no cure is known and hence there is a more restricted set of potential patients for whom *treatment is available,* at least technically speaking. It is an unfortunate fact that not all of those who could be treated are treated, at least not as soon as their condition becomes apparent. Some do not seek medical advice; others do, and are put on waiting lists where they may possibly wait many years. Others are advised by their general practitioners not to bother going on the waiting list because of the time they may have to wait. Thus a still smaller area constitutes patients actually treated. By these steps need may be related to patients treated.

Demand arises in a different fashion as it depends on an individual's own assessment of his need for medical attention and his desire to have treatment. Demand for medical attention almost certainly comes from those who are treated, but it also comes from those not treated for whom treatment is available, from those needing treatment for whom no treatment is available and even from some who are healthy.

The determination of the appropriate level of hospital resources is thus the determination of the size of the treated area. This can be approached either from an assessment of need or an assessment of demand and the two are unlikely to yield the same result.

Need can and has been measured by various morbidity surveys which have estimated the state of health of the community. These studies cannot, however, be easily used to determine the required level of hospital resources for a number of reasons (*see* Chapter 1).

First, many types of facility are available for treating illness (general practitioners, health centres, local authority clinics, in-patient and out-patient hospital facilities). Hospitals, in particular the in-patient departments, are only one of these facilities, that is, only part of the treatment available area. The place of the hospital system, in the context of other health care systems, is a subject for research in its own right. Secondly, we might choose not to treat some trivial ailments, that is, we might choose to make the treated area smaller than the treatment available area. Finally, an understanding of the effect of available treatment on mortality and morbidity may be required, as an increase in the treated area may reduce the size of the area of need. For example, it is possible that some of the more serious cases of a complaint, such as peptic ulcer, may be the result of past non-treatment. The provision of facilities may influence the morbidity pattern itself and hence the need for facilities.

The second approach to the determination of the total level of resources is to base the provision of facilities on demand, assuming that the hospital service is there to provide what people want. Demand is likely to be related to need but is unlikely to be identical to it. Several studies have been carried out, for example, to determine demand, most of which have used some version of the critical number formula.

$$C = \frac{(D + W)\, L\, 1{,}000}{365\, P} \text{ beds per 1,000 of population}$$

where C is the critical number of beds,
$\quad\quad D$ is the discharges and deaths,
$\quad\quad W$ is the increase in waiting list,
$\quad\quad L$ is the average length of stay,
$\quad\quad P$ is the population.

As a result of a number of these studies it became apparent that the number of beds required was always approximately the same as the number available. It appears that the system is self regulating with supply influencing demand, and hence the variables on the right-hand-side of the critical number equation all cannot be considered independent. Since this difficulty was pointed out the method appears to have fallen into disuse.

Both of these methods seem to present difficulties but there are two ways in which these difficulties might be overcome. First, it should be noted that studies of demand have considered only the number of beds. If the clinical condition of the patient admitted was classified by diagnosis and severity it might be possible to determine for any hospital a marginal level of severity below which patients are not admitted. By relating the marginal level to the number of beds per thousand of the population a subjective judgement of the marginal level at which need should be met could be translated into a bed provision figure.

The second approach follows from the observation that studies of both need and demand suggest that provision of facilities is inadequate.

If it is accepted that the provision of resources is constrained by financial allocations made by the government then it might be better to avoid the question of provision and concentrate on the problem of using the resources available in the best way. In order to determine an efficient resource mix it is necessary to understand the way in which hospital resources influence the output of a hospital. This understanding is at present not well developed but the potential for improvement is indicated by the differences in length of stay observed between different countries, different regions of this country, and different hospitals within a region. Representative figures which show up to a 30 per cent range even within one set of data are given in Table 9.7.

Two approaches have been used to the determination of a resource mix, which may be described as optimum in some sense, simulation studies and comparative studies. Simulation studies have already been described. These in general show a surplus of either beds or theatre time when operating for maximum throughput with an existing installation. A mix of beds and theatre time which gives the minimum cost per case may be deduced. This method is very valuable when a mix of beds and theatre sessions is to be determined, but it is not easily adaptable to staff resources and so far this has not been attempted.

TABLE 9.7

Length of Stay of Patients for Appendicitis and Hernia Repair

Reference	Source		Length of stay (days)	
			Appendicitis	Hernia
Forsyth and Logan	Barrow 1957			
	Males		10	11
	Females		9	11
	USA 1957–58			
	Males		7	9
	Females		7	9
Revans	14 hospitals			
	Minimum		9·1	10·0
	Maximum		14·6	13·4
Aldred and Hindle	Hospital	1	8·1	11·4
		2	8·2	10·1
		3	10·0	11·7
		4	10·3	13·3
		5	9·9	15·8
		6	7·7	11·4
		7	7·6	9·6
		8	9·4	11·9

Comparative studies, that is studies which compare the length of stay and the level of resources existing in different hospitals, are the only method so far used to determine a minimum cost per case resource mix incorporating staff. In order to measure throughput its inverse, the length of stay of patients, is used. Also this can be influenced by many factors other than resources of which some of the more important can be corrected relatively easily.

Resources are measured by attempting to determine their availability to the patients. Availability is defined as a measure of the amount of a resource applied to a treatment unit. For resources used directly on patients the treatment unit can therefore simply be a patient (or bed, as there is a simple correspondence). For indirect resources a weighted test is used.

Data for a study of this type was obtained from records of general medical and general surgical patients in eight hospitals in similar towns in one region of the country. Following the determination of values for all the measures for each hospital a series of correlation analyses were carried out. Some of the results of this have already been described (Table 9.3).

The availability of pathology and radiography staff showed no effect on length of stay. A number of complicating effects may explain this. First, the use of mechanical equipment for testing as well as personnel makes resource assessment difficult. Secondly, the time taken to return results is of great importance if the results are to be useful in diagnosis and the relation of this time to work-load may well be complex.

Nursing resources were found to have a significant effect on the length of stay of medical patients, but not on surgical patients. Junior doctors of both specialties were found to have a significant effect on length of stay. For consultant specialists the initial results were obtained by using hospital averages for the consultants of each specialty. This gave confusing results because of differences in average length of stay between patients of different consultants in the same hospital. A second analysis using averages for each consultant separately carried out for each diagnostic group showed a significant effect of consultant availability on length of stay.

Some important differences emerged between the effect for medical consultants and for surgical consultants. In general the effect of consultant availability on length of stay was greater for medical diagnosis than surgical diagnosis. Also if the same complaint may be treated either by a surgeon or by a physician the effect is greater for the physician. Finally, for surgical diagnoses the effect of consultant availability on length of stay is greatest for those diagnoses least likely to require a surgical operation. These results taken together suggest that there is an important qualitative difference in the way resources are used between medical and surgical patients, and hence a different approach may be required for study in the two specialties.

The correlations observed may now be used in some simple models to determine levels of resources which would minimize cost per case. If an increase in the availability of doctors, for example, reduces length of stay and thus the hotel cost more than it increases medical cost per patient, then a net reduction in cost per case will result. This principle has been discussed earlier.

The first model fitted included only consultants as a resource, and is defined by the equations.

$$l - l_0 = \frac{a}{m}$$

$$C = (h + m) \, l$$

where l is the length of stay in days,

m is the consultant availability (consultant cost per day),

h is the hotel cost per day,

C is the total cost per patient.

Values for l_0 and a are estimated from the correlation results. Note that in the correlation results availability is measured as doctor sessions per bed (per week). This is readily translated by a constant factor into doctor cost per day (per patient) using hospital cost data, which is also used to obtain a value for h. More complex models incorporating more resources can be used. For example, the following multiple resource model gave results reasonably consistent with those from the single resource model.

$$l - l_0 = \frac{a}{m} + \frac{b}{n}$$

$$C = (m + n + h) \, l$$

where n is the nurse availability.

The minimum cost per case optima for consultants suggested by these models is shown in Table 9.8. But in interpreting these the reader

TABLE 9.8

Comparison of the Ratio of Beds to Consultants Recommended by Different Sources

Source	Number of beds per consultant
The Development of Consultant Services	130
Platt Report	30–40
Present average	37·3
Present minimum	31·8
Suggest optimum	20·8

should be aware that no sensitivity analysis has been performed on these results, and should remember that other criteria apart from cost per case are relevant in determining staffing levels for doctors and nurses.

The levels of nurse staffing suggested by the model are approximately the same as those currently in use, at least in the hospitals studied. The levels of consultant staffing suggested are considerably above those currently in use and those suggested in various official reports.

Acknowledgement

The study of length of patient stay and resource availability was the subject of a doctoral dissertation of the Department of Operational Research at Lancaster by Keith Aldred. Dr. Aldred is now employed by the Operational Research Group of Civil Service Department.

10—A Practical Approach to Surgical Scheduling

Anthony Hindle

Introduction

A hospital can be viewed as a system having certain resources such as doctors, nurses, beds and operating theatres with which to carry out its task of treating patients. Scheduling decisions, governing the admission, treatment and discharge of patients, are made by medical staff who use mainly medical criteria, i.e. the needs of each individual patient. Yet each such decision is in effect an allocation of certain resources to a specific task, an administrative decision which has administrative consequences — the results of all these decisions taken together will determine how effectively the hospital's resources are being used.

Similarly there are decisions about resources which affect the medical performance of the hospital. These are often taken by senior administrative personnel who do not have the training necessary to appreciate all the medical consequences of their decisions.

The research described here is intended to demonstrate to medical and administrative staff the consequences of their decisions, and the main tool used is computer simulation.

The strategy of the research has been to work towards an understanding of a complete hospital by modelling its component parts. For scheduling purposes a hospital consists of virtually autonomous sub-systems, each sub-system usually corresponding to a *specialty*. Each specialty, such as gynaecology or orthopaedics, consists of one, two or more consultants – experts in the treatment of particular complaints – who head a 'firm' of junior medical staff and who are equipped with resources such as the work of administrative staff, an allocation of time in an operating theatre, a number of beds in a ward and access to various service departments such as radiography and pathology.

This section describes work carried out in three surgical specialties—orthopaedics, opthalmology and ear, nose and throat surgery – and is concerned with scheduling the admission, care and discharge of patients.

The first part of the study involved the development of a simulation of an orthopaedic unit at the Albrough Clinic. The aim was the design of a *single consultant simulation* capable of general application to the problems of the surgeon scheduling resources to patients. The results obtained from the study lead to a revised patient admissions system at the Albrough Clinic. Central aspects of this investigation are studies of consultant estimation ability for patient operation duration and patient length of stay.

Following this the approach was extended to the development of a *multispecialty simulation model.* Models were produced of ear nose and throat and ophthalmology specialties which were considered separately, and then jointly. The models use the *single consultant simulation* as the building block. The simulations enable such questions as the benefits derivable from increased consultant co-operation to be examined. Also they have been used to examine the consequences of timetabling and resource changes.

The results give confidence that a basic approach to the structure of surgical scheduling problems has been successfully developed. The simulations are capable of progressive refinement and can be readily adapted to consider new practical problems, and also certain strategic questions such as performance measurement, organizational changes, and resource allocation.

The work described in this chapter is part of a project, sponsored by the Department of Health and Social Security, which is in progress at the Department of Operational Research at the University of Lancaster. The research was carried out by staff—student teams in the Department.

Systems Analysis

The three surgical specialties reported here are generally similar in the way in which the flow of patients is controlled and managed.

Figure 10.1 describes the flow of patients through these surgical specialties. Nodes D_1 to D_7 form the decision centres which govern the admission, treatment and discharge of in-patients.

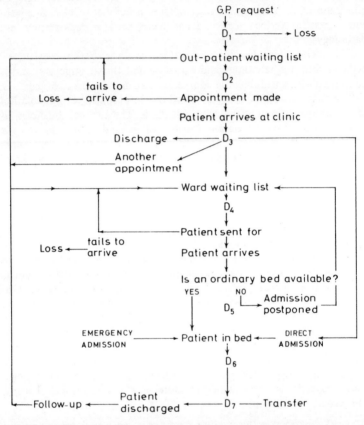

Figure 10.1. Flow of patients through a typcial specialty

DECISION D_1

The consultant surgeon receives requests for attendance at one of his out-patient clinics from a number of sources. Most commonly these originate from a general practitioner but they may come from another consultant in the same or different hospital. The general practitioner's request is usually made in a standard letter in which he describes briefly the symptoms of the patient's illness and may include a provisional diagnosis. The general practitioner is often asked to categorize the patients as urgent or non-urgent. On the basis of this information the consultant decides either to place the patient on his own out-patient waiting list or refer him to another specialty or hospital — 'loss' on *Figure 10.1.*

DECISION D_2

Each week it is decided who to invite from the waiting list to the out-patient clinic. The identity of the people selected will depend on the consultant's estimate of the urgency of the case and, to some extent, the length of time the person has been on the waiting list. Often clinics are divided into new patients and return visits and a specified number of each are taken every week. Some of the people invited to the clinic will not attend and are marked 'loss'.

DECISION D_3

Decision D_3 prescribes the course of treatment to be followed by the patient. It is taken either at the out-patient clinic or, in the case of emergency cases, in the casualty department. Resulting from decision D_3 the patient may be either:

(1) admitted directly to a hospital bed;
(2) have his name added to the ward waiting list;
(3) treated as an out-patient; or
(4) discharged to the care of the general practitioner or transferred to another specialty.

In each case, the patient will require the use of some of the resources of the hospital.

D_1, D_2 and D_3 represent decisions made in the out-patient department of the hospital. Patients requiring in-patient treatment are either admitted directly or put onto the ward waiting list.

DECISION D_4

Decision D_4 is the 'admit' decision. A certain number of people are selected from the waiting list and invited to attend for admission to the ward a few days later. There may be one or more waiting list admission days each week. The people actually selected will depend on a number of factors; medical, managerial and social. At this point in a surgical specialty a definite commitment of the bed and operating theatre resources of the hospital is made.

DECISION D$_5$

If a person arrives at the ward and a bed is not available, decision D$_5$ must be made. He may be refused admission and remain on the waiting list, he may be sent elsewhere for treatment, or a temporary bed may be erected for him in the ward. If the ward is full, the action taken will depend on the urgency of the case and the availability of alternative resources.

DECISION D$_6$

Whilst in the ward, the principal decisions concerning the patient's treatment will be made. Although these will, for the most part, be of a medical nature, they will involve the use of the resources of the hospital.

DECISION D$_7$

Provided the patient does not die while undergoing treatment he will finally be discharged. If he is discharged he may be either: (1) referred back to the care of his general practitioner; (2) asked to attend an out-patient follow-up clinic, or (3) added to the ward waiting list for subsequent readmission.

Alternatively, he may be discharged and transferred either to a convalescent home or to another ward.

The flow diagram portrays the patient's interaction with the surgical specialty. Some or all of the decisions (D$_1$ to D$_7$) have to be made for every person entering the system as each places a different demand on the resources of the system. Clearly the resources must be available to satisfy this demand. Any policy attempting to use the resources effectively must endeavour to regulate the flow of patients through this system; i.e. regulate the demand on the human and physical resources.

Factors Affecting Surgical Scheduling Performance

The resources available to a specialty will affect patient scheduling in two ways. First, with more resources, both human and physical, a specialty will deal with more patients and will be better able to satisfy the need for the particular forms of treatment it can provide. However, there is a second facet to the problem, namely that of the balance of resources available to the specialty. For example, if a surgical specialty is blessed with an abundance of beds it will be inclined to use them as fully as possible, but this may well lead to congestion in the operating theatre; thus the allocation of operating theatre time should be in balance with the bed allocation. Although in surgical specialties the critical balance is likely to be beds in relation to theatre time, similar arguments will apply to the other resources: doctors, nurses, radiograph equipment, pathology services and so on.

Given an allocation of resources to a specialty the next question is that of the efficiency with which they are used. In the previous section a series of decisions were described and discussed. In order to throw light on patient scheduling efficiency it is necessary to investigate the objectives behind this series of decisions. What is the specialty trying to achieve? Unfortunately this question is very difficult to answer. However, certain indices of performance are available.

Perhaps the most often used measure of a hospital's performance is the length of its waiting lists for treatment. This attracts considerable public concern because the effect of a long wait for treatment on the individual patient is direct and obvious. However, this index is extremely difficult to interpret. It has been pointed out many times that the demand on a hospital is a function not only of the basic need for treatment in the community, but also of the level of supply of resources to meet this need. In other words the relationship between supply and demand is complex and waiting list behaviour will reflect this complexity.

The long-term average bed occupancy is often suggested as a criterion of performance for a surgical specialty: but again interpretation is difficult. It can be pointed out that optimum bed occupancy can be achieved by keeping the same patients in the ward as long as possible. High turnover in use of beds conflicts with high bed occupancy. However, in the short term this measure can be meaningful in that a fluctuation in the number of occupied beds implies a variation in the load or demand on the ward. In particular, it may on occasions be necessary to put up highly inconvenient temporary beds. If the bed occupancy index could be combined with a length of patient stay measure this might well yield a very useful yardstick. However, the prescription of correct lengths of stay for patients is clearly difficult and begins to tread on the emotive ground of clinical independence.

Certain measures are available from a study of the behaviour of the operating theatres. If the activities of a surgical specialty are badly planned the operating sessions may be highly variable in length. For example, some sessions may run seriously over time leading to backlogs, a cutting down of cleaning procedures and to dissatisfaction amongst patients and staff.

Operational research, in relation to surgical scheduling, can be defined as a search for a function relating inputs to outputs, or resources to performance where two types of input variable can be recognized; controllable and uncontrollable. Given the discovery of this function the control variables can be set to give optimal performance for the specialty.

Perhaps the most readily controlled variable in surgical scheduling is the case mix of patients − the sex, age and diagnostic balance admitted to the system. The next in flexibility is the timetabling of the specialties' activities, although it would be most sensible to determine an optimal timetable for the hospital as a whole. Finally the allocation of resources between and within the specialties of the hospital can be modified.

Uncontrollable variables occur in many forms. First, a surgical specialty may find it difficult to exercise control of the processes generating the patient demand on the system. This is particularly the case in relation to emergency admissions who may arrive for operation without any prior notice. Also unpredictable effects can arise from private practice activities, day case work on the wards, the disruption of a specialties' work by other specialties and so on. However, a second main area of uncertainty of control arises from the medical treatment variables, principally length of patient stay and operation duration per patient. These factors are not as inviolable as medical staff sometimes maintain; the variability from consultant to consultant testifies to this fact.

A Simulation Approach

Reasons for difficulties in applying operational research in hospitals are not difficult to find. One reason is that the management structure in hospitals is such that a real decision making entity on a given aspect of the hospitals' activity is very often difficult to identify. The formal hierarchical committee structure seems but loosely related to the real influence process. Also there exists a division of responsibility between the administrator and the doctor in hospitals and, since the medical staff are responsible for most patient treatment decisions, control of hospital performance is in their hands. It is only slowly that doctors are accepting their management role and the inability of the administrator to prescribe a role for them makes efficient management difficult. Many previous operational research investigations sponsored by the administrative side of the service have failed to gain the full co-operation of the medical staff, and difficulties have arisen when trying to implement their findings.

However, working with the medical staff of a hospital is also a difficult task for several reasons. First, it is not easy to involve them in management; they are clinicians and medical researchers by training and inclination. Secondly, qualified medical staff (consultants) are used to working in independent spheres. They are all formally equal in status, none are direct employees of the hospital, and they are subject only to the general guidance of their peer group. The result of these properties can be, for example, marked differences in patient length of stay in hospital, but treated by different consultants. Since the concern of operational research is with improving the effectiveness of the hospital's treatment of patients and since the only qualified judges of these factors are consultant medical staff it seems appropriate to regard them as the principal decision makers. Also since consultants operate more or less independently and are of equal status it seems appropriate to undertake, at least initially, a consultant by consultant analysis.

Given these factors, together with the problems of quantification of medical outputs described in the previous chapter, a simulation approach would seem to be an appropriate one.

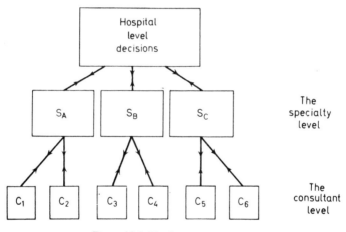

Figure 10.2. The hospital hierarchy

Thus it was decided to regard the hospital as a hierarchy of three levels: consultant, specialty and hospital, as illustrated in *Figure 10.2*. The aim has been to develop computer simulation models appropriate to decision making at each of these levels by using the single consultant model as the basic building block.

In a practical application to a total hospital scheduling problem it would be appropriate to undertake the following analysis.

Consultant level

(1)   Establish constraints on resource utilization at this level.
(2)   Analyse actual and future demand in terms of the number and type of patients.
(3)   Analyse treatment policy in terms of the timing and utilization of resources by type of patient.
(4)   Carry out simulation experiments to evaluate various scheduling systems which satisfy the constraints (1) and requirements (2) and (3).

Specialty level

(1)   Establish constraints on resource utilization at this level.
(2)   Carry out simulation studies to determine a scheduling system for the specialty based on the scheduling systems of consultant level
(3)   Re-examine and adjust the scheduling systems derived in consultant level (4) in light of the results of (2), if these violate the constraints of (1).

Hospital level

(1)   Establish constraints on resource utilization at this level.
(2)   Carry out simultation studies to determine a scheduling system for the hospital if specialties operate the scheduling systems of specialty level (2).
(3)   Re-examine and adjust the scheduling systems derived in specialty level (2) if these violate the constraints of (1).

As a result of carrying out this programme of work a contribution could be made towards the following.

The establishment of a hospital information system operating within and between all three levels.

The establishment of measure of performance for individual decision makers at each level.

The establishment of procedures whereby the effects of changes in procedure and resources on performance can be determined.

An understanding of organizational processes whereby conflicts are or could be resolved.

The research described in this report is a contribution towards this methodology.

The Albrough Clinic

The first surgical scheduling problem tackled, using the simulation approach described above, was a unit for cold orthopaedic surgery at the Albrough Clinic. Two studies were carried out: some preliminary experimental work with one of the consultant orthopaedic surgeons, and then an examination of the total unit.

The orthopaedic ward at Albrough is part of a general orthopaedic unit. It is physically separated from the rest of the unit, draws its patients from its own waiting lists and is, in general, administered as a separate unit.

Three consultants perform operations at Albrough. The 20 beds in the ward are divided into two groups of ten, each in a separate room.* Seven of the first group are allocated to the first consultant, seven of the other to the second consultant, and the remaining three in each group are allocated to the third consultant. Each consultant maintains a separate waiting list. In a normal week there are three operating sessions scheduled. The time available for each session is three hours. At any given time all the patients in the ward are of the same sex. For example, from January to June 1968 the patients were female. The patients were male from June until November, and then were again female. There are, however, facilities for treating two patients of the opposite sex to that currently filling the clinic's main beds.

The orthopaedic ward at Albrough (hereafter this unit will be referred to as the 'clinic') is a cold surgical one — this means that all admissions are from the waiting lists. Emergency orthopaedic cases are treated at the main infirmary as are serious cases requiring special facilities. The majority of patients are from the neighbouring area. They are placed on the waiting list after having been seen by their consultant at the out-patient department. In addition, patients seen at an out-patient department north of Albrough are sometimes placed on the clinic's waiting list. A survey of data on patient admissions also showed that a small number of patients are transferred from the main infirmary, and from other out-patient departments, to the clinic. It should be noted here that not all patients arriving at the clinic have operations.

If it is decided to place a patient on the ward waiting list after he has been seen at the out-patient department, the relevant details of the patient are entered in the waiting list file; that is his name, sex, age,

---

*Each group of ten is further divided into nine and one. The single bed is in a private room.

diagnosis, doctor, date of placement on the waiting list, and any remark which may be pertinent to his particular case; for example, he may be marked urgent or there may be a remark about particular social factors relating to his case. In this way the waiting lists are built up for each consultant so that he can see, at a glance, which patients, and how many, are on his list. The lengths of the waiting lists vary considerably. For example, consultant A has about 500 patients on his list while consultant C has only 50. It should be mentioned that these waiting lists, although they relate to the Albrough clinic, are kept at the main infirmary.

Each week a consultant will examine his waiting list and choose patients to fill his beds. These patients receive written notice, say on Friday or Saturday, to attend for admission on the following Tuesday. At the same time, two lists are made of the selected patients. One is sent to the medical records department so that they can send down the appropriate medical files to the clinic. The second goes to the ward sister. She uses it to make the necessary arrangements concerning admissions.

Occasionally patients do not turn up and may do one of two things. They may write to the clinic, saying that they cannot come, or they may just fail to turn up. In either case, this information is not known until Monday or Tuesday. The ward sister informs the consultant's secretary at the main infirmary, who then tries to get in touch with alternative patients. The patients who fail to turn up are usually put back on the waiting list if they so desire.

The basis for the procedure at the clinic had one fundamental weakness − the time between the decision to call patients and their admission was too short. Other than the failure to show difficulty it gave rise to a problem of radiograph availability.

When the list of chosen patients is sent to the medical records department the relevant material is gathered together and sent to the Albrough Clinic. However, these records may not reach the clinic until four days later, and even then they are rarely complete. In more than 50 per cent of the cases it is necessary to chase up radiographs which may be kept at Albrough or the northern clinic. Their location can sometimes be found from references in the case notes although generally the ward personnel rely on a series of inspired guesses as to where they are. Locating them at short notice has been described by the ward sister as her major headache. The problem is accentuated by two factors.

(1)   The physical separation of the Albrough clinic and the main infirmary.

(2)   The very short time available to locate the radiographs.

Because of these difficulties it is a regular practice at the Clinic to take new radiographs on the day of the operation.

It was fairly easy to see that some of these problems might probably be solved by giving patients longer notice of the date they are required in hospital.

The Ear, Nose and Throat and Ophthalmology Unit

The second study carried out involved ear, nose and throat and ophthalmology specialties at Louphill. The unit concerned with these activities is considerably more complex than the Albrough Clinic. There are two consultants in each specialty. In addition a dental surgeon makes some use of the facilities.

The unit consists of two wards, one male and one female (Table 10.1).

TABLE 10.1

Ward	Ear, nose and throat	Ophthalmology	Dental	Total beds
Male	9	9	2	20
Female	9	9	1	19

In addition, consultants have available a small number of temporary beds which can be erected in these wards to cater for emergencies. Each specialty is allocated a certain number of sessions in the major operating theatre (Table 10.2).

TABLE 10.2

Specialty	Type of session	
	Morning (4 hours)	Afternoon (3 hours)
Ear, nose and throat	4	2
Ophthalmology	1	1
Dental	0	1

The unit contains a minor operating theatre which at the beginning of the study was poorly equipped and used only for one ear, nose and throat session per week. In addition to these resources, each consultant sometimes has beds allocated to him in private wards and the children's wards, these patients taking up time in operating sessions. These admissions are controlled by the sisters concerned, and are rarely predictable by the consultant. Theoretically, the ear, nose and throat consultant is allocated two children's beds and the ophthalmology consultant three. In practice, this allocation frequently does not materialize, as there is a serious shortage of children's bed at Louphill: waiting lists for an operation tend to be much longer in the children's ward than for the same operation in an adult ward, and the time period in many cases is as long as 18 months. Finally, each consultant operates on a certain number of patients as day cases. These day cases are chosen from a waiting list in the same way as in-patients.

The unit had many problems due to the rapid expansion of ophthalmological work at Louphill. The year prior to the start of the project saw the trebling of the consultant surgeon availability to this ophthalmological unit, putting beds and operating theatre time at a premium. Also, of course, the ophthalmology specialty began to squeeze the ear, nose and throat specialty.

The question was whether changes in waiting list admission procedures, the timetabling of the operating theatres, or the organization of the unit could relieve the situation.

The Simulation Models

SIMULATION MARK 1

The first model was intended to clarify ideas and examine certain consequences of the admission decision (decision D_4) on bed utilization. The program (like all the programs described in this report) is written in Fortran IV and is intended for use on the university's I.C.L. 1909 computer.

A general flow diagram is shown in *Figure 10.3*.

The program for the model is divided into several separate sub-routines. These sub-routines correspond to actual events which take place in a surgical specialty, and are listed as follows.

(1)   An out-patient clinic is held.

(2)   A decision is made as to the number of people to admit on the next admission day from the ward waiting list — the 'admit' decision.

(3)   A patient is admitted to a bed in the ward.

(4)   A patient is discharged from the ward.

A general demand on the ward is incorporated in the model. This demand consists of direct admissions, casualty or emergency admissions, and waiting list admissions.

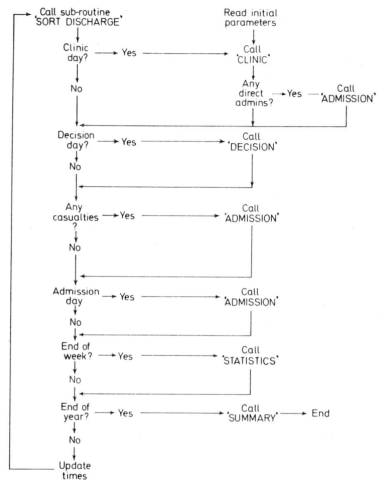

Figure 10.3. Simulation – mark 1.

One object of the simulation is to demonstrate the effect of the 'admit' decision, event (2), p. 210 on bed utilization. The program records relevant statistics such as bed occupancy and number of admissions and discharges.

The simulation goes through a daily cycle of events. At the beginning of each day the simulation tests for discharges, event (4). Thus it is assumed that all discharges occur at the beginning of a day and the bed becomes available immediately for a new patient.

The casualties or emergencies occurring that day are admitted by calling an 'admission' sub-routine, corresponding to event (3). The casualty demand for the model is a daily sample from an empirical distribution.

The 'admission' sub-routine admits patients to the hospital. If there is a bed available the patient is admitted, and his length of stay in the ward is sampled from a probability distribution (assumed negative exponential). However, if a bed is not available the patient is not admitted but is placed on the ward waiting list.

When an out-patient clinic is held a percentage of the people attending are put on the ward waiting list, a percentage are classified as direct admissions and the remainder are discharged. The numerical value of these percentages and the number attending the clinic each week are sampled from empirical probability distributions. If there are any direct admissions sub-routine 'admission' is called as before.

Two days before the admission day the 'admit' decision is made. A certain number of people are selected from the ward waiting list and invited to attend for admission to the ward two days later. It is possible to stop the program at this point and allow the selection to be made by a human operator. Alternatively, an automatic rule can be used which relates the number of people selected to the number of empty beds. An example of a decision rule is as follows.

$$\text{Permissible admissions} = \begin{cases} \text{number of empty beds} \\ plus \text{ number of expected discharges} \\ minus \text{ integer number (NB)} \end{cases}$$

The integer number (NB) is set to a numerical value at the beginning of a simulation experiment.

Clearly a large positive value for (NB) corresponds to a safe or pessimistic rule. It would result in very few people being admitted from the waiting list; and if the casualty demand was low that week, some beds might remain empty all week. However, the chance of having to refuse an emergency admission is very small. A large negative value for (NB) would result in higher bed occupancy and throughout but the number of refusals would also be increased.

An example experiment

The input for the model is generated prior to the simulation by sampling from the appropriate expirical distributions. The input for each week consists of one card containing the following data.

(1)   The number of general practitioner requests received.

(2)   The proportion of out-patient clinic attendances added to the ward waiting list.

(3)   The percentage admitted directly from the out-patient clinic.

(4)   The number of emergencies for each day of that week.

A series of experiments, performed using the decision rule described above with integer numbers $(NB) - 2, 0, +1, +2, +3, +4, +6$, gave the results shown in *Figure 10.4*. This relates the number of refusals to a measure of waiting list length as the integer number (NB) varies.

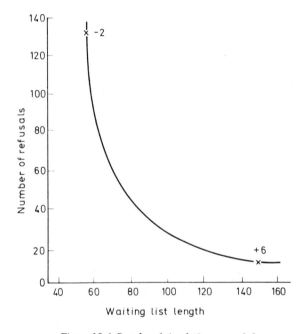

Figure 10.4. Results of simulation — mark 1.

SIMULATION MARK 2

This model introduces an operating theatre scheduling facility. *Figure 10.5* shows the general flow diagram.

The 'patient select' sub-routine selects patients randomly from a sample of past patients of the surgical system simulated and adds them to the waiting list. The number of patients added daily is a Poisson variate with expected value proportional to the current number of patients on the waiting list. The procedure results in a waiting list which is stable.

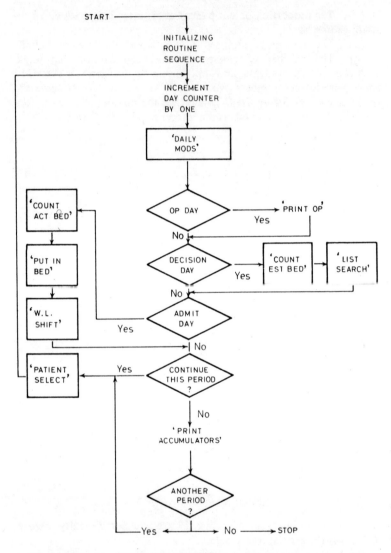

Figure 10.5. Simulation – mark 2

The source data consists of a sample of past patients together with estimates of operation duration and post-operative stay (obtained from the surgeons concerned). At the time of placing patients on the waiting

214

list values of actual operation duration and post-operative stay are generated using statistical methods. The ward occupancy at any time is represented in an array — 'beds'. The information contained in the array for each bed is as follows.

(1) The case number of patient.
(2) Estimate of remaining post-operative stay.
(3) Actual remaining post-operative stay.
(4) Day placed on waiting list.
(5) Actual remaining pre-operative stay.
(6) Estimated operation duration.
(7) Actual operation duration.

The 'daily mods' sub-routine updates and monitors the various pieces of information every day, discharging patients when their stay is complete.

'Count est bed' is called weekly on decision day to estimate the bed availability for the following admission day whereas 'list search' is called each week on decision day to decide which patients to admit next admit day: the number of patients to be selected having been computed by 'count est bed'.

'List search' can operate in a variety of ways and essentially the process attempts to simulate a human planner deriving a session within time limits with a reasonable balance between long and short estimated operation duration patients.

'Count act bed' is called weekly on admit day to count the number of available empty beds.

'Put in bed' is called weekly to execute the admission plan and place the information required in the array 'beds'.

'W.I. shift' is called weekly on admit day; this routine removes patients admitted from the waiting list and restructures it.

'Print op' is called weekly on operation day to compute and accumulate various statistics of interest.

'Print accumulators' is called annually to print out a wide range of statistics and to handle any re-initializing that is required.

An example experiment

With a given 'list search' procedure, it is possible to vary the balance of theatre time to beds and note the consequences for patient throughput, bed occupancy and operating theatre utilization.

The results of an experiment of this type is illustrated in the previous chapter (*Figure 9.18*). It represents the behaviour of a system with one three-hour operating session and a variable number of beds.

Bed occupancy is expressed as a percentage and throughput of patients as an actual number. Operating theatre utilization is expressed as the percentage of theatre sessions taking the correct time ± 10 minutes. The decision rule for admission was attempting as far as possible to fill the beds available and hence an optimal resource balance is suggested.

SIMULATION MARK 3

In order to handle the increased complexity of the ear, nose and throat, ophthalmology system the simulation described above needed to be modified and extended.

Three new programs were constructed.

A two consultant model for the ophthalmology specialty.

A two consultant model for the ear, nose and throat specialty.

A four consultant model for the combined specialties, allowing for interaction.

Each program works through a calendar, the duration of which is input as parameter; each day sub-routines carry out various tasks as appropriate, e.g., 'scalpel' performs operations on patients, 'income' brings patients into hospital.

General concepts of the models

Program parameters

The following parameters are read in as data and so may be easily altered.

(1)   Number of beds in each ward.

(2)   Clinic day each week (i.e., the day on which additions are made to the waiting lists).

(3)   Decision day each week (i.e., the day when next week's admissions are planned).

(4)   Admission days and operating days each week.

On each admission day patients are brought in for a particular operating session, and so admission days are fixed a suitable time before the corresponding operating sessions.

By altering these input parameters the effects of changes in the allocation of beds, operating sessions, and admission days may be tested without difficulty.

Patient populations

Data relating to past ophthalmology and ear, nose and throat patients treated in the unit are read onto magnetic tape for use as data for the simulation programs. Of these some are casualty patients, and others are day case patients. The remainder are used to form the waiting list 'population'.

For each patient the following data are put onto the magnetic tape.

Post-operative stay, i.e., the time the patient stays in hospital after his last operation.

Number of operations (if any).

Pre-operative stay, i.e. the time the patient must stay in hospital before his first operation.

Duration of first operation (if any).

Sex of patient.

Diagnostic category of patient.

Consultant who treated the patient.

Degree of urgency, i.e. waiting list, urgent waiting list, emergency or day case admission, and for those patients requiring a second operation.

Inter-operative stay, i.e. the minimum time which must elapse between the patient's two operations.

Duration of second operation.

Note (1)   For a patient not requiring operation the post-operative stay is equivalent to his total stay.

(2)   No patient required more than two operations.

Generation of waiting lists

Each consultant sees his patients in his out-patient clinics; if they are in need of hospital treatment they are added to the in-patient waiting lists. In the program this is done in sub-routine 'clinic' by selecting at random a given number of patients from the waiting list population. The program categorizes the waiting lists by sex, consultant and diagnosis.

Once added to the waiting list a patient remains there until chosen for admission by sub-routine 'indecision', the planning procedure for the coming week.

At the beginning of each simulation run a realistic waiting list is generated. Using the information obtained from the study of waiting lists the composition of a typical waiting list, categorized as above, is determined. A subsidiary program is used to generate from this the patients who will constitute the initial waiting list, and this is input as data to the simulation program.

Casualties

The patients forming the casualty population come from two sources – accident cases, and patients seen at an out-patient clinic whose condition is so serious as to require an immediate admission. The number of casualties to be admitted to hospital each day of the year is a sample from empirical distributions. The corresponding patients are chosen at random from the casualty population and admitted to hospital by sub-routine 'income'.

The admission decision

Sub-routine 'indecision' in the programs chooses, from the patients currently on the ward waiting list, those to be admitted the following week. It is assumed (and this corresponds with practice) that this is done only once each week, even though there may be several admission days next week.

On the decision day each week the routine first counts, for each admission day the next week and for each of the two wards, the number of beds expected to become free after the admission day previous to this one, and before or on this admission day. This procedure allows not only for patients currently in hospital, but also those patients already chosen for admission later that week who may have been discharged by the admission day the following week. The procedure does not specifically leave beds free for casualty admissions; where necessary temporary beds may be erected for these. However, for casualty patients already in hospital, the counting procedure does consider when these will be discharged.

Having decided how many patients to admit on each of the next week's admission days, the routine then decides which patients are to be admitted. The general method of doing this is to select the patients to be admitted from the diagnostic categories in approximately the proportions that occur in the real system; in doing this one obtains similar distributions of lengths of stay so that valid comparisons can be made between the real and simulated systems.

The admission procedure

The sub-routine 'income' deals with all admissions. The routine locates, for each patient to be admitted, a bed in the appropriate ward. If no fixed bed is empty a temporary bed is put up for this patient.

Operating procedure

The sub-routine 'scalpel' carries out all operating sessions. For each session the following checks are made for each patient in hospital

Is the patient being treated by the consultant performing the operating session?

Does the patient require an operation, and has he been in hospital long enough to be ready for that operation?

If these tests are satisfied the operation is carried out and details recorded.

Discharge procedure

All patients are checked for discharge each day and those ready are discharged. If a discharge vacates a permanent bed and there is a patient occupying a temporary bed, the latter is moved into the permanent bed.

'Stats' and 'summary'

At the end of each simulated week, the sub-routine 'stats' prints out results of the week's admissions, operating sessions, and details of the waiting lists. At the year end 'summary' outputs results of the year's simulation run.

Differences between the models

Ophthalmology specialty

This is the simplest of the three models. It is written to allow each of the consultants just one operating session per week sharing nine beds in each of the two wards.

Ear, nose and throat

This model is similarly written for two consultants sharing nine beds in each of the wards. However, there are more operating sessions per week than in the ophthalmology model; each consultant now has two sessions per week and a fifth is shared between them, each having alternate weeks.

In the ear, nose and throat specialty a not insignificant number of day case patients subsequently stay in hospital for one or more nights. Since such events are unpredictable, patients of this type may be treated in the simulation in the same way as casualty patients. The number of such day case patients in the ophthalmology specialty is so small as to be negligible.

Combined specialties

This model is essentially an amalgamation of the two described above, the four consultants (two in each specialty) sharing 18 beds in each of the wards rather than each specialty having nine beds in each ward. Apart from this, the structure of the program is exactly as in the separate models.

Experiments, Results and Further Research

ALBROUGH

The simulation model used was the Mark 2 version described in the previous section.

Experiment A

At an early stage in the study of this clinic one of the consultant surgeons was experiencing difficulty in controlling operating session duration. He was particularly concerned about session overrun. It was thought that improvement might result from a modification of the patient selection decision. Simulation experiments were carried out examining the consequences of various decision rules for patient admission.

Measurement of performance

Good performance implies that the operating session takes the correct time: in these experiments this time being 200 ± 20 minutes. A measure of performance is the proportion of sessions falling outside these limits.

Sessions can fall outside limits for two main reasons. First, because of the balance between theatre time and bed availability and, secondly, due to inefficient patient selection. The latter problem was the initial concern.

The patient selection decision

In discussing this decision with the surgeon it was clear that he took into account the following factors in selecting a particular list of patients.

Urgency.

Time on the waiting list.

Fitness for operation.

Junior doctor training requirements.

Medical interactions (i.e., clean and dirty operations).

Expected operation durations.
Expected lengths of patient stay.
Bed availability.
Also there were other social and medical factors mentioned.

In examining the parameters most likely to influence the performance of the unit in terms of bed and theatre utilization (expected bed availability, and expected operation duration) it was clear that the surgeon gave these very cursory explicit attention.

It was decided, therefore, to run a simulation experiment to determine the performance of the unit based only on resource use considerations; i.e., ignoring medical and social criteria. In order to do this it was necessary to carry out some resource demand estimation experiments.

Estimation

For the unit to operate ideally and with 100 per cent efficiency it would require that: (1) the exact number of beds that will be empty on a particular admission day be known in advance; (2) everybody requested to come in on a particular admission day actually does so; (3) the sum of the operation durations of patients in a particular session be close to the time allowed.

Clearly, the performance of a real unit could approach the ideal case if the exact bed requirements and operation durations of patients were known in advance. This can never be the case though, and estimates must suffice in place of exact knowledge. The performance of the unit depends on the accuracy of these estimates.

An orthopaedic consultant surgeon at the Albrough Clinic undertook to provide information on which to base an assessment of a consultant's estimating ability.

In April 1968 a recording system was introduced at the Clinic, which kept a record of the duration of each operation performed. For the purposes of comparison the surgeon generated time estimates for 235 of these operations, using all the information that was available except, of course, the actual operation times. These estimates referred to operations performed, not only by this surgeon himself but also by another consultant surgeon at the Clinic. In the presentation of the data those operations which had the same time estimates were grouped together. Five of the groups were sufficiently large to yield meaningful distributions, the distributions being of the actual times for each estimate. These distributions are presented as histograms in *Figures 10.6, 10.7* and *10.8*. *Figure 10.6* refers to operations performed by the surgeon concerned. *Figure 10.7* refers to operations performed by other consultants and *Figure 10.8.* is for all operations.

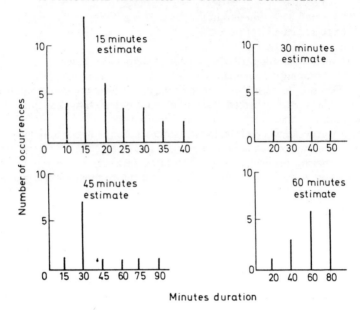

Figure 10.6. Actual operation durations for particular estimate groups: consultant estimating the duration of his own operations

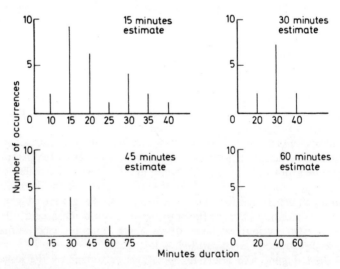

Figure 10.7. Actual operation durations for particular estimate groups: consultant estimating the duration of another consultant's operations

222

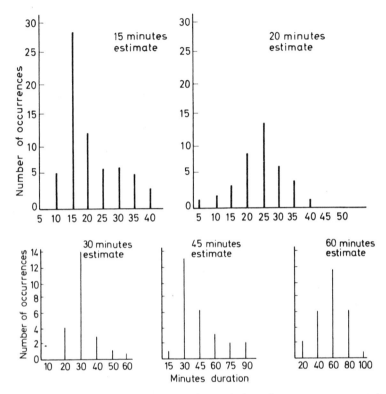

Figure 10.8. Actual operation durations for particular estimate groups: aggregated

The basic data obtained from this exercise has certain obvious limitations.

(1)　The estimates were made retrospectively, and without reference to case notes. The surgeon had only brief diagnostic details for each patient and thus his performance may have been worse than could be expected. He is certain that this factor is important and he feels confident that, in a real situation, his performance would be better.

(2)　Some of the operations were actually performed by other consultants, and it is well established that times for particular operations can vary considerably for different consultants. However, the surgeon in question, when estimating a particular operation time, knew who had actually carried out the operation and made some subjective adjustment in the light of this.

(3)   The consultant was called upon to estimate a large number of operations at one sitting. This undoubtedly had a distorting effect on the results. It is possible to show that his performance deteriorated towards the end of this exercise.

The shapes of the histograms are fairly consistent with one another and with what would be expected in practice, particularly for the ones which contain information on a reasonably large number of operations, i.e., the modal value coincides approximately with the estimated value, and they are unsymmetrical, generally with a tail to the right. There are a number of possible reasons for this.

(1)   The surgeon is exhibiting a consistent bias — in fact he is being optimistic. He is inclined to under-estimate the time an operation will take: a very common human characteristic. This is not unreasonable.

(2)   He had made the estimates on the basis of more limited information than would normally be available to him, so that even in the cases characterized by no unforeseen complications, high variability is to be expected.

(3)   Some of the cases do exhibit complications which would have been foreseen had the patient been examined.

(4)   In a small number of cases complications may have arisen, which, even given the most favourable circumstances, would not have been foreseen.

If an estimating system has been implemented and has settled down, reasons (1) to (3) will have greatly reduced effects so that in assessing the surgeon's innate estimating ability we feel justified in discarding extreme values.

At the Albrough Clinic, at present, it is unlikely that post-operative stay estimation by consultants is carried out explicitly. However, it is certainly implicit in the admission system in that a consultant has to decide how many beds he will have available on his next admission day. Here the estimation is of the form, 'Will patient X be out of the Clinic by next admission day or not?'. The time-span between making the decision regarding a patient and the next admission day for a given consultant is only four days, which means that there is an excellent chance of a consultant being correct.

The major incentive behind an attempt to introduce an explicit post-operative stay estimation system is to extend the span between a consultant deciding on bed availability and its associated admission day. This means that longer notice could be extended to patients. Associated with this, of course, is the requirement that inaccuracy in estimation over a longer span than at present does not lead to either a significant increase in temporary bed usage or a significant decrease in bed occupancy.

Although very little experimental work has been carried out on a consultant's performance as an estimator of post-operative stay, certain models have been developed. In general it is clear that estimating post-operative stays only presents difficulty in the case of relatively long-stay patients.

Simulated estimation

It is assumed that actual operation durations can be generated from estimated values as normal variates with expectation equal to the estimate and standard deviation directly proportional to the estimate. For a particular estimate E the actual duration is drawn from a normal population where $\mu = E$ and $\sigma = C \times \mu$.

Thus the constant of proportionality C reflects the accuracy of the estimates (or, more strictly, their inaccuracy since when $C = 0$, $\sigma = 0$ the estimation is perfect and accuracy decreases with increasing C).

This process, although not very rigorous, is a convenient method for obtaining ideas about the performance of the system. The preliminary experimental work on estimating post-operative stay suggests this presents difficulty in the case of relatively long-stay patients. Patients who stay one or two weeks can be estimated with a very good accuracy. There is also evidence that in the event of error there will tend to be an under-estimation of the actual stay.

For these reasons it was decided to employ the following algorithm to generate 'actual' post-operative stays from estimates.

(1) If estimated length of stay is 7 days or less, set the actual stay equal to the estimate.

(2) If estimated length of stay is in the range 8 to 14 days, the actual stay is generated by adding 7 days to the estimate with a probability of $P/2$.

(3) If the estimated length of stay is greater than 14 days, the actual stay is generated by adding 7 days to the estimate with probability P.

In other words a patient's actual post-operative stay is either equal to the estimate, or 7 days longer. Although somewhat crude, this approach fits in well with what appears to be the case in practice.

Clearly P is used as a measure of estimating accuracy of post-operative stay. For $P = 0$ estimation is perfect and accuracy decreases with increasing P.

The experiment

For various values for bed numbers and operating theatre session duration the simulation was run to obtain the relationship between the

225

operation duration estimation parameter (*C*) and the performance of the unit in terms of operation session control (the proportion of sessions outside limits). The decision rule, under all circumstances, attempted to keep the beds as full as possible, and select patients to fill operating time available using a simple summation of operation duration estimates for individual patients. The sort of result obtained is shown in the previous chapter (*Figure 9.17*).

The results give an indication of the level of performance which might be expected from the unit and of the performance of the unit in relation to the balance between bed and theatre time availability. They also, of course, indicate the gap between current and expected performance. However, in order to obtain these results the consultant surgeon is required to pay explicit attention to the estimation of operation duration per patient and use these estimates in his patient selection decisions.

The effects of medical and social criteria

The results described above are conditional on the resource utilization decision rule being able to encompass all the other factors mentioned previously in 'The patient selection decision'. This hinges on whether or not the waiting list has sufficient variety in terms of operation duration expectations to satisfy medical and social requirements and the resource utilization objectives also.

This was checked by carrying out experiments in which the consultant surgeon studied computer-selected operating theatre lists and modified them to the extent that medical and social criteria were violated. Very little modification was made and where it was necessary it was usually possible to generate an acceptable list with the same bed and theatre time implications.

Experiment B

The simulation model was modified to experiment with the effects of the accuracy of estimation of post-operative stay on Clinic performance. Although the Clinic operated with negligible reliance on post-operative stay estimation, this is not the case with the system altered to give longer notice to patients.

The main changes are that: (*i*) 'count est bed' is modified to estimate the number of beds available on the next admit day but one, two and so on; and (*ii*) 'list search' derives an admission plan for the next admit day but one, two and so on.

In a typical experiment, the simulation was run for one year for 25 values of P between 0 and 0·5 at each of the 8 values of C used in the previous experiment (i.e. 200 simulated years in all).

As previously mentioned the procedure used for generating actual post-operative stays from estimates simulates an observed tendency to under estimate length of stay. This implies that there will be a tendency to over estimate the number of beds that will be available on admit day. Thus the measure of performance chosen was the yearly refusal rate, i.e. the sum over the year of the differences between the estimated beds available and the actual beds available. This is more expedient from a programming viewpoint than to allow for temporary beds in the simulated ward.

For a given value of P there was no significant difference between refusal rates for different values of C so the 8 values of refusal rate for each value of P were averaged. The average refusal rate plotted against P is shown in *Figure 10.9*.

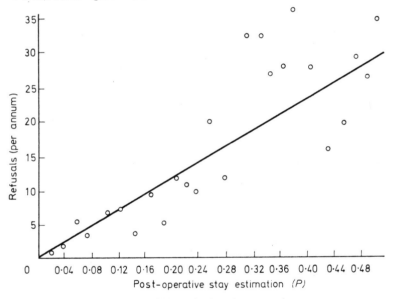

Figure 10.9. Refusals and estimation

It is possible using these results to estimate the disruption to the specialty caused by planning ahead using a booked admission procedure. The operational problem was to determine a mix of planning horizons for the beds in the unit, e.g., some operating under the present system, some on one week ahead and so on.

227

Recommendations

The following are quotations from a paper containing recommendations for the Albrough Clinic based on the simulation experiments described above.

'An effort should be made to give people longer notice. For example, we suggest that, initially, a patient be given one week's extra notice of an impending operation. This means that a surgeon chooses patients, not for admissions five days hence as is now the procedure, but for 12 days hence. This involves allocating beds to patients in advance and it requires a particular type of information – this information can be estimated with considerable accuracy. The system can easily be modified to give longer notice.'

'In many hospital specialties, the introduction of such a system would be fraught with danger, but the Albrough Clinic is particularly appropriate.

(1) Because of the relative simplicity of the structure of the patient intake, i.e. it is a cold surgical ward.

(2) Because of the ease with which post-operative stays can be estimated.

Under the proposed system the consultant would first see his patients at the out-patient clinic as before. However, in deciding to place patients on the ward waiting list, he would provide estimates of their bed requirements (i.e. length of stay) and theatre time requirements. There are two important points here.

(1) Estimates should be made for his own patients only.

(2) These estimates should be made at the out-patient clinic when he is confronted by the patient.

This additional information should be placed on the waiting list slip and filed as before.'

'The ward sister will have a separate file for each bed. Each file will contain particulars of the patient currently in the bed and those of any patient due to be admitted to that bed. In consultation with the surgeon she can decide how many and what beds will be available for admissions twelve days hence. In the case of the long stay patients the consultant will re-estimate their length of stay in the light of their progress and the ward sister can update her files accordingly. This will give the consultant the necessary information to choose his admissions.'

'Patients are chosen, as before, by consulting the waiting list file. The relevant slips are removed from the file and sent to the Albrough

Clinic, where they are placed in the appropriate bed files and used to progress the beds. The list of patients is sent to the medical records department as before. This should allow adequate time for the gathering together of all the relevant case notes and x-rays.'

'In deciding on the number of patients to be sent for at 11 days notice, the consultant should use the following rule.
Number sent for = estimated beds available *minus* one
The consultant will send for one or two cases on a four day basis each week, as at present.'

'Deciding on bed availability is done with the use of a *planning chart*. This will present a visual representation of the bed occupancy on any given day.'

EAR, NOSE AND THROAT/OPHTHALMOLOGY UNIT

Experiments

Five experiments were performed three with the individual specialty models and two with the combined specialty model, to investigate the behaviour of the system as a whole.

The first two experiments were performed to assess the model's accuracy in representing the present system at Louphill. The third was an evaluation of the effect of using a minor operations theatre for cataract cases. The fourth was a direct comparison of the situations arising from running the unit as one specialty of 18 beds per ward or as two specialties each of nine beds per ward. The fifth was an investigation of the effects of an alteration in the weekly timetable of the combined specialties.

Simulating the present system

Ideally the programs ought to choose patients for admission in the same way which they are chosen at Louphill. The people who make the decisions told us that 'usually for each operating session two adult males, two adult females and one child are chosen'. The numbers actually chosen over a period of time do not bear this out. It is probable that the actual selection procedure is more flexible, taking into account bed availability and short-run fluctuations in the proportions of different categories on the waiting list, and that the quoted figures represent a long-run target level. It is also true that some categories receive higher priority than others. A decision rule which reproduced the overall structure of past performance was, in fact, chosen.

229

Ophthalmology – experiment A

The results of experiment A together with an actual year's results are given in Table 10.3. There are a number of criteria by which the two sets of results may be compared.

(1)   The allocation of beds between the consultants is more even than in practice, resulting in a ratio of 1·24 between the numbers of waiting list admissions for the consultants, instead of 1·42.

(2)   The ratio of male to female admissions in the simulation is slightly greater than one. Given wards of equal sizes and identical scheduling policies this is to be expected since the average length of stay is greater for females. The discrepancy in the actual results is due to the fact that for part of the time a side ward (male) was used for female patients because the waiting list for females was considerably longer than that for males.

(3)   On average the annual throughput was 20 higher in the simulation than in practice, though in a total of 545 this is not a great difference. It can readily be explained by the fact that in the last six months of 1967 three scheduled Friday operating sessions did not take place. Allowing for this the agreement is extremely good.

(4)   It is also possible to compare the simulated and actual systems on the average bed occupancy. However, for similar total throughputs and the same number of beds in the two cases, the two systems should be in agreement on this dimension because the average length of patient stay will be the same in the two cases. A more meaningful comparison can be made between the number of nights on which the use of temporary beds was required. Unfortunately the available bed occupancy figures combine the figures for the two wards into a single figure. This could obscure the fact that beds in one ward were overloaded. However some comparison can be made between the number of nights on which the total number of beds used by the specialty exceeded 18 for then at least one ophthalmology patient must have been occupying an additional bed, in at least one of the wards. During the second half of 1967 there were 28 such nights; this compares with a figure of 31 for the average of the two halves of the first year of the simulation.

It would seem then that the model accurately represents the global aspects of the present system, like total throughput of patients and the load placed on the resources by these. It is less accurate in the more detailed aspects of allocating beds between the consultants and allowing flexibility in the size of the wards.

Ear, Nose and Throat – experiment B

Experiment B does for the ear, nose and throat model what experiment A does for the ophthalmology model. The results are given in

Table 10.4. The simulated and actual systems may be compared in the same way as for the ophthalmology model.

(1)   The ratio between the numbers of waiting list admissions for the consultants is 0·80 in the simulation, 0·91 in practice.

(2)   In both the simulated and actual results slightly more female patients are admitted than males. This is to be expected since, unlike the ophthalmology specialty the average length of stay is greater for males.

(3)   The total throughputs in the two systems are almost identical, differing by only six in a total of 958.

The problem of having patients with pre-operative stays of more than one day are not as important in this simulation because the operating sessions are more frequent, though a slightly higher proportion (4 per cent) of waiting list patients fell into this category than in the ophthalmology specialty.

(4)   The number of nights on which the total number of beds used by the specialty exceeded 18 was seven during the second half of 1967 compared with an average of 20 for the two halves of the first year of the simulation.

(5)   A further comparison between the two systems can be made on the proportion of patients in the various categories admitted. The overall proportions of patients admitted were in good agreement with those of the second half of 1967 but the simulation performed less well at a more detailed level. The reason for this is that there are between-sex and between-consultant differences in some categories, e.g. more female tonsil patients than males, consultant 2 treated more ear cases than consultant 1. To reproduce these idosyncrasies the selection rule would have to be very much more complicated; it was felt that for the purpose in mind this complication was not justified. In any event, the discrepancies were not excessive.

As for the ophthalmology model, it appears that the ear, nose and throat model accurately represents the overall aspects of the present system but performs less well in detailed aspects.

Changed use of the minor operations theatre (experiment C)

The experiment was aimed directly at the evaluation of a proposal for upgrading the minor operations theatre, previously used only by the ear nose and throat specialty, for cataract operations under local anaesthetic.

The experiment searched for the best feasible timetable for use of this theatre and also an appropriate allocation of beds between male and female cases. The results are shown in Table 10.5.

It can be seen that the results were highly satisfactory: the throughput of patients treated by the specialty was 15 per cent up on current

TABLE 10.3

Results of Experiment A

| | Admissions | | | | | | | | Nights in extra beds | | Bed occupancy (percentage) | |
| | Consultant 3 | | Consultant 4 | | Male ward | | Female ward | | | | | |
Year	W.L.	Cas.	W.L.	Cas.	Total	Cas.	Total	Cas.	Male ward	Female ward	Male ward	Female ward
SIMULATION												
1	272	37	217	33	282	39	277	31	57	55	77·9	78·6
2	265	26	210	26	274	26	253	26	35	42	76·3	78·3
3	261	23	219	48	284	42	267	29	80	53	80·3	78·9
4	258	31	206	49	283	44	261	36	113	76	79·6	80·9
Average	254	29	213	39	281	38	264	30	71	56	78·5	79·4
ACTUAL Results based on Jul.–Dec. 1967	262	40	184	38	244	44	280	34	Unknown		77·6	

W.L. – Waiting List Cas. – Casualties

232

TABLE 10.4.

Results of Experiment B

| Year | Admissions | | | | | | | | Nights in extra beds | | Bed Occupancy (percentage) | |
| | Consultant 1 | | Consultant 2 | | Male ward | | Female ward | | Male ward | Female ward | Male ward | Female ward |
	W.L.	Cas.	W.L.	Cas.	Total	Cas.	Total	Cas.				
SIMULATION												
1	316	109	416	70	455	81	456	98	23	39	74·3	77·2
2	362	94	438	75	464	85	505	84	26	8	74·7	69·2
3	355	106	446	56	476	79	487	83	5	19	69·8	67·5
4	354	100	438	73	465	84	500	89	20	19	74·3	69·7
Average	347	102	434	68	465	82	487	88	19	21	73·3	70·9
ACTUAL Results based on Jul.–Dec. 1967	354	126	388	90	476	100	482	116	Unknown		70·5	

W.L. – Waiting List   Cas. – Casualties

233

TABLE 10.5

Results of Experiment C

Year	Male ward W.L. admissions Diagnostic category					Female ward W.L. admissions Diagnostic category					Consultant		Total	Total nights in extra beds
	1	2	3	4		1	2	3	4		3	4		
1	94	76	38	16	283	240	63	32	30	388	358	313	671	381
2	101	71	35	36	277	237	56	29	29	377	355	299	654	243
3	105	69	35	35	283	245	56	28	28	380	367	296	663	287
Average	100	72	36	36	279	241	58	30	29	382	360	303	663	241

W.L. – Waiting List

performance. Also most of this increase was accounted for by female cataract cases — these cases being subject to the longest waiting times for treatment.

Separate specialties versus *combined specialty (experiment D)*

Experiment D, the results of which are given in Table 10.6, seeks to answer the question: 'What, if any, are the benefits to be gained from organizing the ophthalmology and ear, nose and throat specialties as one unit sharing common resources?'.

Instead of each specialty having fixed bed allocations as in the separate models, the combined specialty model treated these wards as having 18 beds, access to which was allowed to all four consultants. The timetable was kept fixed and, by use of the same random number streams as in the separate models, the addition of patients to the waiting lists was exactly reproduced, as was the incidence of casualty patients. The three (one for ophthalmology, two for ear, nose and throat) admission vectors remained unaltered from the separate models. In the decision routine however a simple 'evening out' procedure was no longer satisfactory as this was found to admit a disproportionate number of ear, nose and throat patients. Instead a deliberate bias toward the ophthalmology sessions was introduced to restore the balance. The success of this may be judged from the results.

The performance of the combined specialty may be compared with that of its constituent parts on a number of aspects.

(1) The combined version shows no increase in total throughput. Since the balance between patients of the two specialties and the proportions in different diagnostic categories are preserved, this cannot be due to differences in the type of load placed on the resources in the two cases.

(2) In the combined version approximately equal numbers of males and females are admitted. This represents a balance between the extra females admitted by ear, nose and throat and the extra males admitted by ophthalmology.

(3) The combined model shows a considerable saving in the use of temporary beds (from an average of 83 patient-nights to 20). This to be expected, since in this version, if one specialty requires more than nine beds in one of the wards, it may be possible to find an empty bed not required by the other specialty whereas this is not possible when the unit is run as two separate specialties.

(4) The average bed occupancy in the two wards does not markedly differ from that obtained by combining the figures of the separate specialties.

235

TABLE 10.6

Results of Experiment D

	Combined specialties					Separate specialties
Diagnostic category	Year 1	2	3	4	Average	
Consultant 1						
1	57	59	54	50	55	
2	49	43	46	49	47	
admissions 3	14	11	9	14	12	
4	175	195	181	162	178	
5	44	50	52	63	52	
6	0	0	0	0	0	
Casualties	95	85	95	86	90	
Day cases	14	9	11	14	12	
Total admissions	448	452	448	438	446	449
Consultant 2 1	128	124	117	115	121	
2	37	37	42	41	39	
3	10	10	10	10	10	
4	147	159	161	158	156	
5	98	106	108	107	105	
W.L. admissions 6	0	0	0	0	0	
Casualties	60	61	42	59	56	
Day cases	10	14	14	14	13	
Total admissions	490	511	494	504	500	502
Consultant 3 1	140	141	137	137	139	
2	70	71	69	68	69	
3	26	26	30	32	29	
4	24	30	30	31	29	
Casualties	37	26	23	31	29	
Total admissions	297	294	289	299	295	293
Consultant 4 1	101	99	94	93	97	
2	53	55	52	57	54	
3	29	30	33	33	31	
4	28	31	34	31	31	
Casualties	33	26	48	49	39	
Total admissions	244	241	261	264	252	252

TABLE 10.6 continued

		Combined specialties					Separate specialties
	Diagnostic category	Year				Average	
		1	2	3	4		
Casualties	Male ward	120	111	121	128	120	
	Female ward	129	110	112	125	119	
Total admissions	Male ward	740	748	750	751	747	746
	Female ward	739	750	742	754	746	741
Nights in extra beds	Male ward	15	16	20	31	20	90
	Female ward	18	15	30	18	20	77
Bed occupancy	Male ward	77·5	75·7	77·4	77·9	77·1	75·9
	Female ward	78·8	74·0	75·1	75·9	75·9	75·1
Total throughput		1479	1498	1492	1505	1493	1497

The results of this experiment seem to indicate that the benefits to be gained from a combined specialty are somewhat limited. In the present version of the model the extra freedom in the use of beds that is available has been entirely taken up in reducing the demand for temporary beds rather than in increasing the total throughput. If the combined specialty were prepared to tolerate a higher demand for temporary beds, a higher total throughput would be possible.

Timetable alterations (experiment E)

The present structure of the timetable is very awkward as far as the ophthalmology specialty is concerned. Cataract patients are the most common in this specialty and generally stay in nine days. The consecutive operating days available to ophthalmology means that their bed cannot be filled for five days. If all patients were cataracts this would imply an average bed occupancy of only 64 per cent. Similar arguments can be applied to the other classes of ophthalmology patients.

Certain feasible timetable changes were tested one of which amounted to exchanging the Tuesday and Thursday morning sessions between consultants 2 and 3, ear, nose and throat and an ophthalmic surgeon. The results of this experiment are given in Table 10.7. Again, it was necessary to incorporate in the decision procedure some bias towards the ophthalmology sessions to prevent them being swamped by ear, nose and throat but apart from this conditions were exactly as in experiment

237

TABLE 10.7

Results of Experiment E

		Combined specialties (new timetable)					Experiment D
	Diagnostic		Year			Average	
		1	2	3	4		
Consultant 1	1	54	55	53	52	54	
	2	50	44	50	49	48	
W.L. admissions	3	13	11	10	14	12	
	4	184	203	185	190	191	
	5	48	53	57	59	54	
	6	0	0	0	0	0	
Casualties		95	85	95	86	90	
Day cases		14	9	11	14	12	
Total admissions		458	460	461	464	461	466
Consultant 2	1	119	117	120	108	116	
	2	42	41	46	45	43	
	3	11	13	12	12	12	
	4	157	169	158	164	162	
	5	98	107	98	193	101	
W. L. admissions	6	0	0	0	0	0	
Casualties		60	61	42	59	56	
Day cases		10	14	14	14	13	
Total admissions		497	522	490	505	503	500
Consultant 3	1	165	169	160	161	164	
	2	84	84	79	81	82	
	3	30	26	36	31	31	
W.L. admissions	4	27	35	33	34	32	
Casualties		37	26	23	31	29	
Total admissions		343	340	331	338	338	295
Consultant 4	1	106	109	102	112	107	
	2	56	62	60	55	58	
W.L. admissions	3	38	36	41	36	38	
	4	37	38	39	37	38	
Casualties		33	26	48	49	39	
Total admissions		270	271	290	289	280	252

TABLE 10.7 continued

		Combined specialties (new timetable)					Experiment D
	Diagnostic	1	2 Year 3		4	Average	
Casualties	Male ward	120	111	121	128	120	
	Female ward	129	110	112	125	120	
	Male ward	794	791	801	795	795	747
Total admissions	Female	774	802	771	801	787	746
Nights in extra beds	Male ward	53	43	37	62	49	20
	Female ward	45	30	36	40	38	20
Bed occupancy	Male ward	81·6	80·0	80·9	83·3	81·4	77·1
	Female ward	82·7	79·7	80·5	82·3	81·3	75·9
Total throughput		1568	1593	1572	1596	1582	1493

A comparison of the results of these two experiments shows a 2 per cent increase on throughput of ear, nose and throat patients, and a 13 per cent increase for ophthalmology, which combined represents a 6 per cent increase for the unit as a whole. This increase in bed utilization has not been achieved without some cost however, Slightly more than twice as many temporary beds have been used and the ophthalmology operating sessions have been overloaded.

Recommendations

The following three changes considered are all possibilities that were discussed with the consultants involved in the study.

(1) A timetable change (juxtaposing an ophthalmology operating session and ear, nose and throat session).

(2) The conversion of an additional theatre for use by the ophthalmology specialty for cataracts.

(3) Running the two specialties as one unit.

The reaction of the consultants to these possible changes varied widely. In fact, the second change has already taken place, although it is still too early for its effects to be assessed. The other two are unlikely to happen, the first because it is in large part an alternative to the second, the third largely because it would have little effect.

The timetable change consisted of exchanging Tuesday morning's ear, nose and throat operating session for Thursday morning's ophthalmology session. The present timetable, with its two operating sessions on Thursday and Friday is very awkward for the ophthalmology specialty. Running both single-specialty and two-specialty models taking account of this change indicated an increase in throughput of about 15 per cent. This resulted in an overloading of the two ophthalmology operating sessions and an increase in the number of extra beds erected in the wards throughout the year. Naturally, the bed occupancy figures are raised.

Close to one of the wards is a minor operations theatre which was formerly poorly equipped and used only for one ear, nose and throat session per week. Recently this theatre was improved, and it is now possible to carry out ophthalmology operations under local anaesthetic. A proposal was made for each consultant to use the theatre for one additional operating session at the beginning of the week, principally for cataracts.

Running the single specialty model taking account of this change showed that there are more male ophthalmology beds than are really needed, but fewer female beds (since there are more female cataracts than males). At the cost of some inconvenience, this can be overcome because the male ward contains a side ward which can be used for females instead of males. This can be simulated in the model by setting the size of the wards as male: 7 beds and female: 11 beds, instead of nine each. This resulted in an increase of ophthalmology throughput of 15 per cent but a reduction in the length of operating sessions. The adverse effect was an increase in the number of extra beds erected in the wards throughout the year.

Combining specialties might be expected to be beneficial from an organizational viewpoint, provided medical constraints are satisfied. Multispecialty wards, categorized as 'acute' and 'non-acute', are in operation elsewhere. We tried to evaluate the resulting benefits of such a ward in our own situation. Instead of each specialty having nine male beds and nine female beds, the combined model treated the two wards as having 18 beds each, access to which being allowed to all four consultants. The timetable was kept fixed.

A comparison of the results of the combined specialty model with those of the two single-specialty models showed that:

(1)   there would be no increase in total throughput;

(2)   approximately equal numbers of males and females would be admitted (the extra females admitted by ear, nose and throat and the extra males by ophthalmology);

(3)   there would be no significant difference in bed occupancy;

(4)   there would be a considerable saving in the number of extra beds erected throughout the year (from about 150 to about 50).

FURTHER RESEARCH

A start has been made towards the goal of a total hospital model for the patient treatment process, and the results to date are encouraging. Ways in which this work should develop are clear.

(1)   Research into other surgical specialties, i.e. specialties not yet examined. In particular it is essential that an investigation be made of a general surgical specialty.

(2)   Further practical application of the models already developed. Real problems should be tackled in systems similar to the Albrough Clinic and the ear, nose and throat ophthalmology unit.

(3)   Research into the decisions leading up to patient admission to hospital. It is especially essential that attempts are made to model surgical out-patient work.

(4)   Use of the models 'off-line' to throw light on strategic surgical planning questions. Questions such as resource balance, performance, measurement organizational change and so on could be examined.

Eventually, of course, it is tempting to think that the models will form a basis for an effective methodology in the planning and operation of total hospital systems.

11–Financial Management in the Health Service

R.W. Wallis

Introduction

The amount and quality of service any organization is able to provide ultimately depends upon the resources made available to it. Whatever shape the resources take, whether physical items such as buildings and equipment, or the services of doctors, nurses or administrators, they have to be purchased and thus money or finance must first be raised. The economic fact of life, however unpalatable, is that there is never enough finance available to satisfy all our wants, and thus the necessity of rationing it out between competing ends arises. It is vital, therefore, that the limited funds available are used to give the maximum benefits possible; and since it is the physical assets and services which money buys that produce benefits or satisfaction, it is the way these are utilized which determines whether more or less value is obtained from the money provided. Thus everyone in the health services, or for that matter any other organization, has a part to play in financial management, however indirect his or her association with the finance function may be. This is because everyone is involved in the use of real resources, which financial resources or monetary funds are used to provide; whether it is in deciding how they should be used, or actually using them.

Despite this automatic involvement in the use of resources, however, there is a tendency by non-specialist finance staff in organizations to think of the financial problem of 'making ends meet' to be that of the finance officer, treasurer, or accountant alone. Thus financial problems are often viewed as though they are separate and distinctly different problems from those of management in general. In fact the technique of recording various aspects of, and changes in, resources known as double-entry book-keeping, which is the peculiar contribution of the accounting profession to the management process, has had some far-reaching effects upon the administrative structures of organizations and upon administrative behaviour and attitudes.

Broadly, it has ensured that the accountant has become more than a mere book-keeper or data processor. He has become a specialist in analysing and interpreting the organization's activities in terms of money, in advising on how to obtain finance and on the effects of using it. In short, he has become a *financial manager.* At the same time, whilst basically a simple technique, the accountant's work often appears to others to be wrapped in mystery, and his terminology can create a barrier to communication between himself and the non-specialist.

It is the aim of this section not only to indicate how the financial administrator aids the efficient utilization of resources in the health services, but to outline the problems involved in furthering his contribution to the total management process.

The financial specialist cannot work in a vacuum. The extent to which he can contribute to the success of the organization's work depends, in part, upon the co-operation he receives from other members within the service, either by supplying him with information appropriate to his needs or by making the best use of the services he can provide. For this to happen it is imperative that the non-specialist understands the usefulness and the limitations of the techniques of financial management. It is by examining the role of the financial administrator and his techniques that this understanding can best be achieved.

Because of the complex structure of the health services and the space available, it is impossible to do more than provide an introduction to this aspect of management. The manner in which health services are organized affects the way in which finance is raised and the form of financial administration and techniques adopted and used by different sections of the service. Thus the financial arrangements of local authority health services differ from those of the hospital services. Consequently, although practical illustrations will be drawn from different areas of the Health Service, the emphasis will be on general principles and problems of financial management rather than a detailed description of existing practice and procedures. By doing this at least the basis for a mutual understanding between financial specialists and their colleagues may be laid.

Management and the Finance Function

MANAGEMENT IN ORGANIZATION

The essential problem which faces the manager(s) of any organization, or for that matter any individual is illustrated in *Figure 11.1*. Means are limited, ends, in general, are unbounded and consequently the need to choose between competing ends arises. Management thus commences with *decision making*. Moreover, it is concerned with an *input/output system*.

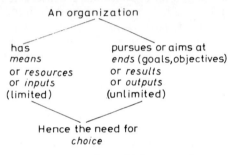

Figure 11.1

The management process, however, involves more than merely deciding which ends to pursue, what sort of resources to acquire, or how to use them to achieve the objective sought. Once decisions have been taken, action is needed to bring about the desired results. Moreover, the action taken, or alternatively the execution of the decision must be controlled to ensure, so far as possible, that the ends are achieved. It is possible therefore to think of organizational activity as being of three types: decision making; executive action; and controlling.

There are dangers in over simplifying the picture in this way, however. First, because it may suggest that some people in an organization are concerned only with management activities, that is, with decision making and controlling, whilst the rest are responsible for executive work only — those who actually do the job, whether this involves physical or mental activities. In fact everyone makes decisions, takes action and controls, although the amount of time spent on these different activities and their relative importance will vary from person to person depending upon his place in the organization or the nature of his responsibilities.

Secondly, it may suggest that decision making ends when action commences. In practice, an initial decision or set of decisions will

244

require innumerable further decisions to be made and stimulate activities of many different kinds so that the whole organizational process is extremely complex and interacting.

Moreover, there is rarely in practice a time limit set to achieving the overall objective, particularly for public sector organizations. Thus, the health services exist to meet human needs not just now but into the future. The relative emphasis which is given to different categories of need will undoubtedly change over time, as will the skills and resources available for meeting them, so that management is faced with a dynamic situation which calls for the continual re-appraisal of the objectives aimed at and the methods of achieving them. Thus, decisions regarding long-term aims may be in the process of formulation at the same time as control is being exerted over action aimed at achieving short-term objectives.

Nevertheless, the distinction made does help to clarify discussion about organizational activity and behaviour. It enables the different roles people play to be identified more easily so that, in particular, managerial or administrative activities on the one hand and technical and professional skills on the other may be distinguished and their relationship analysed. With regard to management processes, it draws attention to the difference between the decision making and the control aspects of management so that their nature and relationship may be examined more critically. It should be stressed, however, that, whilst this distinction helps in understanding the management process, the term control is often used as a synonym for the total management process embracing both the decision making and regulative aspects.

To approach an organization as an input—output system also provides useful insights into the management process and its problems. In particular, this view immediately suggests that by relating input to output some assessment of the organization's efficiency can be achieved, in the same way that the efficiency of other systems can be assessed. For example, a car which does 40 miles per gallon of petrol may be considered more efficient, as regards the output from its fuel consumption, than another which does only 36 miles per gallon. However, the concept of efficiency provides pitfalls for the unwary. It is especially easy to confuse technical and economic efficiency. For example a car which does more miles per gallon may nevertheless be less efficient from an economist's point of view. It may have a higher capital cost, do fewer miles over its life, be less speedy and so on; the overall effect being that it costs more in relation to the satisfaction it provides, whether in terms of money or not, than another which achieves a lower mileage per gallon. The manager of an organization is, of course, in the position of co-ordinating the efforts of people with different types of professional and technical skills, and different concepts of technical efficiency, so as to ensure that the organization achieves its aims regardless of the various techniques employed.

But more than this, his responsibility is to ensure that aims are achieved efficiently from the economic standpoint; that more, rather than less, value for money is obtained from the use of resources. He is thus in the position of having to balance different kinds of technical appraisals of the organization's objectives and activities and reconcile these with the overall aim. There are two main problems from the manager's point of view. First, that of establishing some criterion by which to measure efficiency and, secondly, that of ensuring professional and technical skills are applied with this criterion in mind.

It would be false to suggest that the search for a completely objective measure of economic efficiency has so far been successful. The main difficulty faced by non-profit making organizations is that of converting their output into monetary terms, so as to achieve a comparison between the cost of providing their services with the benefits or satisfactions they provide. Yet the establishment of some criterion of economic efficiency is a prerequisite for the guidance of decision makers and the control of executive action.

In the description and analysis of financial management in the Health Service which follows, the lack or inadequacy of such a criterion of administrative efficiency will emerge as the crucial factor in explaining both the importance of financial management and the limitations inherent in the techniques used.

STRUCTURE OF ORGANIZATIONS

The nature and size of an organization will determine the way in which activities and responsibilities are distributed amongst the organization's members or officers. However, specialization takes two main forms. First, by the amount of authority and responsibility vested in an individual and, secondly, by the type of work or function he or she performs. Thus in local government, authority rests ultimately in the hands of the elected representatives who are the members of the council, though much of this authority may be delegated down through the Health Committee to the Medical Officer of Health, his deputy, and so on down the hierarchy. Similarly, in the hospital service the authority of the Minister, itself derived from Parliament, is delegated to boards of governors, regional hospital boards and hospital management committees and through them to their officers.

By contrast, the work or place of an individual in an organization may be described by reference to the type of work or function he is concerned with. The main distinction, as suggested earlier, tends to be between an administrative function which is found in any organization, whatever its objective, and an executive function whose characteristics are determined by the particular field of activity with which the organization is concerned. For example, all industrial organizations have common administrative problems which are dealt with by secretaries, solicitors, accountants and 'general' administrators, though on the executive side one firm may be concerned with producing chemical products, another with electrical engineering, another with civil engineering and so on, so that quite different skills and qualifications are required by the executives concerned.

In the hospital service the parallel distinction is between the administrative departments, on the one hand, and medical/nursing (or treatment) departments on the other. Similarly, in local government it is possible to identify departments such as the town clerk's, or borough treasurer's, whose function is to provide the administrative services necessary to sustain not only local health services but the whole range of local authority services in their area. Comparison of the hospital service with a local authority service, however, highlights the relationship between administrative and executive functions, and the factors which affect the resultant structure and distribution of responsibilities (whether on a functional or authority basis) in an organization. Thus in the hospital service financial specialists are wholly concerned with hospital administration. By contrast in local government a financial specialist may well serve not only the health department but other executive departments as well. Size, the volume of work, geographical and other factors will determine the extent to which administrators, financial or otherwise, will be wholly concerned with, or attached to, a particular executive department. Thus in a large local authority a finance clerk may be wholly concerned with health service financial matters and be actually attached to the Medical Officer of Health's staff. At the same time, an accountant on the staff of the treasurer's department may be nevertheless employed wholly on health service accounting, and liaise with the Medical Officer's finance clerk. In the hospital service, on the other hand, whilst financial specialists are obviously concerned only with hospital work, different categories of finance work may be performed at Ministry, regional hospital board, hospital management committee (that is, group) or individual hospital levels.

Any appreciation of the problems of financial management clearly requires an understanding of the nature of the finance function itself, the sub-specialities within this function, and its relationship with the other functions of an organization.

FINANCE FUNCTION IN PERSPECTIVE

How organizations may be viewed as input—output systems having a production cycle for which different stages may be distinguished is illustrated in *Figure 11.2*. First of all, monetary funds must be raised and collected. Secondly, these funds are used to obtain real goods and services which must be stored or maintained until they are used to produce the goods or services which comprise the output of the organization concerned.

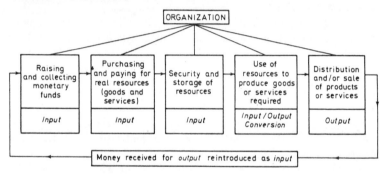

Figure 11.2.

In private commercial organizations the objective will be to convert the physical output into money so as to earn a profit in the process which constitutes the owner's income and which may be used to expand the financial basis of the organization; that is, it may be 'ploughed back'. Public health authorities, at least in the United Kingdom, make few charges for their services so that their production cycle in general excludes the sales function.

The stages shown in the production cycle in *Figure 11.2* relate essentially to the physical activities which different individuals in an organization engage in. It indicates simply that an organization consists of a set of related sub-systems by which resources are converted through time, in successive stages, from the form of money into a final output. Consequently, administrative activities are not separately distinguished.

Delineating the nature and scope of the finance function, or indeed any other function, is no easy matter since there is more to any operation than the physical, observable activities involved. Clearly,

248

however, the finance function is concerned with money, both in raising funds and disbursing them to obtain real goods and services. Money is generally accepted as representing wealth or value and acting as a measure of value. This enables it to act as a medium of exchange and store of value, since people are willing to accept money in exchange for real resources, knowing that they can in turn use it to obtain other goods or services either immediately or in the future. Because it enables the value of real resources to be measured people are willing to give up resources in return for payment in the future, knowing that the amount of the debt can be clearly established. Its use thus permits debtor—creditor relationships to exist. But in particular, the use of money to measure the value of resources provides the common basis for recording, or accounting for, the different resources controlled by an individual or organization. And since, in the production cycle, resources change their form from money or cash into various types of intermediate input and eventually into different kinds of output and possibly back into cash, the ability to record these changes in terms of a common measurement unit provides an objective basis for measurement and control over the use of the available resources, whatever form they take.

Accounting

Accounting for resources is thus an essential part of the finance function, since it is in terms of money that such records are kept. The precise scope and nature of the financial records kept by any organization will depend upon various factors. The law may prescribe that certain records must be kept. But, quite apart from legal requirements, the size and nature of the organization, the complexity of its operations or objectives, its methods of finance, production processes and many other factors will affect the structure of accounting arrangements and the techniques of financial data-processing adopted. In particular, however, much will depend upon the extent to which it is considered that the various activities in the organization need to be translated into terms of money for control purposes.

The basic accounting system, known as the double-entry system, produces four main categories of information. (1) The total amount of funds available to an organization. (2) The extent to which the organization is liable to repay money to those who have provided finance. (3) The way in which funds have been used (or remain unused in the form of money. (4) The amounts of revenue received or earned by selling or charging for goods and services. Some of this information is needed to assess the need for funds either to purchase goods or services, or repay old debts. The rest indicates the value of resources, including cash, under the control of the various members of the organization. Such a system provides the basis for rendering a 'stewardship' account to owners, ratepayers, taxpayers or other interested parties outside the organization of the total amount of funds raised and the way they have been used — information which is used also to assess the organization's dependence upon, and need for, external finance. It also provides a limited amount of information which is useful for planning and controlling the utilization of resources within the enterprise.

The main limitation of stewardship or financial accounting, however, is that it is essentially historical in nature and provides information only upon what *has* happened, not what *ought* to have happened. Moreover, the analysis of financial transactions which the basic double-entry records provide is often inadequate for the needs of internal management.

In consequence, some form of financial budgeting and cost analysis is required if an organization's system of financial control is to be in any sense complete. The techniques of financial accounting, cost accounting and budgeting control are explained at some length later. For now it is enough to recognize that these information systems, their operation and design, are essentially a part of the finance function which thus impinges upon, and for practical purposes is inseparable from, the other functions in terms of which an organization may be analysed. Thus, whilst the primary data from which financial plans and records are built up are for the most part collected from outside the data processing or other sections of the finance department, nevertheless, the task of designing and supervising procedures for the collection of data, which are relevant to the management of financial aspects of the enterprise, almost invariably falls within the finance officer's range of duties. So too does the design and supervision of associated procedures for ensuring the security and proper utilization of the organization's different resources, which necessitates the financial specialist advising upon the way in which the responsibilities for the authorization of the use of resources, their physical control, and the associated record-keeping, are allocated to different individuals within the organization. Matters such as these come under the heading of internal check and internal audit procedures, and are explained later.

To summarize, *Figure 11.3* charts the relationship between different aspects of the finance function. It shows that the finance officer is responsible for advising on the raising of funds and their disbursement, actually controlling the receipt and payment of cash and organizing financial information systems. Its intention is to emphasize that the processing of financial information is independent of physicial cash flows and that, although ultimately actual cash receipts and payments arise out of the raising of finance and its expenditure, financial

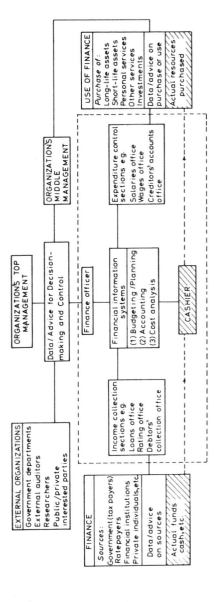

Figure 11.3. The finance function in perspective. (1) The oblong of broken lines surrounds activities concerned with finance functions. This does not imply that these are all necessarily located in a separate finance office. (2) Unbroken lines connecting the various entities or sections, within or outside the organization, are not arrowed since information flows which they represent are generally two-way. (3) The physical flows of cash etc. into the organization, and their conversion into real resources are distinguished from information flows to emphasize the physical and informational aspects of resource utilization

recording involves much more than keeping track of flows of cash. At the same time, it shows that the finance officer's tasks of advising, exercising physical control over cash flows and organizing information systems are all related, however the various tasks may be distributed amongst the members of a finance officer's staff, and emphasizes that financial information systems lie at the heart of the management process.

FINANCIAL CONTROL AND THE ORGANIZATION OF RESPONSIBILITIES

Financial control is fundamentally concerned with the utilization of valuable resources. But it is people who use or misuse resources so that the ability to control the way resources are used depends upon being able to control the actions of individuals. Obviously, therefore, there are various physical, psychological and legal factors which will determine how far individuals can or will comply with requests, instructions or orders so that, ultimately, control problems revolve around human personalities. However, in order to establish any basis for control it is necessary to identify: (1) the extent of a person's responsibility for using resources; (2) the nature or purpose of this responsibility; and (3) the particular kind of resource involved. For example, the Medical Officer of Health in a local authority has overall responsibility for translating the health committee's policies into effect. The extent of his responsibility may be identified in financial terms by the size of the budget approved for his department's work. The nature of his responsibility derives from the particular objectives which the policies of the health committee seeks to achieve, for example, the prevention and treatment of disease and the provision of a health visiting service, for which medical equipment, the services of doctors, health visitors and so on will be required. However imprecise or ambiguous the policies of the committee were, he would clearly not be considered to be carrying out his responsibilities properly if he overspent his budget allocation or used funds to establish, for example, a pharmacist's shop. The real difficulty in establishing a control system lies in defining responsibilities so that it is possible to identify when they are not being fulfilled. This is particularly so where authority must be delegated, because of the size or complexity of the organizational unit, and many individuals are involved in accomplishing its objectives and using its resources. Thus the effectiveness of a control system depends largely upon being able to identify particular individuals' responsibilities and then trace how far they are fulfilling them; and in many cases it is difficult or even impossible, with the techniques at present available, to gain the degree of control which management would consider ideal, at least without the system costing more than the resultant benefits warrant.

There are two main stages in financial control. First, the decision making aspect and, secondly, control in the sense of ensuring decisions are implemented. In both the local authority health service and the hospital service financial plans or budgets are prepared which embody the outcome of policy decisions, indicating the amounts of expenditure approved, in more or less detail, for different purposes. Such budgets set limits to the amount which can be spent on the service as a whole, and on particular aspects of it. The extent to which such plans may be used for control purposes will depend upon how far they identify the particular amounts with the various tasks to be accomplished, or the persons responsible for them. But however constructed, once approved by the appropriate authorizing body, they indicate the amount of the funds which may be legitimately used for the purposes laid down and provide the basis for some degree of financial control.

The second stage of control, once the extent of funds authorized has been established, consists of ensuring they are actually obtained and used for the purposes intended. The finance officer's task is to ensure that (1) monetary funds due to the service are assessed and collected; (2) money is only spent in amounts and for purposes as authorized in the budget; (3) goods and services purchased are actually received; (4) arrangements exist for the security of resources utillized; and (5) goods and services are actually used for the purposes authorized. In order to accomplish this task the finance officer depends upon his accounting records to trace the flows of money and resources into, through, and out of the organization. This means that he must attempt to ensure that the various persons responsible for the physical flows of money and resources can account for the amounts under their control and how they are used. Again the degree to which control can be exercised in detail will depend upon the form of the accounting records kept and the amount and type of information which individuals are required, or are able, to provide relating to the flow of resources.

Control is not, it must be emphasized, simply a matter of keeping records alone. Book-keeping entries merely give a picture of what is happening according to those who have supplied the data for recording in the accounts. It is important, therefore, that there should be some reconciliation of the accounting records with the physical facts of the situation and that, so far as is possible, the method of collecting the primary data ensures its accuracy. Thus (1) internal check and (2) audit procedures complete the arrangements for a system of financial control based upon a financial budget and an accounting system.

The principle underlying an internal check system is that members of an organization should have their responsibilities so arranged that their activities constitute a check upon each other. In particular, no single person should be in a position where he is responsible for *all* of the following aspects of transactions involving the raising or use of scarce resources.

(1)   Authorizing the raising or use of funds, monetary or real.
(2)   Holding or storing funds.
(3)   Actually using funds to provide services.
(4)   Recording transactions relating to such funds.

For example, if an accountant kept records relating to debts owed to his organization, handled cash receipts and was authorized to write off bad debts, he might record debts as being bad which had actually been paid and pocket the cash paid in. Thus, in practice the authority for writing off bad debts usually rests in a senior official, and a cashier's responsibilities do not include keeping the main debtors' records.

Internal check procedures, often laid down in the standing orders or financial regulations of the organization concerned, help to prevent or reveal both deliberate or accidental misapplications of resources *and* inaccuracies in the data processing procedures. Such procedures include not simply the identification of different individuals' responsibilities but authorization, requisitioning, tendering, ordering, purchasing, certification, payment and recording procedures covering all the stages in the raising and use of funds. The size of an organization often makes it impracticable to achieve an entirely satisfactory separation of responsibilities, and the need to secure economies in operation may lead to tasks being combined which, from an internal check point of view, would be better separated. There may thus be, conflict between a principle of financial control and some overriding management principle.

Internal check procedures must not be confused with audit, and particularly *internal audit,* procedures. Audit involves the authentication of an organization's records by ascertaining whether they represent what has actually happened, or what the actual position is. An auditor must, therefore, not merely check the arithmetic accuracy of the records, but reconcile the records with the legal and physical aspects of the transactions they represent. In principle, an auditor must be independent in that he is not himself involved in any aspect of the work he audits. Invariably, local authorities and hospital authorities are subject to some form of external audit by law in the same way that companies must have their accounts audited under the provisions of the Companies Acts. In addition to external audit, however, most organizations of any size employ internal auditors. The internal auditor's task is to maintain a continuous supervision over the system of financial control, regularly reconciling records with the facts of organizational activity and looking out for weaknesses in the internal check arrangements. The internal auditor is usually responsible to the treasurer or chief financial officer, and is a part only of the internal financial control system whose adequacy the external auditor must take into account in performing his own particular duties.

It will be evident that all members of an organization play some part in its system of financial control. For most this often takes the form of initiating, scrutinizing or certifying documents which provide information regarding the use of resources, such as the filling in of time sheets or the requisitioning of materials from stores. Such data form the basis for decision making and control, so that quite apart from the physical use made of resources everyone can play an important part in management by ensuring that information is accurately compiled.

Budgetary Control

Since a budget is a financial plan its form, method of preparation and use will be influenced in two main ways. First, by the sources and methods used to finance the activities of the enterprise for which it is prepared and, secondly, by the purposes for which the money is to be spent, that is, the nature of the enterprise's activities.

Public authorities inevitably raise the vast bulk of money needed to finance their activities either by levying rates or taxes upon the public, or certain sections of it, or by charging those directly benefiting from the services they provide. Even though, initially, public bodies may borrow money to finance their services, sooner or later the repayments of the loans raised, plus interest thereon, must be met by members of the public, either as taxpayers or customers. In order to assess the taxes or charges to be levied some estimate of the total expenditure must be made.

Financial planning, for taxation purposes in particular, has traditionally focused attention upon the need to establish the rate or level of taxation to impose for the year ahead. At central government level, the annual budget embodies taxation proposals for the coming year and the Finance Act gives legal effect to them, whilst local authorities must by law fix a rate for the ensuing 12 months. In order to calculate the rate at which to set taxes or rates, therefore, the authorities concerned are compelled to survey their spending requirements at least one year ahead.

The resources required to sustain most services may be divided into two broad categories: (1) those which once purchased will last several years such as buildings, machinery and vehicles; and (2) those which are used up quickly, especially within one year, such as fuel, power and the services of employees. In fact, the year is adopted by accountants as the basis for distinguishing between *capital* and *revenue* expenditure respectively. It will be apparent that however long an asset may last its cost must sooner or later be met, in the case of public bodies, by levying taxes or charges to cover it. At the same time, since certain assets provide services for several years it makes sense, on the grounds of equity, that the cost should be met by those benefiting from them each year. Yet whilst expenditure may be charged out, or recovered, over several years, it is necessary to obtain finance initially to purchase the assets by borrowing or from some other source. Paralleling the distinction between capital and revenue *expenditure,* therefore, is the distinction between capital and revenue *finance,* so that a budget is ultimately the result of two sets of decisions relating to how much to spend and how to finance the expenditure, both of which are related to each other and for which the time factor plays a crucial role. Thus the stimulus to expenditure lies in the needs of citizens for health services, and these needs change over time for many reasons both as to their kind and their urgency. Similarly, on the financing side, the availability of finance alters over time. In particular, it may be politically inexpendient to raise the level of rates or taxes at a particular time.

One of the fundamental problems, then, in preparing a budget is that of deciding how far to look ahead: should plans be made, and their financial effects assessed for one, five, ten or even more years ahead? This is a question to which attention will be given later. For now it is enough to note that even where expenditure is financed by borrowing initially, the amount of the debt charges and associated running (or revenue) expenses must be assessed at least for the following year ahead.

So far the budget has been discussed as if it were simply a means of assessing the amount of finance required, although this clearly involves some consideration of how the money is to be spent. However, more than just summarizing the financial plans of an authority, the budget has come to be the basis of financial control in providing a yardstick by which to measure how far *actual* expenditure and funds raised conformed with, or departed from, the plans made. More than this, once approved by the relevant body the budget establishes the authority for spending and financing activities and clarifies the limits upon executive action envisaged by the policy makers.

It is important, therefore, to think of the budget in relation to both the decision making and control aspects of management. As a document, or series of documents, the budget simply reflects the final outcome of decisions made regarding objectives to pursue and how to finance them. At the same time, it provides the starting point for controlling administrative action taken to implement these decisions. How far the plans it embodies are capable of fulfilment and thus meaningful, and how far it provides an effective basis for control purposes will depend upon the decision making processes and techniques adopted on the one hand, and upon the form which the budget takes on the other.

BUDGETING IN LOCAL GOVERNMENT

Local authorities vary both in size and in range of functions. Moreover, they are autonomous and have the responsibility not merely for spending but for raising the necessary finance. Nor surprisingly, therefore, there is no uniform procedure of budgeting in local government in the same detailed way as exists in the hospital service. However, the need to comply with the numerous legal requirements with respect to both methods and sources of finance, the objectives on which money can be spent and the organizational structure of an authority have resulted in a distinguishable broad pattern of procedures which run through local government authorities generally.

The timing and mechanics of the estimates procedure

The size and complexity of a particular local authority's organizational structure affects both the time over which a budget is prepared and the procedures adopted. For authorities which are large the compilation of estimates will begin several months in advance of final approval of the rate to be levied.

First of all, it is usual to ascertain the actual expenditure during the current year up to the time of commencing the preparation of estimates. This provides an indication of how far actual expenditure is currently departing from what was previously planned and thus a basis for revising the previous year's approved estimates to show how much will be spent by the end of the current year. Having revised the current year's estimates in the light of the trend of actual expenditure, the following year's estimates may then be more realistically framed and any likely over or under spendings on the current year taken into account in fixing the next year's estimates and rate.

The compilation of revised, actual and estimated expenditure figures usually follows the classification of expenditure in the financial accounting records. In most authorities this classification is based upon the standard form devised and recommended for adoption by the Institute of Municipal Treasurers and Accountants (I.M.T.A). This classification provides for total expenditure to be analysed under objective headings describing a particular service or section thereof, and within these headings on a subjective basis, that is, on the basis of the type of input on which money is expended. Table 11.1 shows the major classifications on the standard form and their relationship to each other. Table 11.2 shows how they are used in considering budgetary requirements.

Naturally, the co-operation of the accountant and administrative officers of the various departments is required in preparing both revised actual figures and future estimates. The accountant is able to

TABLE 11.1
I.M.T.A. Standard Form Classifications

OBJECTIVE CLASSIFICATIONS

(I) *Main service headings*	(II) *Division of service headings*	(III) *Sub-division of service headings*
Health	Administration (Health Office)	
Education	Health centres	
Welfare	Care of mothers and young	
Parks	children	Day nurseries
Highways	Midwifery	Clinics and centres
etc.	Health visiting	Dental care
	Home nursing	Mother and baby
	Vaccination and	homes
	immunization	Other services
	Ambulance service	
	Prevention of illness	
	Care and after care	
	Domestic help	
	Mental health	
	Other health services	

SUBJECTIVE CLASSIFICATIONS

(I) *Standard groupings*	(II) *Sub-groupings*	(III) *Detail headings*
(a) Expenditure classifications		
Employees		Repair etc. of buildings
Running expenses	Premises	Alterations to buildings
Debt charges	Supplies and	Maintenance of grounds
Revenue contributions	services	Fuel, light, cleaning
to capital outlay	Transport and heavy	materials and water
	plant	Furniture and fittings
	Establishment	Rent and rates
	expenses	Contribution to renewal
	Agency services	and repairs fund
	Miscellaneous	Apportionment of
	expenses	expenses of operational
		buildings
(b) Income classifications		
Government grants		Fees, tolls, etc.
Sales		Charges for concerts etc.
Fees and charges		Contributions towards
Rents		maintenance costs
Interest		Contributions by other
Miscellaneous income		local and public
		authorities
		Board and accommodation
		charges (staff)

(1)   The divisions of service headings illustrated relate to the Health Services Act, 1946, and not to other local authority health services such as Rodent Control, Baths and so on which might be added to this list.

(2)   Sub-divisions of service headings are illustrated only by reference to Care of Mothers etc. division.

(3)   In the subjective classification only running expenses is broken down into sub-groupings as an intermediate classification. Other standard groupings (I) nevertheless encompass many detailed (III) classifications similar to that shown for the premises sub-grouping, or fees and charges standard grouping.

(4)   The way in which the I.M.T.A. classifications are applied in local authorities depends upon their range of services, organizational structure, and amount of detail which they wish to produce or publish.

(5)   The classifications adopted attempt to provide for comparability of financial data between different authorities, whilst allowing for flexibility in application to different organizational structures. Comparability is achieved particularly by the standardized subjective classifications.

(6)   This Standard Form of classification for all local authority services has, since 1958, been supplemented by more detailed recommendations for various individual services and designed to allow for the peculiarities of the different services. The health and welfare service forms produced recently, and intended to be adopted from the 1st April 1970, prescribe methods of apportioning such expenses as those of administrative staff and buildings to other divisions of service headings. They deal with problems similar to those discussed on pages 298 to 293 and are intended to ensure that government grant claims and inter-authority comparisons are dealt with on a comparable basis.

TABLE 11.2

Financial Statement for Budgetary Purposes Based Upon IMTA Standard Form

Day nurseries	1970–1 estimate	1970–1 actual expenditure to date	1970–1 revised actual	1971–2 estimate
Employees	30,000	17,000	33,000	35,000
Running expenses				
premises	6,000	2,800	5,900	6,100
supplies and services	4,500	2,300	4,800	4,700
establishment	4,000	1,900	3,700	4,000
miscellaneous	200	120	200	200
	(14,700)	(7,120)	(14,600)	(15,000)
Debt charges	1,000	500	1,000	1,100
Total	£45,700	£24,620	£48,600	£51,100

(1)   The third column shows the actual expenditure as shown in the accounting records up to the date at which the statement is prepared. Where a following year's estimates have to be considered several months in advance only 6–7 months, figures may be available.

(2)   The fourth column shows likely actual expenditure on basis of knowledge regarding trend and pay/price increases.

(3)   Comparison with the first column enables likely over/under spendings to be assessed.

(4)   In practice such statements might show all the detailed headings provided by the standard form, and for other objective headings might have additional subjective groupings, for example, Revenue contributions to capital outlay, or transport expenses.

(5)   Income has been ignored.

(6)   Additional columns might be used to show previous years' figures or over/under spendings.

supply from his accounting records information on what has happened up to date and to advise on such matters as the likely effect of employee's superannuation schemes, insurances and loan charges on a department's expenditure. On the other hand a department's administrator, rather than the accountant, will know of possible expansions in the service, changes in establishment and so on.

It will be apparent that if the effects of new capital expenditure is to be included in the revenue estimates, some examination of intended capital schemes is a necessary part of the revenue estimate procedure. In principle, capital estimates may be related to revenue estimates by approaching the problem in one of two ways. Either, the local authority will have established at some time in the past a comprehensive programme of development as a guide to the commencement of schemes in particular years, in which case the health department will take this into account in formulating its revenue estimates; alternatively, in the absence of any capital programme, the health department will include the effect of schemes which its medical officer and the health committee consider should be included for the year in question. The former approach suggests itself as being more rational, in so far as the overall and long-term effects are considered, and in planning the development of all services the need to co-ordinate the efforts of different local authority services may be made more apparent and taken into account. The absence of some previously determined programme of development inevitably increases the possibility that services will be developed in a haphazard way both as to timing and their effect on other departments. On the other hand a rigidly laid down programme may ignore changes in need or available resources, and in practice some adjustments to a prescribed programme will be necessary.

The arrangements for preparing revenue estimates differ from one authority to the next, and the involvement of both members and officers varies. A typical pattern for health service estimates would be as follows.

(1) Preparation of estimates by health department officials in co-operation with treasurer's staff.

(2) Submission of the estimates to the health committee for approval.

(3) Incorporation of the health services estimates into a preliminary overall budget for the authority by the officers of the finance department.

(4) Consideration by the finance committee of the overall effect.

(5) Return to the health committee for further consideration in the light of recommendations or comments of the finance committee on the availability of funds.

(6)   Reconsideration by the health committee, with the medical officer advising on the effect of deleting particular items of expenditure.

(7)   Final approval of estimates, as amended by various committees, by the finance committee and incorporation into the annual budget to be presented to the council.

(8)   Presentation of the budget for approval by chairman of the finance committee, on the occasion of his budget speech before the council, and the fixing of the rate levy.

BUDGETING IN THE HOSPITAL SERVICE

Whilst in local government the procedure for the preparation of estimates varies in form and timing between authorities due to differences in size, committee structure, departmental organization and the services administered; the hospital service, by contrast, exhibits a much greater uniformity.

The basic reason stems from the organization and financing of the hospital service on a national basis. Thus the Department of Health and Social Security with its responsibility for exercising overall control over the hospital service and obtaining the necessary finance from the Exchequer, lays down uniform procedures for budgeting which are followed by all the executive agencies; namely, the boards of governors of teaching hospitals, regional hospital boards and hospital management committees. Differences stem only from the different functions performed by the three types of body.

Broadly, the boards of governors administering hospitals bearing the responsibility for medical education prepare all the estimates, capital and revenue, required by the Secretary of State, whilst for the rest of the hospital service the budgetary process is divided between the regional hospital boards and the hospital management committees within the areas of the regional boards.

In particular the regional hospital boards, with their responsibility for planning and organizing the development of the hospital service within their regions and exercising overall supervision over hospital services, are concerned with assessing the requirements for capital finance for the region as a whole, since they administer capital spending and the region's hospital building programme. In addition, they co-ordinate, assess the effects of, and control the revenue expenditure estimates of the hospital management committees within their region and incorporate these with estimates relating to the maintenance or revenue expenditure of regional board services, administrative or specialist.

The Department of Health thus deals directly only with boards of governors and regional hospital boards; the latter being responsible for the activities of their hospital management committees, but in both cases capital and revenue requirements are separately presented. The Department, in order to obtain finance, must submit estimates to Parliament, via the Treasury and the Chancellor of the Exchequer, for approval, with or without amendment. Moreover, the Department has the problem of collating not only estimates for the hospital service but for other aspects of its work in applying for its total annual vote of funds from Parliament. In consequence, the processing of estimates has departed from the pattern laid down when the hospital service was first established on a national basis in 1948. Initially, hospital management committees submitted an estimate of expenditure and income for the forthcoming year to their regional hospital board, in a prescribed form, not later than the 1st September each year.

The regional hospital board, after examination of the hospital management committee's estimates with any modifications forwarded these, together with a summary of them and the regional hospital board's own estimates, to the Ministry by the 15th October.

By mid-January the Minister would inform the regional hospital board of the total sum allocated to each region for the forthcoming year, subject to the ultimate approval of Parliament and, after discussions with the hospital management committees, the regional hospital board would notify the total sums allocated to particular hospital management committees. Such sums would be notified in late February; and the hospital management committees were required to re-submit final *detailed* estimates of how the allocations were to be used for approval by the regional hospital board. Such detailed estimates formed the basis for control over actual spending in the year.

The sources of weakness in this procedure were threefold. (1) In order to complete the finalization of the Department's estimates, compilation had to be started at a very early date at the hospital management committee level. (2) The time for examination at each stage was necessarily limited in order to complete the overall process. (3) The estimates related to only one year ahead. The broad effect was that inadequate consideration tended to be given in formulating the estimates to the future development of the service, that is, insufficient attention was given to forward planning.

At the same time, the final allocations made to hospital management committees necessitated a late adjustment of the expenditure plans which had formed the basis of the original estimates.

Subsequent to the Report of the Working Party on Hospital Revenue Allocations in 1961, the budgetary process was changed and is no longer so rigidly geared to the parliamentary vote procedure. Thus, the Department now informs boards of their allocations for a particular year in the preceding August, and of provisional allocations for the year beyond that. Final detailed estimates of the way it is intended to spend the allocations are not forwarded to the Department by the regional hospital boards until about May, after discussion with the hospital management committees. In this way, the detailed use of available funds can be considered more carefully and with prior knowledge of how much is available. It may be inferred from this that the boards' and committees' role is simply to decide how to spend allocations predetermined for them by the Department, and that hence they are simply passive agents in the budgetary process. This is untrue in so far as the Department gains the information on which to base its allocations from statements prepared each year which show, with varying degrees of detail, the following data.

(1)   The actual expenditure for a particular year, for example, 1968/69.

(2)   The revised estimated expenditure for the current year, for example, 1969/70.

(3)   The estimated expenditure for the following year, for example, 1970/71.

(4)   The forecasts of expenditure for two further years, for example, 1971/72 and 1972/73.

Thus, for example, allocations for 1971/72 and provisional allocations for 1972/73, notified in August 1970 by the Department, would be based upon forecasts made in earlier years by the boards, interpreted in the light of whatever subsequent information relating to actual expenditures, revised estimates, estimates and forecasts, becomes available with each year, and with regard to changes of policy and the constraints imposed by central government decisions regarding the rate of growth of public expenditure on particular services and in total.

The effect, broadly, is that the Department decides the total amounts to be included in its Parliamentary estimates at a fairly early date on the basis of forecasts; thus giving boards and committees a firmer basis for deciding their detailed patterns of spending, and a longer time for considering them than formerly. The Department then uses the latest information on actual expenditures, revised estimates and so on, in drawing up the Parliamentary estimates in the detail required for vote purposes. This involves making allowances for salary and price increases, or other factors which have altered or become apparent since the original allocations were decided upon.

The system outlined is but a part of the complicated pattern of control over public expenditure which has developed since World War II and which owes much to the ideas contained in the 1944 White Paper on employment policy and the Plowden Committee's 'Report on the Control of Public Expenditure in 1960'. Thus the annual budget has become an instrument for regulating the economy as a whole rather than just an exercise in assessing the needs and means of financing public services. A system of five-year 'forward looks' attempting to assess the effect of the whole range of public expenditure proposals in terms of their demand on real resources has been developed which extends beyond those which are voted on annually by the House of Commons, thus providing for a more complete and longer-term approach to the planning and control of public expenditure. The pattern reflects the fact that parliamentary control over public expenditure is achieved not so much by the ability of the members of the House of Commons to decide in detail the amounts of public money to be spent, but the extent to which they can in various ways influence the broad policies of the government of the day which set the pattern of public expenditure and attack the way money has eventually been spent as revealed by the Appropriation Accounts laid before Parliament in the year following the spending.

COMPARISON BETWEEN LOCAL AUTHORITY AND HOSPITAL SERVICE PROCEDURES

The estimates procedures in public authorities stem principally from the need to calculate the rate of taxation to be levied in a particular year, yet the method of classification of expenditure adopted in presenting the estimates for approval also provides a basis for exercising control as the money is actually spent.

We have also seen that in the hospital service the complexity, at central government level, of the processes of planning and controlling public expenditure has resulted in the compilation of estimates at committee and board level playing only a subsidiary role in so far as assessing the amount of taxation to levy is concerned. The practical significance of the detailed estimates prepared at the regional and committee levels lies in their usefulness in establishing a set of criteria by which to prescribe and define the authority for spending funds so as to assess whether or not it has been exceeded. In local government, mainly because of the existence of a substantial degree of independence, the primary need to establish the rate levy for the following year is still relatively important, though the significance of approved estimates for control purposes parallels that of the hospital service.

In both types of authority the estimates are, however, built up on a 'subjective' classification of expenditure; that is on the 'line-by-line' or input categorization of expenses rooted in traditional financial accounting classifications. This method of classifying expenditure, together with the manner in which the distinction between capital and revenue items is dealt with in the financial accounting systems of these authorities, needs further consideration if the nature and the problems of financial management are to be fully appreciated.

However, some of the problems of operating financial control on this basis must be highlighted immediately. Where control revolves around ensuring overspendings of authorized amounts do not occur, and authority for expenditure is based upon subjective classifications of expenditure, and, further, capital allocations are treated separately from revenue allocations, the possibility arises that attention in management both in decision making and control will be unduly focused upon particular inputs to the detriment of the outputs, or overall objectives, they are intended, when used in combination, to achieve.

Thus executives may attempt to ensure they get at least the same allocation of resources for particular inputs, for example cleaners' wages or cleaning materials and equipment, as in the current year without giving adequate attention to changing the combination of inputs required to achieve the same end product; for example by using a contractor's services or more expensive equipment but less manpower. Having been given authority to spend on particular headings they may also aim to ensure they spend the full amount authorized, lest subsequent allocations be reduced, regardless of the contribution a particular input makes to the efficient operation of their section or the organization in general. This is especially so where allocations are rigidly tied to particular financial years, and provision for carrying forward unspent authorizations is not permitted by the budgetary regulations laid down.

In practice, of course, a good deal of informal discussion takes place in attempting to relate capital expenditure proposals and the associated revenue implications; and in controlling actual spending, the practice of *virement* seeks to mitigate the difficulties of detailed authorization of expenditure. *Virement* means simply allowing an overspending on one heading of expenditure to be offset against an underspent heading. But this raises further problems. Executives may seek to manipulate their estimates, inflating apparently essential items of expenditure at estimate stage, in the hope of using eventual underspendings for less important purposes; the effect being to reduce the control of those authorizing expenditure over the organization of priorities in the use of scarce resources.

Differences in the procedures for discussion, co-ordination between different participants, and allowing for flexibility in implementing budgetary authorizations in different authorities and at different levels, prevents any general conclusion about the effectiveness of budgetary control in the health services as a whole. Potential sources of weakness emerge more clearly from an examination of the associated techniques of financial and cost accounting.

The Financial Accounts

The double-entry system of recording transactions, and events affecting the wealth of an organization, achieves two distinct ends simultaneously. First, it provides a degree of control over the accuracy with which transactions are recorded, and secondly, and more importantly, it provides for the classification of transactions in a way which enables the different financial aspects of an organization to be distinguished and their effect on the organization to be clearly displayed.

Whatever techniques of data processing are used, from pen and ink manual records to modern electronic computers, the double-entry system, like any other form of data processing, has both inputs and outputs. Inputs take many forms such as time-sheets, salary registers, stores requisition and issue notes, receipts, cheque-book counterfoils, minutes and so on, and these different sources of information are referred to as 'primary' data. The output of the double-entry system takes the form of two main financial statements: the income and expenditure (in commercial undertakings, profit and loss) account and the balance sheet, though this is not to say that other statements may not be produced. In practice, various methods of collecting and organizing the primary data for classification are adopted. Thus memorandum books or journals, and specialized books or ledgers dealing with only one type of transaction, such as debts owed to or by the organization, are used to achieve a preliminary classification or summary of numerous detailed transactions. But however many subsidiary records or manipulations of primary data are involved, and however many individuals initiate or process the primary data, the end result is that a complete record of the organization's financial transactions, arising from dealings with other parties, is available in the form of a set of 'ledger' accounts. In other words, the information required to prepare an income and expenditure account and a balance sheet will, at any time, be available in the double-entry system, though it may need adjusting to make the statements comparable with those for other organizations or periods.

Suppose, for example, a private nursing home is set up by a group of people on a commercial basis. They would contribute funds which may be labelled or classified in two ways if the view is taken that the nursing home is in some way an enterprise or entity separate from that of its managers or owners. First it can be said that the entity owes its owners the amount they have contributed in order to finance its activities, or alternatively that the entity's source of funds is ownership or 'equity' capital. Secondly, the funds may be described by their physical characteristics, for example, buildings, land, fixtures or cash. Similarly, any other funds placed under the control of the home's managers could be so classified as to their *source* and the *form* they take. The records showing the amounts at which these funds are valued in money terms are simply classified into as many headings or 'accounts' as is necessary to show: (1) the forms of the wealth; and (2) the source(s) of the wealth at the disposal of the enterprise.

The 'balance' under a particular classification is simply the amount remaining on an account after allowing for all the transactions which increase or decrease a particular category. If, in addition to subscribing funds of their own, the proprietors of the nursing home raised a bank loan and bought supplies on credit from various suppliers, their 'balance sheet' at the time they commenced operations would follow a particular pattern (Table 11.3).

TABLE 11.3
The XYZ Private Nursing Home Balance Sheet as at 1.1.70.

Forms of wealth		Sources of wealth	
Property	6,000	Owners' capital	8,000
Equipment	2,000	Bank loan	1,000
Stores	1,000	Creditors	1,000
Cash at bank	1,000		
	£10,000		£10,000

The 'forms' and 'sources' are shown on the opposite sides from the presentation usually adopted in the UK. The treatment here is more useful for explaining the process of accounting.

From this it can be seen that the home's *assets* equal its *liabilities* to: (1) its owners and (2) outsiders (the bank and suppliers). It is important to realize the 'double-entry' relationship of these figures. For example, if cash (£1,000) is used to pay off the creditors this single transaction would have, from a recording point of view, the *dual* effect of eliminating both the cash *and* the creditors balances. Or alternatively if

267

it were used to buy more stores one asset balance would be increased (stores), and another (cash) eliminated or reduced depending upon the size of the transaction. Thus if, in recording, the same numerical value is not entered correctly in the two accounts affected, the error shows up in the shape of an imbalance. To this extent the system contains a check on the recording process itself.

More important than this in-built checking device, however, is the fact that the dual effect on the financial position of the organization is registered for each single transaction. Thus any transaction will have one of the following effects.

(1) Both an asset and liability will come into being.

(2) One asset will be exchanged for another.

(3) One liability will replace another.

(4) Both an asset and a liability will be extinguished.

Broadly the effect in terms of a balance sheet of a particular transaction will be either to show an increase or decrease in total funds available, or simply a change in the composition of the assets, or liabilities with the total available funds unchanged. A balance sheet extracted from the accounting records at any time, therefore, will give important information relating to: (1) the total funds available; (2) the extent of indebtedness to third parties; and (3) the form in which the funds are held. In particular for commercial organizations it will give an indication of the liquidity position of the organization: that is, the availability of cash or near cash assets from which to meet the demand of creditors.

It will be clear that the information contained in a balance sheet relates only to the overall position at a particular *point* in time. In order to know this, it is necessary to establish two measures. First, one which shows the total expenses, or funds used up in producing products or services during a period, and another showing the amount of revenues or funds arising from the sale of these products or services to customers. The double-entry system, by establishing account classifications for expenses and revenues as well as for assets and liabilities, allows for the effect of transactions to be related to particular periods of time as well as at points of time. A simple example will show what is involved.

Suppose, the XYZ Nursing Home uses its cash over a particular period a 'year' to pay the salaries and wages of staff and other expenses of running the home, and that it sends bills out to patients charging them £3,000 for its services. Cash would decrease, and a balance of expenses would build up of equivalent amount. Similarly, it would record the debts of its clients as assets showing an equivalent balance on a 'revenues' or 'sales' account, to indicate that the source of the new assets was from selling operations. The effect of these transactions in terms of a balance sheet at the end of the period, assuming no other transaction, might follow a particular pattern (Table 11.4).

However, the expenses represent assets which have been used up during the period and are of no further benefit to the organization, and the revenues show the monetary benefits arising from the period's activities alone. It is usual, therefore, to separate these 'revenue' transactions into a separate income and expenditure (or profit and loss) account or statement (Table 11.5).

TABLE 11.4
The XYZ Private Nursing Home Balance Sheet as at 31.12.70.

Forms of wealth		Sources of wealth	
Property	6,000	Owners' capital	8,000
Equipment	2,000	Bank loan	1,000
Stores	1,000	Creditors	1,000
Expenses	1,000	Revenues	3,000
Debtors	3,000		
	£13,000		£13,000

TABLE 11.5

Income statement for the period 1.1.70—31.12.70			
Expenses	1,000	Revenues	3,000
Net profit	2,000		
	£ 3,000		£ 3,000

Balance sheet as at 31.12.70			
Forms of wealth		Sources of wealth	
Property	6,000	Owners' capital	8,000
Equipment	2,000	Net profit	2,000
Stores	1,000		10,000
Debtors	3,000	Bank loan	1,000
		Creditors	1,000
	£12,000		£12,000

In the actual records, therefore, the expenses of a period are 'matched' against the revenues by transferring individual account balances to a summary account, and the net balance resulting — profit or loss — reflects the increase or decrease in total wealth over the period concerned in running the business. Of course, if the proprietors introduce more capital during the period or raise funds from other sources such as creditors or lenders, the total wealth at the disposal of the business will increase in any event. But these sources must not be confused with earnings resulting from actual operations. Equally, the proprietors might withdraw funds, either their original capital* or the profits, or repay third parties, thus reducing the total funds (from both the asset or liability point of view) connected with the business entity. However, their ability to withdraw funds and repay debts will depend upon the availability of liquid resources (that is, cash or near-cash assets). Thus, in the example, although revenue has been *earned*, it is still in the form of debts since the debtors have not yet paid cash. This emphasizes the point that the calculation of income is not measured by simply matching *cash* payments against cash receipts.

The two statements which the 'double-entry' system is devised to produce highlight two interdependent aspects of finance: the measurement of *income* and *capital*. Thus the income statement shows the income produced during a period of time, whilst the balance sheet shows the capital employed at a particular point of time. The problem of measuring income and capital is, however, much more difficult than the illustrations given so far suggest.

If expenses are to be assessed correctly, and these are defined as the value of assets used up in earning revenue, then any stores used to this end or loss in the value of such items as property or equipment should be included as expenses just as much as items such as salaries and wages, or heating and lighting expenses.

Suppose, in terms of the XYZ Nursing Home, £800 worth of stores were used up during the 'year' and that property and equipment declined in value by £200 and £100 respectively; these amounts must increase the expenses shown in the income statement and reduce the assets figures shown on the balance sheet (Table 11.6).

This simple example shows the importance of ensuring that all types of expense are accounted for in measuring the income of a period. Not only is income overstated unless expenses are fully accounted for but in the balance sheet capital employed is shown at a figure in excess of its true value. There is thus a danger that proprietors will take out of the

*The legal form of the enterprise might present obstacles to the withdrawal of capital originally subscribed; for example, in the case of a limited company.

business profits calculated at too high a figure and thus in effect take out funds which constitute the capital base of the organization.

TABLE 11.6

Income statement for the period 1.1.70–31.12.70

Expenses	1,000	Revenues	3,000
Cost (or expense) of stores used	800		
Depreciation expenses			
(a) Property	200		
(b) Equipment	100		
	2,100		
Net profit	900		
	£ 3,000		£ 3,000

Balance sheet as at 31.12.70

Forms of wealth			Sources of wealth	
Property at cost	6,000		Owners' capital	8,000
Less depreciation	200	5,800	Add net profit	900
Equipment at cost	2,000			8,900
Less depreciation	100	1,900	Bank loan	1,000
Current assets			Creditors	1,000
Stores		200		
Debtors		3,000		
		£10,900		£10,900

At this point, some of the main concepts and conventions which underlie double-entry accounting may be summarized as follows.

(1) Accountants distinguish an 'entity' separate from its owner(s). This enables them to relate the recording system to the objectives of the organization alone and show the financial consequences of money invested towards a particular end.

(2) By adopting a dual classification of financial transaction and events, not only is an arithmetic check built into the recording system but different financial effects can be displayed clearly.

(3) By adopting the year as a conventional period for assessing the results of operations, transactions may be classified as to whether they are

of a capital or revenue nature, and expenses may be matched against revenues on the basis of a standard time period, thus facilitating comparisons between other time periods and organizations using the same convention.

(4) In measuring income by matching expenses against revenues, rather than cash payments against cash recepts, income measurement is made less arbitrary and recognition is given to the fact that the time when goods and services are produced or used may be quite different from the time when money is paid or received for them.

APPLICATION OF DOUBLE-ENTRY ACCOUNTING IN LOCAL AUTHORITIES

Local authorities distinguish between capital and revenue transactions. Further, local authorities show detailed classification of expenses and revenues for a financial year on the lines indicated in Table 11.2. Such statements are analogous to the income statements and balance sheets prepared by private sector commercial organizations and are derived from the double-entry records of the local authority which accumulates and classifies primary data on the same lines as private organizations.

Differences in the application of the technique and the presentation of financial information stem mainly from differences in the methods of finance and the nature of the objectives of public authorities compared with private enterprise concerns. Yet the differences are one of emphasis rather than in any way absolute.

First of all, whereas a private firm has a voluntarily subscribed fund of capital which is used to finance capital and revenue expenditure alike, a local authority tends to raise finance specifically for one purpose, and thus maintains the distinction between capital and revenue classifications on the financing side more rigidly.

A particularly interesting feature of local authority accounts is that capital expenditure is retained in the records at the initial cost of the assets involved instead of the asset values being depreciated each accounting period. At first sight this practice suggests that the income and expenditure account and balance sheet of a local authority cannot show either the full expense of running its service, or realistic asset values in its balance sheet. In fact, what happens is that a local authority charges as an expense in its income and expenditure account the cost of repaying loans, or setting funds aside for their repayment, and shows the corresponding amount of loans redeemed in the balance sheet. To the extent that the amount of the loan charge for repayment of principal shown as an expense in the income and expenditure account is equivalent to the amount by which the asset bought from the loan has depreciated in value during the period the expenses shown in a local authority's records parallel the amount of expenses which would be shown by a private firm. The deduction of the amount of loan redeemed from the historical cost of the assets in the balance sheet would give a figure corresponding to the written down values of assets in a private firm's accounts.

It is, of course, unlikely for various reasons that the two methods of displaying the expense arising from the use of capital assets would coincide, except by chance. A local authority's loan charge (expense) would depend very much upon the period of the loan sanction for the particular asset concerned and upon its financing policy; for example, whether it repaid within the maximum period allowed. A private firm's charge for depreciation would depend upon which method of depreciation it employed. For example, an asset costing £1,000 might be expected to last ten years and have no scrap value at the end. Quite apart from the fact that its useful life might turn out to be either longer or shorter than this period, and it might have some scrap value when sold finally, it is possible to allocate the £1,000 over ten years in a variety of patterns: by a straight line (annually uniform); an increasing; a decreasing; or a variable charge. There is, therefore, an element of arbitrariness in both methods of calculating the expense of running the service involved if the underlying purpose is assumed to be the statement of the value of resources used up. In fact, local authority accounting aims at ensuring that an account of how far the amounts of taxation and expenditure authorized in approving the budget are actually raised or incurred, rather than any precise allocation of costs or benefits to particular accounting periods. The emphasis, that is, is upon preparing accountability or 'stewardship' accounts, which serve to show how those responsible for raising or disbursing public funds have carried out their responsibilities.

For this reason, the original cost of assets purchased is retained in the balance sheet and the original sources of finance are detailed so as to show how far the assets have been paid for, or the extent to which debt is still outstanding. This rationale also justifies the treatment of charging the costs of certain assets as expenses in the income and expenditure account, which according to a strict interpretation of the term 'capital expenditure' would be 'capitalized' in the accounts, and then shown as fixed assets in the balance sheet. Thus the cost of such assets as furniture, typewriters and the like, which obviously benefit more than one financial year, are shown as expenses of the year in which they are incurred. At least this is the case where the items are accepted as being ones which should be paid for out of the normal yearly income. In a fairly large authority with many such items there will be a tendency for a proportion to need renewing or replacing each year. In such a case, the cost of such items charged to the rates will tend to average out from year to year, and the replacement policy adopted may well be aimed at producing such a result.

Occasionally, where it is decided to finance a large item of expenditure of a capital nature from the revenue of a particular year, rather than borrow, the asset is capitalized in the accounts and shown on the balance sheet. But the income and expenditure account shows as expenditure the amount of this charge against revenue. This treatment may seem inconsistent, but it does underline the fact that local authority accounts aim particularly to reveal how money has actually been spent and raised.

The way the double-entry records are manipulated in local authorities is of concern to the financial specialist only, but the statements produced by his technique provide much of the basic data used in administering the various services. To illustrate the form of those statements we may use the example of the XYZ private nursing home, varying the assumptions made in that illustration to fit the local authority situation.

Suppose the AMC Local Authority establishes a mental health hostel; it needs the same amount of equipment and has the same pattern of expenses as the private nursing home. However, it charges no fees, the cost of the service falling upon the ratepayer. Table 11.7 shows the income and expenditure account and balance sheet which show the financial effect of running the home for the 'year' in question and the final position. It can be seen that expenses are the same as for the private organization, with the exception of the items labelled 'loan charges (principal)' and 'revenue contributions to capital outlay' which take the place of depreciation expense. The figure of £450 for loan repayment is based upon the following assumptions: (1) that the local authority has financed the purchase of the property costing £6,000 by raising a loan at the beginning of the year, repayable in equal instalments over 20 years; that is, at £300 per annum; (2) that the equipment costing £2,000 is financed partly by raising a loan for £1,500, repayable over 10 years, and partly by a revenue contribution of £500 from rates in the first year. The revenue contribution charge shown as an expense reflects the effect of this latter decision.

The total amount needed for the year's activities is thus £2,750, and this is shown as the amount of income raised from ratepayers to finance the service. It should be noted that it is shown as coming from the general rate fund since the different services are financed from such

THE FINANCIAL ACCOUNTS

TABLE 11.7
AMC Local Authority Hostel – Balance Sheet at Year's End

Capital outlay		Loans outstanding		7,050
Property	6,000	Current liabilities		
Equipment	2,000	Creditors		1,000
	£8,000	Capital discharged		
Current assets			300.	
Stores	200	Loans redeemed	150	450
Cash	800	Revenue contributions to		
		capital outlay		500
	£9,000			£9,000

Income and expenditure account for year

Employees		Income from rates (via	
Salaries etc.	1,800	general rate fund)	2,750
Running expenses			
Stores etc.			
Loan charges			
Principal	150		
	300		
Interest	–		
Revenue contributions to			
capital outlay	500		
	£2,750		£2,750

Cash account
(as shown in the actual records – not presented with the above statements)

Receipts		Payments	
Loan	7,500	Loans repaid	150
			300
From ratepayers	2,750	Salaries	1,000
		For property	6,000
		For equipment	2,000
	10,250		9,450
		Balance in hand	800
	£10,250		£10,250

275

a fund*, and in this example, in the absence of any income from other sources such as fees paid by the residents or other authorities using the service, it represents the net charge to the ratepayers for the year for this particular service. This figure of income represents the amount required to finance the cost of resources used up in providing services for the year. It says nothing about whether the authority has: (1) purchased more resources than it has used, (2) paid for them or (3) actually received cash from the ratepayers. Thus, in this example, it purchased £1,000 of stores but only used £800 worth. It did not pay for any of the stores purchased; hence the creditors still outstanding at the year end. It is assumed, however, that cash equivalent to the income required from the general rate fund has been received. Thus the balance sheet can be considered to consist of two sections: a capital and a revenue section. The capital section shows that capital outlay, amounting to £8,000, has been financed in such a way that by the end of the 'year' £7,050 is still owed to lenders, whilst £450 of original debt has been redeemed and £500 was contributed from revenue thus avoiding recourse to loan or other financing methods. The revenue section shows that the authority still owes £1,000 for goods purchased, of which £200 has still not been used, and the cost of the rest has been provided for and is shown as a cash balance.

By contrast, the figures charged as 'depreciation expense' in the private nursing home's accounts amounted to only £300. The assumptions implicit in this figure might be that the property (£6,000) will last 30 years and contribute equally to each year's services, and similarly that the equipment (£2,000) will last 20 years. These are obviously arbitrary assumptions, but they serve to highlight the fact that the expenses in the private commercial accounts, may be defined and measured in a different manner than in a public authority. Moreover, different assumptions and conventions may be employed in different organizations within either sector in classifying and measuring the effect of financial transactions upon the entity concerned, so that in either field the financial statements produced from the double-entry system need to be interpreted with care in drawing conclusions from them. In particular it should be recognized that such statements, or the individual figures contained therein, might be used for quite different purposes, and that whilst they may be quite appropriate for one they may be unsuitable for another. Thus for certain 'stewardship' purposes they may be invaluable; for example, in showing how money has been spent, or what cash balances are available for meeting debts. But for assessing how much a particular asset is worth, in the case of 'selling

---

*The number and description of 'funds' or accounts used in a local authority depend upon its functions and accounting arrangements.

it off' immediately the value shown in a balance sheet might be less useful since the depreciation written off, or loans redeemed since it was purchased, may be quite out of line with its real depreciation.

APPLICATION OF DOUBLE-ENTRY ACCOUNTING IN THE HOSPITAL SERVICE

Prior to 1948 the majority of hospitals were administered by local authorities and thus their financial accounting procedures and conventions resulted in the production of financial statements discussed in the previous section.

The main financial effect of the transfer of hospitals to the central government was that the financing of both capital and revenue expenditure became the responsibility of the National Exchequer. Thus regional hospital boards, boards of governors and hospital management committees are the agents in a principal/agency relationship with the Department of Health and Social Security. Accordingly, their financial accounting procedures reflect this relationship; their basic purpose being to show how funds received from the Department have been used.

Accounting for capital expenditure is dealt with at the regional hospital board level. Since there is only one* source of funds, namely, the Department, capital accounting resolves itself simply into showing how money provided for capital development have been spent in a particular year. No traditional balance sheet is prepared showing the total outlay on fixed assets under the control of the regional board, or board of governors, at a particular year end, though accounts of how allocations have been spent must be kept.

The effect of these arrangements at the hospital management committee level is that the hospital management committee's finance officer is left to account for revenue expenditure and income only. Thus the income and expenditure account and balance sheet he prepares differ from those prepared in a local authority. The income and expenditure account differs in that it contains no provision for either: (1) debt charges; or (2) revenue contributions to capital outlay.

Nor is the I.M.T.A. classification of expenditure and income adopted. The balance sheet differs in that it is composed only of revenue account balances. There are five possible balances which might be shown at a 'year' end; on the assets side – the cost of *stores* still on hand; any *debts* owed by, for example, private patients, and *cash* balances – and on the liabilities side; the amount(s) owed to *creditors;* the remaining

---

*In practice, certain 'non-exchequer' funds exist, for example private endowments, but these are relatively insignificant.

balance representing the amount which is owed to or by the Department of Health and Social Security, either because it has provided funds in excess of the amounts spent for the period, or because it has not provided sufficient. This balance in effect shows the amount owed to or by the principal in the agency relationship, from the point of view of the agent, the Hospital Management Committee, the accounting entity concerned. These two statements are the ones which are analogous to those discussed previously in relation to a private nursing home and a local authority hostel, and show the effect of the bulk of financial transactions affecting a hospital. In addition, accounts are kept relating to relatively minor activities, which need to be kept quite separately, such as the recording of monies belonging to patients brought into care and area nurse training. Also, it is necessary to account for other 'non-exchequer' funds. These are funds provided from private sources, for example, endowments and donations. Often such funds are invested in land, property or negotiable securities, only the income from them being used to provide benefits to the hospital(s) from year to year. Consequently, it is necessary to provide a complete set of capital and revenue accounts in respect of such funds.

Appendices A—E show the type of statements which must be forwarded to the Department*. Only those statements are shown which have the effect of summarizing the whole of the transactions dealt with at Hospital Management Committee level. It should be clearly recognized that many supporting statements accompany these which provide more detailed analyses of some of the items making up these 'final accounts'.

Perhaps the most obvious difference between the local authority's and the hospital service's form of accounts is that, for the latter, the classifications are completely uniform, whereas the adoption of the I.M.T.A form of accounts by a particular local authority is dependent upon the treasurer's discretion. Moreover, whilst the hospital service revenue expenditure includes items of a renewal and replacement nature which will benefit more than one year, just as a local authority's does, there is nothing otherwise comparable with the depreciation expense found in private sector accounting as is the case with the local authority which shows debt charges and revenue contributions to capital outlay.

USEFULNESS AND LIMITATION OF FINANCIAL ACCOUNTING DATA

Having shown the way in which the accountant keeps track of financial transactions and indicated the main differences between the financial statements which the different types of organization prepare, it is

---

*Minor modifications are made to these forms from time to time as the need for particular classifications arises.

necessary to consider the extent to which this recording technique provides a satisfactory or sufficient basis for financial management.

The first point to make is that the financial records provide data which is vital for management purposes at the most basic level. Any organization must keep track of the debts owed to or by it. It must also be able to establish how far its funds are in a liquid rather than illiquid form. Even if the problem of remaining solvent is not urgent because taxes or rates can be adjusted to meet deficiencies, it is still necessary to know how much must be raised to meet commitments, and what funds are available from time to time. The second point is that the financial records provide a stewardship account of how funds have been used or raised. The detailed character of the classifications of revenue expenditure in particular, found in both the local authority and hospital service final accounts, points to the importance attached to the concept of 'public accountability' in public institutions, that is, the need to trace every penny of public money spent by those entrusted with its control. As regards this, it is important to recognize that it is natural that the initial classifications of expenditure should be orientated towards the type of input purchased rather than the ultimate use to which the input is put. Thus expenditure is classified as to whether it is on wages or salaries, fuel or cleaning materials, rather than whether these different inputs are for the benefit of, for example, the in-patient departments rather than the out-patient departments of a hospital. A particular input may be used to achieve a variety of objectives. The account classifications adopted in both local government and the hospital service in producing final accounts, in general reflect the mainly 'subjective' or 'input' emphasis in the classification of the financial accounting records although, as shown earlier, the I.M.T.A. standard form of accounts is a compromise between the 'subjective' and 'objective' forms of analysis. The overall effect of such a system is that the financial accounts prepared tend to emphasize the overall effect of the year's activities rather than enable the full cost of particular activities, departments or processes within the organization to be identified.

Thus, for example, the total cost of running the AMC hostel (Table 11.7) amounting to £2,750 is presented in such a way that, although the individual inputs may be shown in more or less detail, it is impossible to establish without further analysis how much it costs to feed the inmates, or maintain the grounds or gardens, bearing in mind that, for example, the total cost of catering is made up of many individual costs including those of administration as well as obvious activities such as the cook's wages and so on.

The general point regarding the limitation of financial accounting statements, for even stewardship purposes, may be made most strongly by an illustration from the private sector accounting in Table 11.6.

Assume that the XYZ Nursing Home has two categories of client, men and women, or elderly and young people, whose needs or treatment are different. It is quite possible that the net profit figure of £900 conceals a loss on one activity; one 'department' having made a profit of, for example, £1,100 and another a loss of £200. Similarly, in public authorities different departments or activities may be more or less costly than others, and subjectively classified financial statements do not reveal these differences nor do they necessarily enable expenditure to be identified with the particular individuals who are responsible for incurring it.

Clearly the information provided in the financial accounts may not satisfy the needs of the administrator without further manipulation. From a decision-making point of view, it would not be possible, for example, to answer such questions as below.

Would it be cheaper to contract out for cleaning or catering services?

Would it be more economical to use a different mixture of capital and revenue resources?

Is a particular service or activity within the organization too costly?

From a control viewpoint it would not necessarily be possible to ascertain: (1) who was responsible for incurring certain expenditures; (2) whether high costs were due to price increases or mismanagement; (3) how much individual activities or departments cost to operate.

The financial accounts thus need to be complemented by some form of 'cost analysis' designed to provide a firmer basis for answers to such questions.

It should be remembered, however, that local authority and hospital service budgetary classifications of expenditure are based upon those of financial accounts. The implications of this for decision making and control are discussed later.

Two final points may be made. First, the information contained in the financial accounts is essentially historical; it shows what has happened in terms of prices current at the time of the transaction. This must be borne in mind in using the data as a guide for decisions about the future. Secondly, such information is often used in order to compare the activities of one organization with those of another. To the extent that different definitions and measurement conventions are adopted by different bodies, comparisons must be made with care.

Costing in the Health Services

The limitation of financial accounting for management purposes led to the development of cost accounting, but before describing the methods of cost accounting used in the health services some concepts of cost are explained.

The total cost of conducting some enterprise is the value in money terms of the resources used up in seeking to attain its objectives. There are difficulties in defining and measuring the total cost of a year's activities even, and some indication of these has already been given. But, assuming this figure of total cost has been determined, the components may be classified in quite different ways depending upon the purpose in mind or viewpoint adopted. First of all, it is useful to distinguish the different *elements of cost.* Thus, total cost may be broken down into three main elements: labour costs, materials costs and service costs. This is the type of classification achieved in the financial accounts with salaries, provisions, and electricity charges being examples of these different elements respectively. This subjective classification has its uses in budgeting, particularly where price or wage increases affect the same element whatever it is used for. Thus the effect on total costs of a 5 per cent price rise for a particular element can be easily established where accounts are classified by types of input. Next, *fixed* costs may be distinguished from *variable* costs. Thus whilst a hospital, for example, may deal with more cases in one year than another, some costs will remain fixed; for example the matron's salary, in relation to the work done or output achieved whilst others will vary, for example, the cost of food. There is often ambiguity in discussing this distinction. It is one which revolves around the relationship of output to a particular expense, that is, it describes a particular element of cost as a function of output. Of course, fixed costs may alter in the sense that, for example, a matron may be given a pay rise. The important thing is that given a commitment to pay a fixed cost the higher the output achieved the lower is the cost per unit of output. The distinction does not exclude, of course, the possibility that some costs may be fixed only within certain ranges of output and some costs are, in fact, sometimes described as semivariable.

Fixed and variable costs, respectively, are often confused with *indirect* and *direct* costs. A direct cost is an element of cost which can be wholly identified with whatever is being costed, whether it is a department, activity, process or unit of output. For example, radiograph film used in the radiograph department of a hospital would be a direct cost to that department, so too would be the radiologist's salary; but one is variable in that it depends upon the output of the department, whilst the other is fixed. By contrast, many of the costs of administering the radiograph department are indirect. Such costs as those of the finance office in dealing with the accounts relating to the radiograph department, or a stores section in handling materials for it, are not so directly identifiable with it, yet they are nevertheless a part of the total or 'full' cost of running the department.

It is appropriate to deal with the concept of a *cost centre* at this point. It may be described as an area of organization, or an aspect of the organizations activities to which costs may be attributed. Thus the whole of the annual expenditure in running a hospital can be attributed to the different departments of the hospital even if this means setting up some miscellaneous account or cost centre to accommodate the elements of costs which are difficult to identify with, for example, the wards, the radiograph department, or whatever, and may not be directly identifiable with any of the more obvious centres of activity. In short, initially all expenditure may be considered the direct cost of one cost centre or another. But as indicated above, the *full* cost of running the radiograph department is not limited to those costs which can be directly identified with it. It is necessary, therefore, to allocate or apportion some of the direct costs of the other cost centres to that of the radiograph department to ascertain *its* full cost.

Next, a distinction may be drawn between *controllable* and *non-controllable* costs. Controllable costs are those which are subject to the control, or which can be influenced by a particular individual, whilst non-controllable costs are those which the individual cannot affect. For example, a laundry manager can influence certain costs of laundry operation such as the amount spent on power, materials and so on. The rent or rates paid on the laundry may be beyond his control. However, this distinction must be interpreted carefully and with reference to a particular situation. Thus, a particular element of cost may have both controllable and non-controllable aspects. For example, a laundry worker's wage rate may be based upon national agreements, and thus be beyond the manager's control. The time the employee works, and his productivity, may be subject to the arrangement and scheduling of work by the manager. This distinction underlies the concept of 'responsibility' accounting which is concerned with classifying costs so as to relate them to managerial responsibilities.

It is important to recognize that the distinction made between different elements of costs, fixed and variable costs, direct and indirect costs and controllable and non-controllable costs, are made for different purposes and to emphasize different aspects of cost. It is, therefore, pertinent to ask what purposes does cost analysis serve and what sort of information is required.

The broad purpose of cost analysis is to determine the cost of resources used up in attempting to achieve a particular objective, as a basis for decision making and control. Total cost is clearly relevant in considering the consequences of running a hospital. Given that, it is:

(1) useful to relate this to some indicator of the benefits received from this total outlay; and (2) important to assess the contribution made by different activities towards the overall process.

The problems of quantifying the value which attaches to public services are well known, but it is reasonable to assume that where more physical and identical units of output are made available with a given amount of resources rather than less, more value for money has been obtained. So that, for example, the number of patients cared for in a hospital gives some indication of the benefits produced by such an organization. The qualification is that the units of output or service measured are identical in quality. For example, differences in length of stay and the type of case involved make the number of patients dealt with an imperfect indicator of a hospital's output, and in practice care is needed in establishing measures of service. Nevertheless, even if a crude method, it is possible to devise *cost units* with which the value of resources used up in producing different kinds of output or service can be identified.

The cost per patient week (or day) or the cost per case provide examples of cost units related to the end product of hospital activity. Similarly, it is possible to establish cost units for individual activities or departments within the hospital. Examples are the cost per operation, or per operating hour, for an operating theatre, or the cost per 100 lb. weight of laundry washed or per 1,000 articles laundered. In other words, cost units may be established in relation to each of the cost centres into which an organization may be divided. The usefulness of these indicators depends very much upon the accuracy with which costs can be identified with such centres and the purpose for which they are used.

Unit costs may be used for the following main purposes, depending upon whether they are estimated or actual figures.

(1)　As a basis for deciding whether to provide a service because of the cost involved, or alternatively whether to provide it by using organizational resources as opposed to contracting for it.

(2)　As a basis for establishing charges (for example, for private patients).

(3)　As a basis for distributing resources (for example, allocating more funds to high cost areas).

(4)　To establish a standard against which to compare performances in other periods of time or other organizations.

Whether a particular unit cost figure will serve any of these purposes satisfactorily will depend, in part, upon the way costs are attached to the unit of output selected and upon the way it is interpreted. Often a unit cost figure is simply the result of dividing the total costs, fixed and variable, of a period by the number of units of output produced. In particular, it is important to establish what are the *relevant* costs in a particular decision making problem, and a historically-derived average unit cost may well be inappropriate. Suppose, for example, an administrator is trying to decide whether it would be cheaper to contract out for laundry services and an outside firm quote a price which, on the basis of existing laundering requirements, would work out at £20 per 1,000 articles laundered. Possibly his existing costs work out at £25 per 1,000 articles laundered but this does not mean that contracting out will be more economical. First, the present cost of £25 per unit of output will probably include an amount for the use of equipment which is already paid for, a *sunk* cost, and the equipment will bring only a negligible sum if sold for scrap. Moreover, contracting out may not reduce administrative or other fixed costs included in the present average unit cost, since even if these are no longer apportioned to laundering they will still have to be met. An administrator must, therefore, identify the *avoidable* costs which can be saved by adopting an alternative method and compare these with any quotation. Often in decision making incremental costs and not full costs are relevant. Thus if, for example, a laundry is operating at less than capacity, the cost of laundering an extra unit of output (for example, 1,000 articles) will involve incremental costs such as those of a variable nature, for example, overtime payments, cost of washing materials and power. In another case, extra production may involve the installation of extra machinery so that incremental costs may be high.

By contrast, a *full* cost, that is a cost for a unit of output which includes both fixed and variable cost factors, indirect or direct, may be useful where it is necessary to charge for the use of a service, since an organization may wish to recoup an amount which will help to meet overhead expenses.

The problems of analysing and using costing data are further considered after a description of existing costing practice in the health services.

HOSPITAL COSTING SCHEME IN ENGLAND AND WALES

The existing pattern of cost accounting in the hospital service was introduced on the 1st April 1966. There is now a single standard scheme applicable to all hospitals within the service in contrast to the 'main' and 'alternative' (or 'modified') schemes previously operated, which distinguished between hospitals, on the basis of their size, in terms of the total expenditure involved. It must be pointed out immediately that the scheme described serves two broad purposes, First it produces costing data on a uniform basis in respect of the running of hospitals throughout the service. Such information provides a part of the information deemed necessary for decision making and control by regional and departmental authorities. Secondly, the scheme is designed to serve the needs of internal management at the hospital or group level itself. No single scheme is likely to serve the purposes of both internal and external control with the same degree of adequacy and, inevitably, the information produced must be limited. It is not intended, however, that a hospital shall limit its cost accounting simply to that arising from the need to conform with the national scheme. Hospital authorities are open to develop their costing procedures to suit their needs provided they produce the basic information required under the scheme.

The way the costing scheme works is shown in very broad terms in *Figure 11.4*. The total expenditure shown under various 'input' or subjective headings in the financial accounts, and amounting to £200,000 is this example, is reclassified for costing purposes according to the activity or objective it promotes. There are two broad stages. First, all expenditure is identified with one or other of 22 cost centres grouped under three broad headings: non-treatment departments, medical service departments and patients departments.

The identification of individual items of expenditure with particular cost centres is eased by use of a standardized and detailed classification of expenditure, for both financial and cost accounts, which is applied throughout the hospital service to minimize ambiguity of treatment between different hospitals. The individual centres to which costs are allocated are as follows.

Non-treatment	*Medical services*	*Patients*
Nurses in training	Operating theatres	In-patients (wards)
Catering	Radiotherapy	Out-patients
Staff residences	Diagnostic radiography	
Laundry	Pathology	
Power, light and heat	Physiotherapy	
Building and engineering	Pharmacy	
maintenance	Ancillary medical service	
Medical records	departments	
General administration		
General portering		
General cleaning		
Maintenance of grounds		
Transport		
Other services		

The total costs may, at this stage, be thought of as direct costs of these individual cost centres. They may be either fixed or variable costs and, to a varying degree, subject to the control of a member of staff responsible for the activities of the cost centre concerned.

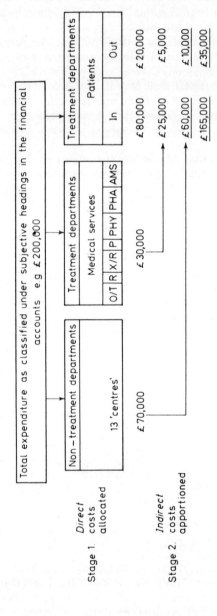

Figure 11.4. Stages in the hospital costing scheme

This primary analysis of costs enables cost statements to be produced showing the main direct expenditure initially associated with the various cost centres other than the in-patient and out-patient departments. Such statements have three main sections. The first gives details of the output of the centre or department; the second shows the main elements of the total direct costs for the department, which is divided by the total units of output (where there is an appropriate output measure) to give a unit cost. The third shows a summary of clearance, that is, how the total cost has been apportioned between in-patients, out-patients and other users of the cost centre's services. Table 11.8 is the form of cost

TABLE 11.8

COST STATEMENT FOR THE YEAR ENDED 31st MARCH 1969

I. HOSPITAL .... TYPE ....

BOARD OF GOVERNORS .... R.H.B.No .... H.M.C.No ....

DIAGNOSTIC X-RAY

Cost Unit - per 100 units weighted points value

1967/68	STATISTICS	1968/69

	No. of weighted points
	  - In-patients
	  - Out-patients
	  - Other Users
	  - Total
		2
		3
		4
		5

1967/68		EXPENDITURE AND UNIT COST	1968/69		
Expenditure	Unit Cost	DESCRIPTION	Expenditure		Unit Cost
£	£		£		£

		Pay - Medical
		    - Nursing
		    - Professional & Technical
		    - Other
		Students' Training Grants
		Drugs and Dressings
		Equipment - X-Ray Film
		       - Major
		       - Other
		Contract Services
				6
				7
				8
				9
				10
				11
				12
				13
				14
				15	

		TOTAL 17		16	

SUMMARY OF CLEARANCE	£
In-patients Out-patients Other Users	
TOTAL	

statement produced for the diagnostic radiograph department, whilst Table 11.9 shows the summary of unit costs statement, which lists the main items contained on all the individual cost statements produced.

TABLE 11.9

SUMMARY OF UNIT COSTS FOR THE YEAR ENDED 31st MARCH 1969

I. HOSPITAL.. TYPE ....

BOARD OF GOVERNORS .... R.H.B.No .... H.M.C.No ....

AVERAGE No. OF AVAILABLE STAFFED BEDS ....

Reference		DESCRIPTION	No. of Units (Whole Numbers)	1968/69		1967/68
Form	Line			Expenditure £	Unit Cost £	Unit Cost £
A	42	In-patients - per in-patient week				
	43	- per case				
	87	Out-patients - per 100 attendances				
	88	- per new out-patient				
AI	37	Day patients - per attendance				
B	15	Operating Theatres - per operating hour				
	15	- per operation				
C	14	Radiotherapy - per course of treatment per day (excluding Medical Pay)				
D	16	Diagnostic X-Ray - per 100 units weighted points value				
E	24	Pathology - per 100 weighted requests (excluding Medical Pay)				
	35	- per in-patient case				
F	14	Physiotherapy - per 100 units weighted points value				
G	10	Pharmacy - per in-patient week				
	16	- per 100 out-patient attendances				
H		Ancillary Medical Service Depts.				
	52	- per in-patient week				
	53	- per 100 out-patient attendances				
I		Catering - per person fed per week				
	12	(i) Provisions				
	16	(ii) Total cost excluding service				
	20	(iii) Staff Dining room service				
	21	(iv) Total cost in Dining Room	—	—		
J		Laundry (a) Operating costs				
	15	- per 100 articles laundered				
	16	- per 100 lb dry weight				
	17	(b) External service - per 100 articles laundered				
	18	- per 100 lb dry weight				
K	19	Boiler House - per 1000 lb of steam raised from and at 212° F				
L	20	Power, light and heat - per 1000 cu. ft. of buildings				
M		Building and Engineering maintenance per 1000 cu. ft. of buildings:				
	8	(i) Supervision				
	12	(ii) Painting and Decorating				
	16	(iii) Other Building Work				
	20	(iv) Engineering				
	21	(v) Total				
N	12	Medical Records - per 100 weighted units				
O	11	General Administration - per weighted occupied bed				
P	68	Other Services - per in-patient week				
	69	- per 100 out-patient attendances				
—		Staff Residences - Total expenditure and average cost per resident per week				
—		General Cleaning - per 1000 sq. ft. of floor area (i) residual areas				
		(ii) whole hospital				

The second stage of the costing process requires that the direct costs of the non-treatment and medical service departments be apportioned to the two 'end-product' departments, namely, the in-patient and out-patient departments, so that a cost summary statement (Table 11.10) showing the overall cost of these departments may be compiled. It should be noted that the direct costs of non-treatment and medical service departments are, from the point of view of the patients' departments, indirect costs. The basis of apportioning these indirect costs to the patients' departments varies, depending upon the type of expense involved and the ease with which it can be identified with the in-patient or out-patient departments. In many cases the cost unit of a particular cost centre also provides the basis for apportioning expenditure. For example, the cost unit of the diagnostic radiograph department is 100 units weighted points value – different types of radiograph having different weights – and the apportionment of the net expenditure on this department, after allowing for that which is attributable to outside users, is made on the basis of the number of units of work done for in-patients and out-patients respectively. The *cost unit* of a cost centre and the basis by which its expenditure is apportioned to a final location of cost must not be confused however. The former provides a basis for assessing the relationship between the activities, or outputs, of the cost centre and their cost, the latter for attributing the cost of these activities to the centres which derive benefit from them.

It must be emphasized that only the main expenses relating to a particular cost centre are initially allocated to it and that cost units are not always set up for particular cost centres. Moreover, the apportionment of cost is based upon fact so far as is possible. Thus, for example, timber used to repair or convert furniture and fittings will be initially charged to the 'other services' cost centre, even though it may be possible to identify, for example, 80 per cent of the total cost of this item with the in-patients department because of work specifically done for this department. When the total costs initially allocated to 'other services' are eventually apportioned to the patients' departments, this 80 per cent timber cost will be charged to the in-patients' department, since this fact can easily be established. The remainder of the cost of timber which may have been used to repair furniture in various departments will be apportioned between in-patient and out-patient departments on whatever basis seems suitable, in the light of any available information on how the timber was used. It will be clear that under this system some expenditure 'leap frogs' a cost centre with which it could be identified as an intermediate step in the costing process. Indeed it is in this way that the existing costing scheme simplifies the allocation (and re-allocation) of costs procedure which the former 'main' scheme had as one of its more complicated features.

TABLE 11.10

COST SUMMARY STATEMENT FOR THE YEAR ENDED 31st MARCH 1969

I. HOSPITAL.. TYPE ....

BOARD OF GOVERNORS .... R.H.B. No. .... H.M.C. No. ....

IN-PATIENTS			OUT-PATIENTS		
1967/68	1968/69	Statistics	Statistics	1968/69	1967/68
	2	Average No. of available Staffed beds	Attendances — O.P. Depts.	45	
	3	Average No. occupied beds	Attendances — Accident and Emergency	46	
%	4 %	Occupation of available Staffed beds	Total attendances	47	
			New Out-patients	48	
%	5 %	Long stay cases % of occupied beds	New Acc. and Emergency	49	
			Total New	50	
	6	No. of In-patient days	Ratio O.P. attendances / New O.P.	51	
	7	No. of Cases	Ratio Accident and Emergency / New A and E	52	
		Av. stay per case — days			

EXPENDITURE AND UNIT COST

IN-PATIENT COSTS			DESCRIPTION	OUT-PATIENT COSTS		
1967/68	1968/69			1968/69		1967/68
Per I.P. week	Per I.P. week	Expend-iture		Expend-iture	Per 100 attend.	Per 100 attend.
£	£	£	Wards — Out-Patients	£	£	£
	8		Pay — Medical		53	
	9		— Nursing		54	
	10		— Domestic		55	
	11		— Other		56	
	12		Drugs		57	
	13		Dressings		58	
	14		Patients' Appliances		59	
	15		Equipment — Major		60	
	16		— Other		61	
	17		Contract Services		62	
	18		TOTALS WARDS — O/P DEPTS.		63	
	19		Operating Theatres		64	
	20		Radiotherapy		65	
	21		Diagnostic X-Ray		66	
	22		Pathology		67	
	23		Physiotherapy		68	
	24		Pharmacy		69	
	25		Anc. Med. Service Depts.		70	
	26		TOTAL TREATMENT DEPARTMENTS		71	
	27		Nurses in Training		72	
	28		Catering		73	
	29		Staff Residences		74	
	30		Laundry		75	
	31		Power, Light and Heat		76	
	32		Bldg. & Eng. Maint.		77	
	33		Medical Records		78	
	34		General Administration		79	
	35		General Portering		80	
	36		General Cleaning		81	
	37		Maintenance of Grounds		82	
	38		Transport		83	
	39		Other Services		84	
	40		GROSS TOTALS		85	
	41		DIRECT CREDITS		86	
	42		44 NET TOTALS 89		87	
	43	—	Cost per Case	—	—	—
—	—	—	—	Cost per New Out-Patient	—	88	

The former scheme is of historical interest only, but certain qualifications to the broad outline of how the existing scheme works must now be made, if some of the practical difficulties surrounding its operation and the significance of the information it gives rise to are to be appreciated. First, it has been suggested that the total expenditure in the financial accounts is simply reclassified in the cost accounts, implying that the total in each accounting system, financial and costing, is the same in amount. This is broadly true, but in both systems account is taken of 'direct credits', that is reduction of expenditure arising from recoupments of costs, for example, charges to staff for accommodation and so on, and profits on trading services such as hospital shops or farms. In the cost accounts, the cost statements show the costs before any credits, and depending on the type of credit involved various adjustments are needed in compiling the final cost summary statement.

Secondly it is important to remember that the cost accounts are compiled from financial account data, and that these contain items which in a private sector undertaking would often be treated as capital items benefiting more than one year. Since cost data is used to make comparisons between different hospitals and different years, difficulties arise where a cost is charged to a particular period simply because it is incurred in that period. Here the distinction often made between a cost and an expense is important. A cost is the price paid for an item, expense is the proportion of this cost used up in a particular period. For many items of expenditure the two terms are synonymous since all the benefit derived from the purchase of a factor of production is gained in the period during which it is paid for. But the essential feature of capital items of expenditure is that their cost is not fully 'expensed' within the year of purchase. The financial accounts shown earlier contain such items. Where these tend to be replaced in similar amounts each year (for example, minor items of furniture and equipment), no distortion of costs is likely to occur. But where, for example, a hospital buys major items of equipment for particular departments infrequently cost statements could easily fluctuate considerably from one year to the next. To counter this the costing scheme allows for an average cost to be substituted for certain kinds of expenditure on major equipment used in laundries, radiograph departments and so on. The effect is similar to that of providing for the depreciation expense on a fixed asset in business accounting. But it must be emphasized such adjustments do not allow for the depreciation on many costly assets, such as buildings financed via the capital allocations of Regional Boards.

A related problem arising from the method of financing such items arises where non-exchequer funds, for example, a private endowment, are used to finance a major item of equipment. Such expenditure will not be charged in the hospital's financial revenue expenditure accounts at all for that hospital; yet another hospital without such monies available will have such a charge in its normal accounts. Again, the costing scheme provides for an appropriate portion of the cost of such non-exchequer expenditure to be brought into the costing records so as to make the data for different hospitals more comparable.

Thirdly individual hospitals depend upon the services of the group's administrative and other services, and upon services based upon particular 'parent' hospitals but shared by other hospitals in the area. Again, this necessitates adjustments between the financial accounts and cost accounts relating to particular hospitals to ensure that there is neither double counting nor any understatement of the full cost of providing a particular hospital's services. For example, radiography may be performed by one hospital on behalf of another. The former will compile a cost statement for this department showing the unit cost irrespective of who the users are. But it must make allowance, as suggested earlier, in compiling its cost summary statement so that only radiograph work in respect of its own patients is charged. The latter hospital will, however, need to include such costs on its cost summary in order to indicate its total costs. A complication arises because charges to outside users include a figure for 'overheads', that is, expenditure not directly charged to the radiograph department of the hospital providing the service. Thus such transactions lead to adjustments to the costs of the 'overhead' departments of the 'parent' hospital in apportioning these costs between the patients' departments of the servicing hospital since a portion of such costs as general cleaning, general portering, general administration and so on are recouped from other user hospitals, and these must be allowed for in completing the cost summary statement.

Finally, a few words are necessary regarding the way in which costs are, in practice, collated and the extent to which they are re-allocated between cost centres before their final apportionment to the patients' departments. As regards collation, there may be small departments, such as a printing shop or an electricity generating plant, to which it is convenient or necessary to allocate costs prior to any of the main cost centres. For example, where a hospital generates its own electricity it will be necessary to summarize the wages and other costs involved in producing electricity before the cost of electricity can be allocated to other centres. Consequently, cost suspense accounts are used to assemble cost data prior to the main allocation of costs to the standard cost centres detailed earlier.

An important example of this kind of account is that relating to the boiler house (steam production). It is also peculiar in that for this account the standard scheme requires that a cost statement must be compiled in the same way as for the other cost centres. The costs of this department are then allocated to the laundry and the power, light and heat cost centres.

Moreover, the second stage of the process depicted in *Figure 11.4* is complicated by a certain amount of re-allocation of costs between the non-treatment departments before they finally are apportioned to the patients' departments. This re-allocation is now limited to charging a due proportion of the expenses of three departments to staff residences. These expenses relate to: (1) the laundry; (2) power, light and heat; and (3) building and engineering maintenance cost centres.

In the light of these qualifications, it will be appreciated that the costing process is no simple matter, and that in view of the many individual costs which have first to be identified with individual cost centres, and ultimately attached to the two main patients' departments, some element of arbitrariness must enter into the costing process despite the issue of detailed and standardized instructions regarding the classification of costs and methods of apportioning them. Ultimately, the usefulness of comparisons of the cost figures produced for different hospitals must depend upon the way in which the costing instructions are interpreted, the care with which they are implemented, and the extent to which it is possible to achieve an identical treatment in the processing of costs. The extent to which this latter condition applies must itself depend upon the existence of similar organizational arrangements and measurement techniques.

LIMITATIONS OF COSTING DATA AND THEIR USE

Costing data may be used to answer three main questions. (1) What is the cost of a particular product, process, operation or activity? (2) Why is it different from that originally planned or of another period or organization? (3) Who is responsible for a cost or for its variation from some comparable data? Taking each of these areas in turn, some of the problems a cost analyst encounters may be identified.

The need to assess the cost of a product or service from the point of view of decision making arises basically because it is necessary to decide whether it is worthwhile committing that amount of resources to its production. To compare this cost with an alternative method of achieving the same end, and to establish the price or charge, it is necessary to fix or levy in order to finance or recoup the expenditure involved. However, the processes involved in producing a service from many different inputs, or using a combination of inputs to produce quite different outputs or services, make it difficult to identify particular input costs with particular outputs especially when some of them, such

293

as fixed assets, contribute to the productive process over a long period of time. Thus plant and medical equipment may last many years, but at the time they are purchased no-one can accurately assess how long they will be serviceable nor how many people will become patients and use them. Clearly, the more patients there are during their life the lower will be the cost per unit of service they give over their life. Thus in attributing a part of the cost to the number of patients they have served in, for example, their first year of use, some assumption must be made which subsequent events may prove false. In this example some patients may or may not use the services a particular asset provides; for example, the radiograph equipment. The 'outputs' or services provided by a hospital are often different depending upon the needs of individual patients, and ideally it would be desirable to identify the cost of caring for each patient depending upon his or her needs. In other words, the social services, in general, are heterogeneous products or outputs rather than homogeneous products like bottles of milk or bricks each of which is identical. Because of the difficulties of assessing costs of services without prior knowledge of the types and quantities of each which will be required in a particular time period, it is impossible in practice to establish with precision how much a particular unit of service will cost. The same proposition applies to the assessment of the various units of service of the different departments or activities which contribute to the end service.

In fact the costing procedures in the health services are basically historic costing procedures designed to establish what a unit of output has cost, and the methods of attributing costs to different departments and outputs have been outlined. The usefulness of such data for the decision making process obviously depends upon the extent to which the assumptions made in collating the costs and attributing them to particular outputs are valid for the purposes of the decisions to be made. Clearly, the cost per patient week, for example, shown in one year is unlikely to indicate the cost for a subsequent year, if only because the prices of input may change. Moreover, the existence of fixed costs means that this historic unit cost is, in part, a function of the output of the year in question; and output may vary in the future. Next, the cost per patient week is an average cost in the sense that it assumes all patients make equal use of the various services provided irrespective of their particular needs. Where a hospital (or hostel) caters for patients of a similar category this assumption may approximate to reality. But where a case mix varies significantly from year to year costs are likely to vary more widely depending upon whether the treatment required is more or less expensive. Consequently, an administrator cannot point to the cost per patient week as being the cost which would arise from accommodating an extra patient for a week since fixed costs would not alter; and variable costs might be different because of price changes relating to the variable inputs required and only the treatment required by an extra patient would determine which individual variable costs were increased. Similarly, the total cost per unit, historically derived, of any of the various services which contribute to the final output is of limited value to the administrator in decision making.

What then of the use of such data for control purposes? Control mechanisms essentially embody some criterion by which to assess whether the activity to be controlled is conforming with what is required of it. Control, therefore, depends upon comparison of what *is* happening with that which *should* happen, and there are three main ways of comparing cost data. First, with similar data relating to a previous period; secondly, with those for other organizations and, thirdly, with some previously established standards. Cost comparisons in the social services are largely of the first and second types, and the validity of such comparisons depends upon the data having been compiled on the same basis for each period or organization. Where, because of the time of compilation, such comparisons only become available after the end of the period concerned, there is no possibility of influencing the course of events; and their usefulness in indicating a divergence from what might be considered a 'normal' pattern of costs depends upon the extent to which they reveal the various factors giving rise to any differences observed. Moreover, much depends upon whether the costs of other periods or organizations can be considered suitable indicators of what ought to happen.

The main factors which are likely to be responsible for a change in unit costs between periods for the same organization are as follows. (1) Changes in the prices of inputs. (2) Changes in the level of output or amount of services provided (because of the effect of fixed costs). (3) Changes in the efficiency with which the inputs are used at any given level of output. A simple example will indicate the costing problems involved in identifying the causes of cost variance.

Suppose there are only two costs in catering for patients or residents of a hostel: a fixed cost (the cook's wage) and a variable cost (the cost of food). Table 11.11 shows what happened last year (Period I) and what has resulted in the current year (Period II).

Such a statement shows the combined effect of different variables upon the cost per unit of output; namely, a rise of 3p. per meal. It does little to identify the causes. The statement for Period II (Table 11.12) presents the informaton so as to achieve this aim.

Table 11.12 shows that although the cost per meal has risen by 3p. various factors working in different directions have produced this result. Thus although the fixed cost per unit remains the same, this has only been achieved because more use has been made of the cook's services thus offsetting her rise in wages. Care is needed in interpreting

TABLE 11.11
Specimen Costs in Catering for Patients or Residents in Hostels

Data	Period I	Period II
Number of meals served	1,000	1,200
Fixed cost: cook's wage	£100	£120
Variable cost: provisions	£200	£276
Therefore cost per meal	30p.	33p.

TABLE 11.12
Catering Cost Statement (for Period II)

Data	Period I	Period II
Number of meals served	1,000	1,200
Fixed cost at Period I wage rate	£100	£100
Fixed cost per meal at Period I wage rate	10p.	8·3p.
Increase in wage rate	–	£20
Effect on cost per meal	–	1·7p.
Current fixed cost per meal	–	10p.
Variable costs at Period I prices 20p. x 1,200	£200	£240
Increase in variable costs based on Period I's use of provisions 5p. x 1,200	–	£60
Decrease due to better utilization	–	£24
Actual variable costs Period II	–	£276
Variable cost per meal	20p.	23p.
Total cost per meal	30p.	33p.

the variation in cost due to greater use of a fixed cost resource element however. It is tempting to infer that this favourable variance is due to increased efficiency. It is in the sense that more use (or output) has been derived from the provision of the same amount of input as before.

However, the improvement has not necessarily been achieved by any change in the way the cook organized her work or operates, but simply because previously she was underworked and is now being stretched to capacity. This improvement, therefore, may have been achieved because of factors outside of the control of either the cook or the organization. It may simply be the result of increased use of available capacity. On the other hand, if the cook was fully stretched in Period I and, for example, meals were limited to 1,000 units because of the inability to serve more without having extra help from another cook, the extra output coped with in Period II may have been due to improved efficiency in the use of the cook's time due to modified work methods. Ideally, the cost statement should enable a distinction to be drawn between the effects on costs arising from simply utilizing the capacity of resources more or less fully, and those which arise from the manner in which resources are exploited. The development of the analysis of variances in this way depends upon defining 'normal' capacities and measurement standards for fixed asset utilization.

The analysis of variable costs in Table 11.12 uses Period I's figures as a standard for distinguishing between variations from price-level changes and efficiency in the use of provisions purchased. Thus by showing the cost at £240 the statement assumes that similar amounts and qualities of provisions are used in Period II per meal as in Period I and shows the result which might have been expected without a price change since the increase in meals served. The effect of the price increase (£60) is then shown assuming that amounts of provisions used vary directly in proportion to meals served; prices have risen by 25 per cent or 5p. per amount used in Period I. Since actual provisions have only cost £276, the difference due to the more efficient use of provisions emerges as £24. Thus a general price increase has been partially offset by the more efficient use of the variable cost resource. Again the interpretation requires care. The 'efficiency variance' may be the result of different factors. Bulk buying of provisions may have produced better discounts or there may have been less waste due to more skilful use of the provisions by the cook, either of which have been achieved without any alteration in the type of provisions bought compared with Period I or in the quality or calorific value of the meals served.

This simple illustration is indicative only of the approach to compiling cost data required if the causes of cost variations are to be revealed as well as the effects. It exemplifies the kind of data produced in a system of *standard* costing where standards are predetermined as a basis for comparing actual performances with them, and cost statements are prepared frequently during the accounting period to enable remedial action to be taken. The obstacle to the development of standard costing systems in the social services lies, of course, in the establishment of acceptable standards in a field where needs and outputs typically lack the uniformity exhibited by industrial products. Given the number of inputs, fixed or variable in nature, which are needed in the provision of health services, and the ways in which they must be combined to produce different kinds of service, the difficulties of the cost accountant become readily apparent. But even when the causes of cost variations are disentangled the question of whether they are controllable or not remains, and who is responsible. Thus in the example given above, the cook might not be responsible for purchasing provisions, or storing them, so that several people may contribute to the overall variation in cost. The extent to which cost classification and analysis is carried must depend upon whether the benefits obtained offset the time, effort and cost involved. These benefits depend very much upon whether, once produced, the costing data is placed in the hands of those who can use it to the organization's advantage and if they so use it.

Certainly, the compilation of historic cost data, for control purposes within a financial year, can only be of use if it is produced at frequent intervals and while there is still time to discern the emerging pattern of costs and take remedial action. Its usefulness also depends upon the existence of some standard(s) by which to assess the nature of the pattern emerging and thus judge the type of action required.

There is little doubt that existing costing procedures are deficient in that they do not provide information which would be potentially useful for managers to have. Nor is there any reason to suppose that yard-sticks for assessing performances are entirely satisfactory. The problem is whether remedying the deficiencies would produce a net benefit compared with alternative ways of improving management techniques.

The Development of Financial Control

A CHANGING APPROACH

In describing the techniques of budgeting, financial accounting and cost accounting which provide the information necessary for financial control, various limitations in the types of information traditionally produced have been indicated. In some cases the way financial information is classified or produced is defective from the point of view of the decision maker; in others from the control viewpoint.

Financial accounting, whilst it produces basic information for day-to-day control, is geared ultimately to the needs of accountability, that is, to providing data which serves as a basis for internal check, internal audit and external audit procedures. It is input orientated and historic in nature, serving in particular the needs of stewardship. Traditional budgetary procedures, too, are geared to the financial accounting classifications of data, and seek especially to establish regularity or legality in the use of public money. Cost accounting has largely been developed from the same mould.

The limitations of the data generated by these systems have been highlighted by the approaches adopted by economists, econometricians, operational researchers and others concerned increasingly with the solution of, or enquiry into, management problems. The broad effect of these different approaches has been to engender a more analytical and rational approach to management problems generally. More particularly emphasis had been laid upon viewing an organization as a system whose parts must be related to the whole, and whose inputs must be related to its outputs. The need to be *rational* in decision making and to be *efficient* in implementing decisions is emphasized.

This has led in the area of financial management to the development of programme and performance budgeting. Neither of these techniques is yet widely applied, and where they are they must be regarded as being in the embryonic stage of development. Their development reflects mainly the acceptance of the need for a more systematic approach towards management and to take advantage of the techniques developed by various disciplines in producing information for decision making and control purposes. To assess the potential of these two techniques and the problems they raise, it is necessary to consider briefly the concepts of rationality and efficiency, and techniques which have stemmed from a more scientific approach to management.

RATIONALITY, COST–BENEFIT ANALYSIS AND DISCOUNTED CASH FLOW

Intuitively, it is reasonable to assume that in using a given amount of resources an organization will seek to achieve more rather than less value or benefits in return for the sacrifice involved. Given various possible courses of action, that is, it will choose that combination which seems likely to produce the maximum benefits possible, and thus act rationally. To select a course of action which seemed likely to produce a smaller return would be irrational. The problem of rational choice lies, first, in identifying and quantifying the relationships between input and output variables and, secondly, in establishing some criterion by which to choose between different relationships. For example, suppose a local authority seeks to ensure the elderly are well fed and cared for. It may do this by arranging for home helps and health visits, or by transferring old folk to hostels. Both will tend to have different costs and benefits associated with them. The important thing is that in any appraisal of the two methods all costs and benefits should be included. In order to identify and quantify the costs and benefits, it is necessary to clarify who bears the costs or receives the benefits. Thus, the local authority in this example will, depending upon which method it adopts, bear the financial costs of providing home helps or hostel accommodation and so on. There may also be external or spillover costs affecting other services. For example, the need to extend water, sewage or other services where a new hostel is built may result in costs being incurred on these services which are not directly charged to the health service account.

The patient too may be involved in different financial costs, if he remains at home rather than lets or sells his house and transfers to a hostel. So, too, will the relatives or friends of the patients who may, for example, be faced with extra travelling expenses in visiting if the patient is accommodated in a hostel.

Finally, society at large, that is all other persons and organizations, may incur different costs depending upon how a patient is treated. For example, voluntary organizations may be relieved of a financial burden by providing care in hostels.

Paralleling these financial costs, whether direct or of a spillover nature, each of these groups may receive different financial benefits. There are obvious difficulties in identifying and quantifying all these financial costs and benefits. An even more difficult task is that of allowing for *intangible* costs and benefits; that is, those factors which present advantages, or disadvantages, gained or lost by the adoption of one method rather than another. For example, the loss (or gain) for a patient of companionship by being treated in one environment rather than another.

Intangible gains or losses provide a particular difficulty when it comes to establishing a criterion by which to select one course of action rather than another, or to rank projects in order of priority. Financial costs and benefits, assuming they can all be identified and measured are, by definition, in terms of money and thus directly comparable. Intangibles, if they are to be allowed for in an appraisal, must either be translated into a monetary measurement or taken into account in some other way. In any event, the appriasal of intangibles is likely to be open to bias and arbitrariness, and since such factors in social services are likely to be very important to the success of a particular policy they need handling with extreme care.

It is beyond the scope of this section to deal with the technique and problems of cost–benefit analysis which is a subject in itself. Since the essence of the technique is to obtain a rational appraisal of different courses of action and the identification and measurement of *financial* costs and benefits plays an important part in this process, it is necessary to consider the role placed by financial techniques. Briefly, an administrator undertaking a cost—benefit analysis will need to obtain monetary measures of costs and benefits. The sources of such measures may usually be traced to accounting records, and thus the administrator must be aware of the limitations of historic cost data and average costs and the arbitrariness of accounting conventions in attempting to use accounting data to predict the consequences of future actions.

Moreover, allowance must be made for the time value of money. This means that money paid out or received in the future is worth less than similar amounts paid out or received in the present. Thus, £1,000 received now is worth more than the same amount to be received in a year's time simply because interest could be earned on money available in the present. Since different projects, or ways of providing a service, have different cash flows both in and out, and the timings of these flows are different, the amounts involved must be discounted to achieve comparability in appraising different alternatives. Investment appraisal by discounted cash flow techniques raises the following problems — whether in cost benefit or less extensive appraisals.

(1) Ascertaining the *amount* of the cash flows.

(2) Ascertaining the *timings* of the cash flows.

(3) Deciding upon an appropriate rate of discount to apply.

Moreover, these problems are intensified where the different projects to be compared have different time-spans and are subject to different degrees of uncertainty regarding the amounts and timings of the cash flows associated with them.

To summarize, rationality in decision making demands that all *relevant* costs and benefits be taken into account in comparing alternatives and that due weight be given in any appraisal to the effect of time and uncertainty. The challenge to financial managers is to supply relevant information and moreover the accountant must be prepared to utilize the techniques of other disciplines to enable him to do this where traditional accounting classifications of data are not appropriate for the purposes required. In particular, the application of mathematical and statistical techniques is important in processing accounting data into a suitable form for management purposes.

PROGRAMME BUDGETING

Programme budgeting is the term which has been adopted by the Institute of Municipal Treasurers and Accountants in the United

Kingdom to describe the planning–programming–budgeting systems (P.P.B.S.) about which a great deal of current literature concerned with the financial management of public sector organizations revolves. A P.P.B.S. was introduced by the Department of Defence of the United States of America in 1961 and since then a great deal of effort has gone into applying the concepts which underlie it to other governmental agencies at different levels: central, state and local.

The essential feature of such a system is that it aims to ensure rationality in the use of scarce resources so that the fullest benefits possible are achieved from public expenditure. Major criticisms of traditional budgeting procedures have been that existing patterns of expenditure have been accepted as 'normal' or 'correct' with little regard to the ultimate aims they are intended to serve, that budgets have been compiled on departmental lines with little regard to the interdependence of different departments or their overall goal(s), that the implications for future years have been given only a limited consideration and that the search for alternative methods of achieving objectives has been unsystematic. Such criticisms must be aimed more at the approach and attitudes adopted by managers in decision making than at the techniques they have used, although their techniques may well have influenced their approach. Any technique is, in a sense, neutral in that it may be correctly used, misused or applied in the wrong context depending upon the person or organization using it. Yet there is always a danger that familiarity with tools or techniques designed for one purpose may result in their being used for quite different purposes uncritically.

The programme budgeting approach towards resource management requires that: (1) the public authority concerned identifies its basic objectives regardless of which section or department of its organization carries them into effect; (2) the future year implications of policies are explicitly identified; (3) all pertinent costs and benefits are considered*; and (4) alternative methods of achieving objectives are identified and analysed systematically.

In practical terms this approach involves the creation of a programme structure, the adoption of a time-span as a basis for planning, and the analysis of the alternative ways of achieving the various programmes.

A programme structure means the identification of the major programme areas and sub-programmes or distinguishing between the main objectives and sub-objectives of the authority so as to reveal the relation-

---

*This requirement raises a crucial problem; namely, that of identifying and assessing the often far-reaching effects of a particular policy or programme where many interests are affected. The problem of the analyst is thus initially one of defining *whose* costs and benefits are to be included in the appraisal.

ship between different programmes or objectives. For example, in the case of a local authority, the major programme areas might be identified as shown in *Figure 11.5*.

The aim is to distinguish the different needs of individuals as a basis for formulating clear policies for meeting them. There is no one way of making these distinctions, and much will depend upon the particular needs of a community, their interrelationship; its range of functions and so on in creating the programme framework. Obviously, in policy making for a particular programme area attention will have to be paid to other areas. Thus, the physical development of the community, the nature of its transport services and the way other programmes are executed all have implications for the health programme.

A programme structure goes beyond this however. The next stage is to identify the different activities and sub-activities which contribute towards achieving these programmes. Essentially, the approach is one of working backwards from ends to means to ascertain what is required in the shape of resources. By way of illustration *Figure 11.6* shows how part of a 'tree' might be developed in attempting to relate the objectives of a local health service to the work activities required to achieve these. This simple partial example highlights both the problems faced in developing a programme structure and its power in emphasizing alternative means to achieve ends. Thus at different stages the policy maker is faced with choices. For example, by spending more on prevention of disease the need to expend resources on cures may be reduced. The need to consider long-term needs is emphasized by this example, and points to the need for the assessment of future year implications. Again, the level of health education expenditure may affect the need for other preventive measures and so on. These alternatives are not, of course, clear-cut. It is not a question of spending on *either* prevention *or* cure, on health education *or* other measures, but of achieving the right balance. The need for the assessment of *incremental* costs and benefits in developing alternative services is emphasized. It is the extra or marginal costs and benefits which are important in considering alternatives since resources are not, typically, used exclusively for one purpose rather than another, but finely balanced to achieve some combination of objectives. The obvious problem in developing a programme structure is deciding upon what range of alternatives to consider. At some stage the alternatives must be appraised in terms of the costs and the benefits associated with them. One aspect of this problem is that of selecting a time-span for which to assess the programme. Moreover, a set of programmes when adopted, after appraising the potential costs and benefits of different possibilities, must be translated into a financial plan embodying the fiscal implications of the policies adopted, so that methods of financing may be considered.

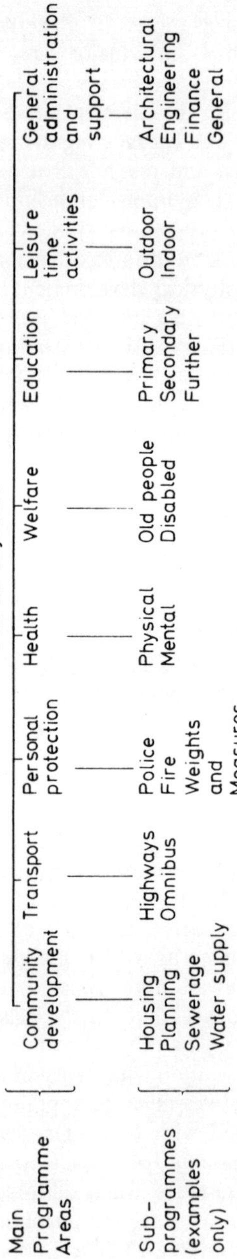

Main Programme Areas	Community development	Transport	Personal protection	Health	Welfare	Education	Leisure time activities	General administration and support
				Overall objective				
Sub-programmes (examples only)	Housing Planning Sewerage Water supply	Highways Omnibus	Police Fire Weights and Measures	Physical Mental	Old people Disabled	Primary Secondary Further	Outdoor Indoor	Architectural Engineering Finance General

Figure 11.5. Programme structure. First stage

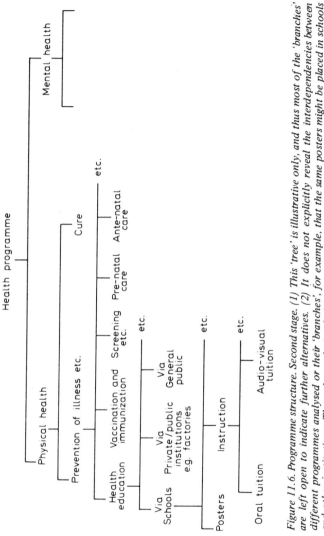

Figure 11.6. Programme structure. Second stage. (1) This 'tree' is illustrative only, and thus most of the 'branches' are left open to indicate further alternatives. (2) It does not explicitly reveal the interdependencies between different programmes analysed or their 'branches', for example, that the same posters might be placed in schools and other institutions. Thus, the analysis of objectives and alternative ways of achieving them does not of itself provide the solution to problems of organizing resources to achieve the objectives decided upon

Five years appears to be the maximum period suggested as practicable for the programme planning horizon. This does not mean that individual programmes, or projects within a programme should not be evaluated for longer periods since different needs have varying durations. It does mean that the effects of different programmes should be compared as to their overall effect over a period long enough to assess their implications for longer than a single fiscal period; and it means that the effect of capital and revenue expenditure proposals must be appraised in conjunction, rather than considered in artificial isolation.

The time-span adopted for a programme structure imposes a constraint upon the alternatives which may be considered. Any further reduction in the possible alternatives to be appraised will be dictated by a host of practical constraints and factors which the building up of a programme structure will help to expose. Thus certain needs will be recognized as more critical than others, alterations to existing methods of work may be impractical for political reasons, and the non-availability of certain types or resources, for example manpower, may rule out some theoretically possible alternatives. Financial constraints particularly may make their presence felt at an early stage in the development of a programme structure.

Finally, the programme budgeting approach requires the analysis of programme areas so that policy makers can be supplied with information on the costs and benefits which may be expected to result from alternative ways of attaining the organization's objectives. The difficulties of cost—benefit analysis were indicated in the last section and the expense and techniques required to perform an in-depth cost—benefit analysis either for a whole programme area or a particular part of it make it certain that less rigorous analyses will constitute the main way of appraising programme areas for the foreseeable future.

The difference in approach between programme and traditional budgets and the problem of manipulating decision making information to serve the needs of operational control, both arise in part from the way an organization is organized to carry out its objectives. In constructing a programme and identifying different activities it becomes apparent that some resources contribute to quite distinctive ends. For example, a Medical Officer of Health administers both physical and mental health programmes, or a nurse may help in both preventive or curative aspects of illness. It may thus be easier to identify a cost with a department than an objective. Yet cost—benefit analysis, however crudely performed, requires that costs and benefits must in some way be distinguished and related to particular programmes. Traditional budgets are built up on a departmental basis; programme budgets on the basis of objectives regardless of which departments contribute to their achievement. Yet, assuming the programme budget is adopted, it is desirable for control purposes to be able to identify the cost and benefits with the departments through which the policy will be implemented and day-to-day control exercised. The reconciliation of data for decision making with that required for operational control thus provides a further problem in establishing a management information system capable of meeting the varied requirements of the management process. The nature of this problem emerges from a consideration of performance budgeting.

THE MEASUREMENT OF EFFICIENCY

The aim of management as distinct from the aim of the organization it serves is to achieve objectives efficiently. However rational the process of decision making, it is the way policies are executed which will ultimately determine the degree of success achieved. The measurement of organizational efficiency is difficult. It depends upon relating input to output. There is also the problem of measuring the efficiency of different parts of the organizations work as well as the whole in order to exercise control at different levels. An essential feature of the measurement of efficiency for control purposes, however, is the establishment of some standard against which to compare performance; and comparisons imply that like is compared with like if they are to be meaningful.

The comparison needed for control purposes is that between what is happening and what ought to happen. Thus standards should be evolved at the planning stage of the management process. The organization must prescribe what output it aims to achieve and what the costs will be.

The difficulties of identifying and measuring costs and benefits have been noted at various points. In particular the translation of benefits into terms of money so as to obtain a measure of economic efficiency has been stressed. Thus hospitals with the same costs per patient per week are not necessarily equally efficient in the sense that the value of the services they provide are the same, and the subjective element in the valuation process is increased where an organization's outputs are not exchanged for cash.

However, the difficulty, or even impossibility, of measuring output values does not prevent the establishment of some assessment of operational efficiency. Provided outputs can be measured in some way, standards can be set up against which to compare performance. Possible ways of expressing the efficiency relationships are as follows.

(1) $\dfrac{\text{Actual output}}{\text{Maximum (or standard) output obtainable}}$ for a given input

e.g. $\dfrac{3,000 \text{ vaccinations}}{4,000 \text{ vaccinations}}$ for a cost of £1,000 i.e. only 75 per cent efficient

(2) $\dfrac{\text{Minimum (or standard) cost}}{\text{Actual cost}}$ for a given output

e.g. $\dfrac{£250}{£275}$ for 1,000 windows cleaned i.e. 91 per cent efficient

(3) $\dfrac{\text{Actual output}}{\text{Actual cost}}$ compared with $\dfrac{\text{Standard output}}{\text{Standard cost}}$

e.g. $\dfrac{10{,}800 \text{ meals served}}{£6{,}000}$ compared with $\dfrac{12{,}000 \text{ meals served}}{£6{,}000}$ i.e. £0·6 per meal compared with £0·5 per meal

These expressions suit situations where (1) a fixed budgeted amount is provided and management hope to achieve as much as possible with it; (2) a given task must be performed, and the aim is to ensure its achievement as cheaply as possible; and (3) where needs are variable. In any event, it is necessary to establish some standard as a basis for comparison and the quality of performance required. Thus if the meals actually served vary in quality from the standard prescribed, the comparison is invalid. A higher cost per meal may simply reflect a better quality of service than originally aimed at; an 'improvement' in effect gained by denying other areas of the organization the extra resources used up.

In dealing with cost accounting the difficulties of establishing standards and analysing the cause of variations of cost where output varies and fixed costs are incurred were indicated. The existence of both controllable and non-controllable factors, affecting both costs and outputs, makes the pinpointing of personal responsibility for efficient operation difficult, especially where several persons contribute to a paritcular performance. Yet if detailed analysis of all the factors affecting performance is practically impossible, it must be recognized that *any* step towards measuring efficiency depends upon achieving some kind of standard and, in particular, relating input to output ahcieved. This is the aim of performance budgeting.

PERFORMANCE BUDGETING

This technique must not be confused with programme budgeting. Whereas the programme budget analyses resource requirements by reference to programme areas or the objectives of an authority, and expresses financial needs from a decision making viewpoint, a performance budget is control orientated. It seeks to identify the performances or outputs required from the different sections of the organization and the costs involved, so that actual performances and costs may be compared with those aimed at.

Like the traditional budget it is framed on departmental lines, but it differs in that it establishes output as well as input or cost criteria as the basis for operational control over departmental activities. It represents an attempt to assess departmental activity involving public expenditure not merely by the regularity or legality of their expenditure but by relating this to units of output and is essentially the basis for an exercise in standard costing, and assessing the efficiency with which operations are conducted.

The implementation of a performance budgeting system involves the establishment of output measures for the various sections of the organization as well as the whole, rather in the way that the hospital costing scheme does. The difference is that outputs are estimated in advance for the year ahead and serve as a standard against which to measure variations in the costs/performances achieved.

The important difference between the programme budget and the performance budget lies in the data on which the two are built up. Thus in choosing between one programme or another the alternative advantages and disadvantages are compared. The assessment of these involves a consideration of direct costs and benefits, spill-over effects and intangible factors which may not be always quantifiable. The criteria on which programmes are selected are thus likely to be complex, a reflection of the numerous factors affecting the decision and the complexity of the objectives aimed at. By comparison, since the performance budget seeks to obtain an indication of operational efficiency and thus relates costs to some measure of performance, the criteria adopted are simple numerical standards which must relate to the actual areas of activity, namely, the department or sections through which work is organized.

For example, in deciding to provide a home nursing service for certain categories of patient rather than hospitalization, many factors would be considered in reaching a decision, including, for example, the potential effect on dependents and other parties, whose eventual response to a policy may be outside the authoritative control or the authority or department initiating or implementing the service. An assessment of the work of home nurses in relation to their cost might be expressed, for example, in terms of the cost per patient (or 100 patients) visited. Such a figure would indicate whether more or less visits were being achieved for a given amount of expenditure than was budgeted for, and would suggest the need for investigation into the causes of any variation. This measure would not, however, necessarily indicate any variation in the relationship between actual costs and benefits compared with those aimed at since it does not attempt to incorporate the numerous factors involved. In particular, it would be difficult to assess in any measurable way the actual side effects of such a social policy even assuming some weight had been attached to these in selecting a policy of home nursing.

The development of appropriate performance standards lies in work, and time and motion, study exercises and organization and method surveys of the various aspects of organizational activity. But in translating programme requirements into performance budgets as a basis for executive control, or using performance orientated data in assessing the merits or otherwise of alternative courses of action when programmes themselves are being considered, the differences in the significance of the data used must be fully appreciated.

THE FUTURE OF FINANCIAL MANAGEMENT

There can be little doubt that the programme and performance budget approaches to financial management will be increasingly adopted in public authorities, that they reflect a realization of the need to view organizational problems in a broader and more systematic manner, and in consequence will demand closer co-operation between the different participants in an organization. Nevertheless, new approaches do not automatically provide solutions. They may identify problems more clearly, but their solution demands changes in attitudes or techniques which may or may not be forthcoming.

The programme budgeting or management by objectives approach depends in part upon the success with which such techniques as cost–benefit analysis are developed. Performance budgeting depends for its success in part upon the establishment of output or performance indicators which reflect as nearly as possible the results required by the authority concerned. The crucial problem here is that illustrated in the last section, namely, that unit costs may not reflect the cost–benefit criteria used in formulating policy. In simple terms, the measures adopted to assess execution of policies may not be adequate guides by which to judge the merits of overall results of these policies, and might result in efforts being misapplied and goals distorted. For example, a visitor aiming to appear efficient might seek to accomplish a target figure of visits and reduce the quality of her work in the process. This points to the need for extreme care in the establishment of performance indicators so as to ensure there is some correspondence between the criteria used in formulating programmes and those used to assess operational performance. It underlines the need to give adequate weight to specialist and technical advice in establishing criteria. Moreover, it emphasizes that quantitative controls must be complemented by quality control, for example, the assessment of the technical aspect of performance by a health visitor's supervisor or inspector.

Establishing criteria for policy formulation and operational control, formidable enough, is only one facet of the overall problem of management. Policies must be actually adopted and then implemented. Ignoring political considerations such as the effect of pressure groups and the difficulties of allowing for flexibility in the timing and introduction of accepted or new policies, effective operational control will depend upon performance indicators being compiled sufficiently quickly for deviations from plans to be remedied. Moreover, not only must management information be placed in the hands of those who can take remedial action but they must actually take that action. In a performance budget system the responsibility for producing control data lies not only upon the finance officer to accumulate up-to-date information on costs but upon the executive department to collate output data, and for the two sets to be related and used effectively. This poses two related questions regarding data collection, processing and supply.

First, the one noted in discussing cost analysis of how far it is either possible or economical to distinguish between the various causes of variation from standards and identify individual responsibility; that is how detailed should control be? Secondly, how should data production be organized?

The use of computers opens up new horizons regarding the type, detail, speed and cost of data production and its effects upon organizational structures. In particular, the possibility of classifications and analyses of data which overcome some of the limitations already noted in existing financial information systems arises, as well as making them available at the various points of decision making and control.

Improved analytical techniques and data processing technology provide grounds for a belief that the programme—performance budgeting approach to financial management will have a material impact upon public administration, including the health services, in the very near future, not least in the amount of effort devoted to the design and establishment of improved information systems. It is pertinent therefore to conclude with some comments which are in part of a cautionary nature.

First, all the variables management seeks to control cannot be expressed in terms of simple numerical indicators and accordingly, such data can play only a part in decision making and control. The use of financial data for management purposes, or indeed any quantitatively expressed data, can lead to it being given too much weight in decision making and control. In contrast, because some factors cannot easily be quantified and thus compared in considering alternatives, it is possible to allocate resources to the production of detailed and sophisticated management data which are simply ignored and thus an unproductive exercise.

Secondly, the establishment of procedures for collating and producing information, and the criteria adopted for management purposes, may have unintended results. The way in which individuals react to control mechanisms, and changes in them, is little understood. For example, performance standards pitched too high may adversely affect motivation. Human reactions must therefore be envisaged and allowed for in introducing more systematic techniques.

Thirdly, the availability of computers capable of producing data in forms and at speeds formerly impossible and broader approaches to management problems, whilst opening up the path to the production of more relevant information and hence effective management, involve, or at least provide arguments for, the reorganization of administrative structures especially the creation of larger authorities. There is a consequent danger that ultimate objectives will be lost sight of in the eagerness to obtain the ostensible benefits of improved managerial technology.

Finally, the ever increasing contributions, both by theoreticians and practitioners from different disciplines, towards the solution of managerial problems demand that attention be given to assessing what sort of priority should be given to introducing new techniques.

The questions are, for example, in terms of financial management, whether emphasis should be given to improving internal or external control techniques, to establishing simple performance indicators or complex control mechanisms, to improving decision making or operational control, and which emphasis will make overall management more effective. The answer to such questions can only emerge from a continuing dialogue between the various participants in the health service whatever their specialist interest may be, and from closer co-operation and understanding of each other's techniques and problems by the various specialists involved.

Bibliography

Abernethy, W.L. (1957). *Internal Audit in Local Authorities and Hospitals.* London; Shaw

Control of Public Expenditure (1961). Cmnd. 1432. London; H.M.S.O.

Cranston, D.G., Butler, P.J., Harty, B.P. and Stares, S.H.E. (1969). *Programme Budgeting.* I.M.T.A. Midland Associates Study Group Report

Doodson, N. (1962). *Local Authority Borrowing.* I.M.T.A. Research Study

BIBLIOGRAPHY

Feldstein, M.S. (1964). 'Cost—Benefit Analysis and Investment in the Public Sector.' *Public Administration* **42**,

Form of Published Accounts of Local Authorities: General Principles, The (1958) I.M.T.A.

Hepworth, N.P. (1970). *The Finance of Local Government.* London; Allen and Unwin

Marshall, A.H. (1960). *Financial Administration in Local Government.* London; Allen and Unwin

McKean, R.N. (1958). *Efficiency in Government through Systems Analysis.* New York and Chichester; Wiley

Milne, J.F. and Chaplin, N.W. (Eds.) (1969). *Modern Hospital Management.* London; The Institute of Hospital Administrators

Montacute, C. (1962). *Costing and Efficiency in Hospitals.* London; Oxford University Press

N.E.D.C. (1965). *Investment Appraisal.* London; H.M.S.O.

Normanton, E.L. (1966). *The Accountability and Audit of Governments.* Manchester; University Press

Patrick, E.J. (1965). *Basic Accounting Principles as Applied to Municipal Accounts.* I.M.T.A. Students' Society Study Booklet

Peters, G.H. (1966). *Cost—Benefit Analysis and Public Expenditure.* Institute of Economic Affairs, Eaton Paper No. 8

Prest, A.R. and Turvey, R. (1965). 'Cost—Benefit Analysis: A Survey.' *Econ. J.* **75**, 683

Report of the Bristol Conference (1969). *The Control of the Trends of Public Expenditure.* I.M.T.A.

Report of the Cambridge Conference (1968). *Local Government Administration in the Future.* I.M.T.A.

Report of the Harrogate Conference (1968). *Productivity in Local Government.* Local Authorities' Conditions Service Advisory Board

Report of the London Conference (1969). *Programme Budgeting: The Concept and Application.* I.M.T.A.

Report of a panel established by I.M.T.A. (1969). *Allocation of Central Administrative Expenses*

Report of a Working Party on Hospital Costing (1955). London; H.M.S.O.

Report of the Working Party on Hospital Revenue Allocations (1961). Ministry of Health. London; H.M.S.O.

R.I.P.A. (1959). *Budgeting in Public Authorities.* London; Allen and Unwin

Rose, K.E. (1969). *Towards Multi-purpose Budgeting in Local Government.* I.M.T.A. Report

Sidebotham, R. and Page, C.S. (1960). *Accounting for Local and Public Authorities.* London; Gee

Solomons, D. (1968). *Studies in Cost Analysis*. London; Sweet and Maxwell

The Health and Welfare Services (1969). Standard Form. I.M.T.A.

Stonefrost, M.F. (1965). *Capital Accounts of Local Authorities*. I.M.T.A. Students' Society Study Booklet

Wallis, R.W. (1965). 'A Critique of Financial Administration in Local Government.' *Local Government Finance Journal* (June)

— (1970). *Accounting – A Modern Approach*. New York and Maidenhead; McGraw-Hill

Wood, F. and Townsley, J. (1970). *Accounting – A Programmed Text*. Stockport; Polytech Publishers

Wright, M.G. (1967). *Discounted Cash Flow*. New York and Maiden-Head; McGraw Hill

APPENDIX A

HMC/BG/RHB

STATEMENT OF BALANCES AT 31st MARCH, 19 ...

Main Code 10

LIABILITIES	Sub code	£	s.	d.	ASSETS	Sub code	£	s.	d.
				HOSPITAL REVENUE AND CAPITAL ACCOUNTS					
Department/R.H.B. Account	001				Department/R.H.B. Account	101			
Sundry creditors (including patients' monies held in bank accounts)	002				Stock in hand	102			
					Sundry debtors	103			
					Cash in hand/at bank	104			
				AREA NURSE TRAINING COMMITTEE					
Area Nurse Training Committee	011				Area Nurse Training Committee	111			
Sundry Creditors	012				Sundry debtors	112			
Cash overdrawn	013				Cash held for A.N.T.C.	113			
				PATIENTS' MONIES					
Due to patients: from hospital Revenue accounts	021				Cash held in hospital Revenue accounts	121			
from other accounts	022				Cash held in other accounts	122			
Sundry Creditors	023				Sundry debtors	123			
				HOSPITAL TRUST FUNDS					
Capital held in perpetuity	031				Properties	131			
Other Funds Account	032				Investments—narrower range	132			
Sundry Creditors	033				Investments—wider range	133			
					Investments—special range (incl. Charity Commission Inv. Fund)	134			
					Stock in hand	135			
					Sundry debtors	136			
					Cash in hand/at bank	137			

I certify that this Statement of Balances and the attached Tables, Statements and Memorandum Trading and property accounts were adopted by the Board/Committee at their meeting held on the ....

Secretary/House Governor

I hereby certify that the Statements of Accounts (as listed below) of which the foregoing is the Statement of Balances are, to the best of my knowledge and belief correct.

Chief Financial Officer/Treasurer

	£	s.	d.
Revenue Cash & Expenditure Reconciliation			
Table A—Central Administration Expenditure			
Table B—Hospital Maintenance Expenditure			
Table C—Other Hospital Expenditure			
Table D—Hospital Maintenance Income			
Capital Cash and Expenditure Reconciliation			
Table F—Capital Expenditure			

Table E
Table X
Table Y
Losses and Compensation Statement
Memorandum Farm Trading Account
Memorandum Market Garden Trading Account
Memorandum Property Account
Memorandum Canteen Trading Account
Memorandum Shop Trading Account

APPENDIX B

Year ended 31st March 19............   TABLE A—CENTRAL ADMINISTRATION EXPENDITURE ....HMC/BG   Main Code 01

Previous Year £	Head of account	Sub code	£	s.	d.
	1. Members of the Committee—travelling and subsistence expenses, payments for loss of remunerative time ...	101			
	2. Salaries and wages (including employer's and employees' contributions to National Insurance and Superannuation)—staff ...	102			
	3. Fuel, light, water and cleaning ...	103			
	4. Structural repairs and renewals ...	104			
	5. Furniture and equipment ...	105			
	6. Rent and rates ...	106			
	7. Printing, stationery, postages, telephones ...	107			
	8. Travelling and subsistence expenses—staff ...	108			
	9. Miscellaneous (a) (b) (c) (d) (e)	109			
	10. Services received from other hospital authorities:—				
	(i) the R.H.B. or other H.M.C.s in the Region ...	110			
	(ii) H.M.C.s in other Regions ...	111			
	(iii) Boards of Governors ...	112			
	(iv) other Regional Hospital Boards ...	113			
	11. LESS Services provided for other hospital authorities:—				
	(i) the R.H.B. or other H.M.C.s in the Region ...	114			CR
	(ii) H.M.C.s in other Regions ...	115			CR
	(iii) Boards of Governors ...	116			CR
	(iv) other Regional Hospital Boards ...	117			CR
	12. LESS Direct Credits (a) (b)	118			CR
	TOTAL—(To agree with item 8 of Revenue, Cash and Expenditure Reconciliation Statement) ...				

APPENDIX C (a)

Year ended 31st March 19 .... HMC/BGRHB

TABLE B—HOSPITAL MAINTENANCE EXPENDITURE

Main Code 02

Previous Year £	Main Heading	Sub-heading	Sub code	Amount £ s. d.	Amount £ s. d.
	1. Salaries and wages:—				
	(a) (i) Medical and dental ...		101		
	(ii) Consultants (Boards of Governors only)		102		
	(b) Nursing ...		103		
	(c) Building and Engineering ...		104		
	(d) Administrative and clerical		105		
	(e) Other staff ...	(i) Professional and technical ...	106		
		(ii) Domestic ...	107		
		(iii) Catering ...	108		
		(iv) Laundry ...	109		
		(v) Trading Services ...	110		
		(vi) Boiler House ...	111		
		(vii) Grounds and ornamental gardens...	112		
		(viii) Other...	113		
		TOTAL OF SALARIES AND WAGES			
	2. Provisions (including contract catering expenditure)		214		
	3. Staff uniforms and clothing ...		215		
	4. Patients' clothing ...		216		
	5. Drugs and dressings	(i) Drugs...	217		
		(ii) Dressings	218		
	6. Medical and surgical appliances and equipment ...		219		
	7. General services (power, light, heating, water, cleaning and laundry)	(i) Boiler fuel ...	221		
		(ii) Other fuel, light, power and water...	222		
		(iii) Laundry materials ...	223		
		(iv) Other cleaning materials and equipment ...	224		
		(v) Laundry—contract ...	225		
		Amount carried forward ...			

APPENDIX C (b)

TABLE 8 (continued) .... HMC/BG/RHB

Main code 02

Amount brought forward ...

		HMC/BG/RHB	Main code 02
8.	Maintenance of buildings and engineering services	226	
9.	Maintenance of grounds and ornamental gardens	227	
10.	Domestic repairs, renewals and replacements		
	(i) Furniture and fittings	228	
	(ii) Hardware and crockery	229–	
	(iii) Bedding and linen	230	
11.	Rents, rates and tithes	231	
12.	Office equipment, printing, stationery, advertising, postage, telephones, etc. ...	232	
13.	Transport ... ... (i) Vehicles	233	
	(ii) Patients' travelling expenses ...	234	
	(iii) Medical staff travelling expenses ...	235	
	(iv) Other staff travelling expenses ...	236	
14.	Trading services	237	
15.	Patients' allowances	238	
16.	User agreements	239	
17.	Miscellaneous ... ... (i) Occupational therapy	240	
	(ii) Other	241	
18.	Services received from other hospital authorities:—		
	(i) the R.H.B. or other H.M.C.s in the Region	242	
	(ii) H.M.C.s in other Regions	243	
	(iii) Boards of Governors	244	
	(iv) other Regional Hospital Boards	245	
19.	Less services provided for other hospital authorities:—		
	(i) the R.H.B. or other H.M.C.s in the Region	246	CR
	(ii) H.M.C.s in other Regions	247	CR
	(iii) Boards of Governors	248	CR
	(iv) other Regional Hospital Boards	249	CR
			CR
	GROSS EXPENDITURE—Carried Forward ...		

APPENDIX C (c)

TABLE B (continued)

.... HMC/BG/RHB

Main Code 02

DIRECT CREDITS				
	Amount brought forward ...			
20. Income from Local Authorities				CR
	(i) User agreements	301	CR	
	(ii) Other income...	302	CR	
21. Staff rents, board, etc.		303		CR
22. Trading Services		304		CR
23. Miscellaneous				
	(ii) Occupational therapy	305	CR	CR
	(iii) Other	306	CR	CR
	TOTAL DIRECT CREDITS ...			
	GROSS EXPENDITURE less DIRECT CREDITS ...			

(To agree with item 9 of Revenue, Cash and Expenditure Reconciliation Statement)

APPENDIX D

TABLE C—OTHER EXPENDITURE (H.M.C.s & B.C.s only)

Main code 03

		£	s.	d.
1. Allowances to patients on licence and/or patients not resident in the Hospital	701			
2. Cost of maintaining patients in hospitals not vesting in Secretary of State (B.G.s only)	702			
3. Other expenditure (specify)				
(a)				
(b)				
(c)				
Total Item 3	703			

TOTAL (to agree with Item 10 of Revenue, Cash and Expenditure Reconciliation Statement)

APPENDIX E

Year ended 31st March, 19...... .... TABLE D — HOSPITAL MAINTENANCE INCOME .... HMC/BG

Main code 04

Previous Year £	Head of account	Sub code	£	s.	d.
	1. From patients — supply of drugs and supply and repair of appliances				
	(i) for appliances more expensive than prescribed — under Section 3 (2) (a) of N.H.S. Act 1946	401			
	(ii) for the repair and replacement of appliances necessitated by lack of care — under Section 3 (2) (b) of N.H.S. Act 1946	402			
	(iii) for dental and optical appliances — under Section 1 (i) of N.H.S. Act 1951, as amended by N.H.S. Act 1961	403			
	(iv) for drugs and appliances — under Section 1 of N.H.S. Act 1952	404			
	(v) for prescriptions on form E.C.10(HP) (to agree with item 3(f) of Revenue Cash and Expenditure Reconciliation Statement)	405			
	2. From patients — accommodation in single rooms or small wards (Sec. 4 of N.H.S. Act 1946) ...	406			
	3. From patients — private accommodation and treatment (Sec. 5 of N.H.S. Act 1946)				
	(i) In-patients	407			
	(ii) Out-patients	408			
	4. Under the Road Traffic Act 1960	409			
	5. Miscellaneous				
	(i) Rents (hospital land and premises)	410			
	(ii) Sale of inventory items and equipment	411			
	(iii) Maintenance charges, working patients	412			
	(iv) Other income — major items to be specified				
		413			
	Total hospital maintenance income (to agree with item 3 (a) of Revenue Cash and Expenditure Reconciliation Statement)				

12—Behaviour in Organizations

F.J. Glen

Introduction

The purpose of this chapter is to present a field of study which is possibly the oldest and the newest of the several approaches to the understanding of the management function. It is old in that it has been implicitly recognized since co-operative activity became a part of human behaviour and since men began to direct and co-ordinate the activities of their fellows. It is new in that the study of behaviour in organizations as a separate field has arisen within the last two decades, following upon the rapid development of applied psychology during World War II.

Organizational psychology has been described as allied to classical industrial psychology and to human relations psychology, but differing from both of them in its greater concern with descriptive and experimental research (Leavitt, 1964). The study of the interactions between individuals, organizations and the environment can extend to include many additional concepts drawn from sociology, anthropology, economics, political science and other disciplines, laying emphasis on the need to understand the total dynamics of the organization in which behaviour is observed rather than on attempts to assess or modify isolated elements of that behaviour.

Many techniques which have been developed as tools of management are of specialized application, or are such that they may be adopted or rejected in accordance with what an individual manager feels to be the demands of particular problems. The study of behaviour in organizations presents a different situation in that it is invariably relevant to the co-ordination of the activities of individuals towards the achievment of a goal — the common characteristic of all management processes. It is not a question of whether this study is of relevance to the manager, but rather whether it is explicitly recognized as a factor in his decision processes or whether he evaluates such factors subjectively and intuitively.

An organization has been defined as 'the rational co-ordination of the activities of a number of people for the achievement of some common explicit purpose or goal, through division of labour and function, and through a hierarchy of authority and responsibility' (Schein, 1965). Such a definition could be applied not only to the activities of an industrial or commercial concern, a government department or a hospital, but equally to units within such systems and to less formally organized activities such as team games. It might be considered that such examples are unrelated, but they share the essential characteristics of the definition and are capable of being studied by similar methods. To acknowledge that hospitals are a special category of organization is not to invalidate the methods of study which have been applied successfully elsewhere. The management problems of a hospital have much in common with those of other hierarchical structures — its activities are a function of the behaviour of individuals within it and of its interactions with the environment in which it operates.

The growing awareness in industry of the human aspects of management problems is reflected in the increasing frequency with which advice is sought from departments and schools of business, management and organizational studies, in universities and elsewhere. It is generally accepted that, although some larger organizations have developed internal departments of management services, few are so large that they can afford to retain a staff of specialists sufficiently comprehensive to deal with every type of internal problem which may arise. When investigating decision processes, communications, efficiency, selection and training and so on, it is frequently an advantage to employ independent specialists rather than for the investigation to be undertaken by individuals who are themselves a part of the organization being studied.

Difficulties can arise from the assumption that a particular problem can be treated in isolation. The internal investigator may find himself in a situation where a full examination of what initially appeared to be a problem at lower staff level begins to involve him in the evaluation of communication difficulties and role relationships at levels senior to his own. Particularly when the organization is not committed to a programme of self-appraisal such a situation can lead to incomplete or abandoned investigations.

The situation can also arise where a consultant's report or recommendation, however valid, is read, accepted, but never acted upon. This may be the result of a deliberate decision on the part of management but, not infrequently, it is the consequence of a study which analyses and evaluates the problem area concerned but does not deal with the actual process of effecting change within the organization. Although it is quite possible to produce a methodologically sound report based upon a series of systematic observations, the value of such studies to management is limited if they do not extend to the actual problems of implementation. Similarly, the value of focal studies is limited unless their effect within the total context of the organization is understood.

Investigation in a hospital setting is complicated by the structural organization. In place of the usual pyramidal structure of an industrial organization we find three main distinct but interacting hierarchies — administrative, medical, and nursing — and a number of related sub-systems of specialist departments and ancilliary services with varying degrees of functional autonomy. In the psychiatric hospital there may well be a complete duplication of the nursing hierarchy for separate male and female staffs. Consequently one finds both the usual problems of a large organization composed of several sub-systems — delay in decision, ego-satisfaction problems for the majority of the people concerned and problems of bureaucratic power for the subordinate (Anderson and Warkov, 1961) — and further problems of communication between professional groups and between status groups within each profession (Revans, 1962).

The difficulties of management when a highly traditional and hierarchial structure becomes subject to pressure from social changes in its external environment are considerable. Application of modern management techniques to the formal aspects of the structure can provide only a partial answer. More important to identify and more difficult to approach are the informal structures existing within the system: problems of communication, of status, prejudice and personal satisfaction must be examined and, as far as possible, understood if technical developments in management are to be maximally effective.

Additional difficulty arises in comparing hospitals with other types of organizations. Perhaps the closest parallel likely to be perceived by the management specialist is a public service, with the function of maintaining the health of the community which it serves. It is unlikely that the idea of responsibility to the community as 'customer' with the patient seen as the 'material to be serviced', would be acceptable to either hospital staffs or to patients.

The patient would, perhaps, prefer to see the hospital as providing a personal service with himself in the role of customer. The staffs of hospitals, however, although they might accept that their role was, at least in part, to provide help to the sick, would be unlikely to accept the premise that their function involved responsibility to satisfy customers in the same sense as would be applicable to other personal service exterprises. Medical services are perceived as being qualitatively different from, and implicitly superior in status to, other forms of service enterprise. The patient might be said to occupy a dependent role in relation to the service, superior to that of material to be serviced but, in terms of this capacity to influence the situation, inferior to that of customer.

PSYCHOLOGY AND ORGANIZATIONS

The study of organizations would be considerably simplified if the formal organization chart provided some indication of the individual characteristics of those whose names appear upon it and of their function within it. At best, however, such charts give a simplified picture of the formal roles within the organization and of some of their inter-relationships. They do not indicate anything of the ways in which similar roles may be differently interpreted by the individuals occupying them, or of the ways in which each member of the organization perceives the roles of others.

The formal organization charts of two institutions may show many points of similarity — similar titles and similar hierarchical relationships. Although it may be obvious, it still requires to be stated that similar roles can be occupied by very dissimilar individuals and that any real understanding of an organization must take account of the individual differences which each member brings to his role. His relationship with colleagues, with superiors and with subordinates, both on a group and individual basis, will be determined not only by his formal role but also by his personal characteristics.

As has been stated above, the role of the research worker or the consultant in this field is not that of providing ready-made answers to stated problems. In many instances the true nature of the problem is not known; there is only a realization that something is wrong. The manager or administrator concerned may have attempted to apply symptomatic remedies on the basis of what he believes to be the problem, and may have met with some measure of success. Often, however, such measures serve to obscure the true nature of the problem and to produce an organization which has added a series of iatrogenic disorders to its original complaint!

Even when a particular problem is stated, it is necessary to ensure that it has been fully defined. Such definition calls for co-operative effort from the manager and from the consultant concerned. The former is usually too closely involved in the situation to appraise it objectively, and the latter cannot be sufficiently familiar with the structure, practices and traditions of the organization concerned to be able to make a fair appraisal alone. As has been noted in other contexts, the first observed presenting symptoms may be a poor guide to the eventual diagnosis, and an observed series of events can be misinterpreted in the absence of some understanding of the total context of the situation in which they appear.

The manager can take the decision as to whether investigation should be undertaken only after the problem has been defined and he is aware of the possible consequences of the course of action being contemplated. It is unlikely that a successful investigation can be carried out within predetermined limits. If certain areas of an organization's functioning, or certain members of it, are to be excluded from the process of evaluation, the available sources of evidence may be so restricted as to invalidate the investigation. Ideally, the organization should be prepared to look at itself 'warts and all'.

It is possible to describe organizations and their corporate activities in general terms and to apply a variety of economic and mathematical systems of analyses to their functioning. It is doubtful, however, whether an organization can be understood in such terms without making many assumptions as to the uniformity and interchangeability of its constituent parts. In analyses of this type measurement of change may be in terms of production or profit, in some directly quantifiable form.

In situations where such criteria cannot readily be identified, or where it is necessary to examine the internal working of the organization rather than its overall efficiency, a more detailed form of examination is necessary. This is particularly true if one wishes to study the ways in which individuals perform their several functions within the structure of the organization. On this level of description it is necessary to recognize that the human components of the structure are far from uniform, and that the efficiency of their functioning is determined to a significant degree by their individual characteristics.

Levels of Variables Studied

INDIVIDUAL PROCESSES

The choice of a hospital service career is unlikely to be determined by chance, particularly in the case of the medical and nursing fields. The individual embarks upon a relatively lengthy training during which his motivation must be sustained by the eventual prospect of professional qualification rather than by any immediate reward either in financial terms or in conditions of work. Particular career choices may commit the individual to further study and training well beyond the point of initial qualification which could arise from a desire to exercise a particular skill or to ensure advancement in the chosen career − goals which are not necessarily identical.

A career in hospital administration need not involve the same degree of commitment in its initial stages, nor does the training and attainment of qualifications limit the individual to a hospital-based future. To a considerable degree the skills associated with hospital administration are equally relevant to the administrative and management functions of other types of organization. The advantages of this greater degree of freedom in individual career development may be somewhat offset by the tendency for a lesser degree of obvious commitment to be associated with lower perceived status within the hospital hierarchy. The administrator may, on occasion, be criticized by his hospital colleagues for showing a greater concern for balance sheets and records than for people: should he show an inclination to concern himself directly with the welfare of patients, however, he may be seen by the same colleagues as stepping outside his proper role.

The extent to which a chosen career provides personal satisfaction will be determined partly by the role in which the individual finds himself and partly by the personality of the individual concerned. In general and possibly rather over-simplified terms, the individual is likely to remain in a particular role and be capable of functioning effectively in it if it provides a sufficient degree of satisfaction, or the prospects of such satisfaction. If the satisfaction is lacking he may abandon the role or seek some form of substitute satisfaction within it which may or may not be compatible with effective performance. If satisfaction is lacking and no substitute is available, but he is obliged by external constraints to continue in the role, his performance is likely to become unsatisfactory and his morale is likely to be low.

The above outline applies most directly in the lower levels of a career hierarchy: at more senior levels a further opportunity for personal satisfaction becomes available. As seniority increases the possibility of interpreting one's role, in terms of personal predisposition, increases correspondingly. The student nurse must attempt to meet the role demands determined for her by her senior colleagues. A ward sister, although limited by the formal constraints of her role, can interpret it in such a way as to impose some of her own standards upon it. A matron can, through time, so introduce her personal standards into the interpretation of her role as to substantially influence the working environment of a hospital.

The latter situation is illustrated by two responses to an enquiry into the recruitment and wastage of student nurses in which brief questionnaires were sent by a regional hospital board to a number of matrons. In the case of one hospital, with an excellent recruitment record and low wastage rate, the enquiry produced a detailed reply from the matron accompanied by her own evaluation of recruitment and wastage problems, and an invitation to visit the hospital and interview any of the nursing staff. A letter also arrived from the principal tutor of the same hospital pointing out that the excellent record of the hospital in nurse recruitment and training was largely due to changes in nursing administration and a policy of consultation introduced by matron. The other reply enclosed the uncompleted questionnaire and a two-page hand-written letter from the matron pointing out that she had not time to deal with frivolous enquiries, and that the question of nursing recruitment and wastage was solely the concern of herself and of no-one else either inside or outside her hospital. This hospital had the highest rate of wastage of student nurses in the sample.

Although Ministry of Health Circular HM(60) 66 provides that it is for the hospital authorities to decide what the duties of a superintendent should be if one is appointed, the interpretations of the role seem to be determined rather more by the personality characteristics of the individual in the posts than by other factors. Some different interpretations of the role in psychiatric hospitals are suggested below.

THE SUPERINTENDENT ROLE

The managing director

In this instance the medical superintendent seems to have found considerable satisfaction in the role of chief executive of a complex organization. His aim is to maintain the efficiency of his hospital as a working unit and to co-ordinate the activities of its component parts to this end. He receives regular reports from all departments within the hospital, and involves himself in planning and decision making at various levels. He has retained little or no direct clinical involvement in the hospital but monitors the work of the clinical firms.

The clinician

Here the physician superintendent appears to regard himself primarily as a practicing clinical psychiatrist. He may retain the leadership of a clinical firm, or may pursue research interests. It is probable that as much as possible of the routine management responsibilities will have devolved upon the lay administration and, possibly, the medical advisory committee. The success of this type of approach is dependent upon the pattern of relationships existing between the internal hierarchies of the hospital and, in particular, between the medical superintendent and the senior members of the administration. In a situation where working relationships are good and communications are effective, this style of approach can produce a good working environment.

The father figure

The situation can exist in which the medical superintendent seems to take a general, but detached, interest in the running of the hospital. He may be very concerned with the pattern of relationships within the hospital, anxious to reduce tensions and avoid conflict, but rarely involving himself directly in the management role. The clinical activities of the hospital may be effectively shared by the other consultants, and the nursing and administrative systems may function with a high degree of internal autonomy. The extent to which this approach will work in practice is largely dependent upon the success with which the management role is discharged by a process of delegation. In the absence of good communications between the medical, nursing and administrative hierarchies, such a system can result in a hospital in which no one is effectively in contact with more than his own section of the organization.

The dictator

This style of approach shares with the previous one the characteristic of considerable personal involvement with the hospital as a closed community. In this case, however, it is often made clear in every possible situation that authority rests with the physician-superintendent. Characteristically, a greater proportion of letters leave this hospital over the signature of the physician-superintendent than in any of the other cases. He is closely concerned with the direction of the hospital's activities but, unlike the managing director in the first example, he may be unable to delegate effectively or consistently.

The situation is illustrated by the case in which, during the absence of the physician-superintendent, a problem arose. The deputy decided that action should be deferred until the return of the physician-superintendent and was subsequently criticized by his chief for lack of initiative. A similar situation arose during a later absence when the deputy took appropriate action -- he was again taken to task, this time for exceeding his authority.

Such examples rarely occur, as it were, in pure culture, but individual approaches to a role which are capable of being characterized in this way are not hard to recognize. The examples tell us only a little about the strengths or weaknesses of the individual concerned but sufficient to suggest that such approaches to the role could have a substantial effect upon the working environment in the hospitals concerned. The advantages of strong directive leadership in this role should not be under-estimated,, however, as it has been pointed out that many progressive regimens in mental hospitals have been pioneered by medical superintendents of this type (Brown and Wing, 1962).

INTERPERSONAL PROCESSES

The primary form of interaction in a study of behaviour in an organization is the pattern of interchange and relationship between two individuals. It is a very common piece of human experience to find that what appear to be similar situations can elicit very different responses from the individuals concerned. Some of the factors which can influence an interpersonal exchange are readily recognizable — facial expression, tone of voice, manner of speech; others are less readily identified but can colour the interchange by introducing elements of positive or negative affect — 'I don't know why, but it was clear from the start that we would/wouldn't get on well together'.

The formal aspects of a working relationship will usually impose a superficial structuring upon the pattern of interactions between two individuals at different levels within the hierarchy. This is most marked in the more rigid types of organization and may actually be codified in the regulations of such bodies. An army private, for example, should, when addressing a non-commissioned officer, stand to attention and address him by his rank; when addressing an officer he should stand to attention, salute (traditionally showing respect for the Queen's Commission rather than the individual) and address him as 'Sir'. Failure to observe such rules could be a chargeable offence under military law. In a working unit, however, the formalities would give only a partial indication of the working relationship between different hierarchical levels. In spite of the formal overlay, observation over a period of time would show that the actual interpersonal relationship in the group could still range from strongly positive to strongly negative.

Such observations might give a better indication of the working efficiency of the unit than could be deduced from the pattern of formal discipline.

Where interpersonal relationships are poor, the attitude could readily arise that: 'I will do what I am ordered to do and what the regulations say that I must do — but that's all!' In effect, a 'work to rule' determined by interpersonal reactions rather than by trade union instructions.

For situations where an individual appears to rely heavily upon the formal structure of rules which regulate relationships within the organization, the question may arise as to whether he has become dependent upon the rules in discharging his role. When an individual feels that his security and authority depend upon the formal structure within which he works, and upon the system of rules which supports this structure, he is in a vulnerable position and likely to see any minor breach of regulation as a personal threat. The rules become important to him not as guiding principles but as protection, and increasing insecurity will tend to produce a correspondingly increasing rigidity in his observance of rules.

The situation can arise when, after a number of years spent in adjusting to the demands of a highly authoritarian system in the way suggested, the individual experiences extreme difficulty in responding effectively in interpersonal situations which are not specifically provided for in the regulations. His attitude to work relationships becomes increasingly rigid and his capacity to adjust to change becomes progressively less.

Although an important element of work behaviour at all levels, interpersonal relationships can exert a wider influence on the total work situation as the seniority of the individuals concerned increases. As indicated above, the effectiveness of different individual approaches to a management role may depend upon effective delegation and shared responsibility. The nature of the interpersonal relationship of the senior members of an organization can substantially effect the interpretation and implementation of policy and the nature of communications within the organization. The effect is not confined to the individuals concerned, but will be found to influence the performance of their respective staffs in varying degrees.

Where the success of an enterprise depends upon effective co-operative activity rather than individual levels of skills, it may be more important to entrust the joint direction of a task to individuals who are technically competent and capable of working together effectively, rather than to those who are technically brilliant but incompatible as personalities.

There is no ideal approach which could constitute a general rule in situations of this type. There is reason to suppose that different types of organizational goal require different patterns of interpersonal relationships and different leadership styles (Roby, Nicol and Farrell, 1963). Similarly, it has been suggested there are individual differences in preference for different types of leadership (Forehand and Gilmer, 1962).

GROUP PROCESSES

The examination of individual and interpersonal behaviour are necessary steps towards the understanding of the working organization, but the relationship of the individual and the organization is also affected by a series of intermediate social processes which exert a considerable influence upon the work situation. Each member of an organization is simultaneously a member of a variety of groups, both formal and informal, some of which are recognizably a part of the total organization while others, at first sight, may seem unrelated to it.

Formal groups are readily identifiable in terms of professional classification, levels of seniority within such classifications, place of work, type of work and so on; also in membership of professional associations and trade unions resulting in groups which have an existence both within and outside the organization concerned.

Informal groups may be less readily recognized but can, nevertheless, exert considerable influences upon individual behaviour. Individuals may be linked by common interests which cut across the boundaries of formal groups and hierarchical levels. Social, religious, political and recreational activities, educational or cultural backgrounds could produce group allegiance of this type.

Groups are important in that they exert influences upon the behaviour of their members which may encourage or inhibit a wide range of individual activities. Belonging to a group implies, in varying degrees, the acceptance of what are seen to be the norms of that group. These may be explicitly stated as standards of professional conduct or in a codified set of rules, or they may simply be tacitly accepted as things which are generally 'done' and 'not done' in certain situations.

Further, informal group membership may facilitate communications between individuals to a greater extent than the formal communications system of the organization. In one hospital a marked reduction in the efficiency of inter-unit communication and co-operation was found to be due to a recently introduced change intended to improve efficiency. It had been decided that the practice of meeting in the common room for morning coffee involved an unnecessary waste of medical staff time, and that the coffee should be provided at the place of work. It had not been realized that this meeting had provided the only regular contact between certain members of staff and that it had provided a main point of exchange of information between units. In that situation, 'mentioning it at coffee time', had been a more effective system than inter-unit telephone calls or letters.

Until recent years the norms of the nursing and medical groups were such that industrial action was not felt to be an acceptable course for their members. A number of social pressures have had, and are continuing to have, the effect of modifying group norms in this area, giving rise to internal pressures within the professional groups to use methods which are seen to be successful elsewhere in raising salary levels and improving conditions of work.

To suggest that a nursing career results from a sense of vocation and that it is consequently different from other career choices is no longer seen as a justification for wages and working conditions which are seen to compare unfavourably with those elsewhere. Restrictive regulations are less likely to be accepted because they are 'traditional' aspects of nurse training, particularly when the traditional practice can no longer be shown to be a necessary part of the training situation. The number of formal rules which exist in any organization, and particularly the number of rules which continue to be applied after they have outlived their usefulness, can often be an indication of the rigidity of the organization itself.

The situation is further complicated in the case of the medical profession by the conflict arising from the wish to retain the advantages of high status and independence as a unique group within society and, at the same time, to obtain the benefits of an organized professional group negotiating with employing authorities over salary and conditions of work. It is difficult to argue claims on the usual grounds of comparability, responsibility, work-load and efficiency, and simultaneously to retain the wide range of personal discretion which a consultant can exercise in the discharge of his duties. The usual bargaining procedures of uniform acceptance of changes or objective assessments of working efficiency are unlikely to be readily accepted.

Typically, indication of dissatisfaction with working conditions tends to arise most frequently from the lower levels of the organizational hierarchy. As has been found elsewhere opportunities for personal satisfaction tend to increase with seniority (Porter and Lawler, 1965), and the disadvantages of being a member of a large organization decrease as one rises within its structure (Forehand and Gilmer 1964). In the hospital setting this type of observation tends to be supported by the emergence of separate bodies representing the interests of the junior levels within professional groups.

It might reasonably be expected that the individuals who find themselves most in conflict with the organization in which they work will tend to leave it if the reasons for their dissatisfaction continue. There will be a corresponding tendency for those who most readily accept the value systems of the organization to become a more selected group as they rise to senior level; acceptance of the standards of the organization being associated with promotion prospects with the result that the characteristics of the structure tend to be perpetuated.

Those who remain within the organization without reaching the most senior levels will show differing patterns of adjustment to the social and administrative demands of the situation. They may form sub-groups within the structure according to whether their work adjustment reflects, for example, active co-operation, passive co-operation or resignation. The relative sizes of such sub-groups within an organization may give some indication of the characteristics of the organization itself and of the approaches of those responsible for the direction of its component units. In some situations it is possible that loyalty to such informal sub-groups could be greater than loyalty to the organization itself.

The existence of such groupings contributes to the informal structure of the organization. In the hospital situation the processes and composition of this informal structure may be, at best, only partially accessible to the senior members responsible for the implementation of policy.

ORGANIZATIONAL PROCESSES

During the past decade the study of work situations has tended to extend beyond the traditional examination of variables which have long been recognized as of importance to management – supervision, participation, leadership, etc. and the question has been raised as to whether those are the most valid categories for the study of behaviour in organizations (Mechanic, 1963). To a considerable degree the interactions between the individual and the organization are determined by identifiable characteristics of the organization itself, and models have been described in which the unit of study is the organization itself with the examination of specific individual and group situations contributing to an understanding of the total situation rather than constituting ends in themselves (Kahn and colleagues, 1964).

Some hospitals, or organizations, may show many of the characteristics of a bureaucratic structure as defined by Hall (1963). At the other extreme considerable efforts may have been made to minimize the effect of formal structures in the creation of a therapeutic community. Formal hierarchical structure is characteristic of the majority of hospitals, however, and the staff will tend to regulate their behaviour in formal situations in terms of the expectation appropriate to that type of organization. This process of adjustment to the environment, created by the organization, has been regarded as an adverse aspect of the effect of the organization upon the chronic patient in a psychiatric hospital (Barton, 1959).

In order to understand the patterns of behaviour within an organization it is necessary to consider the goals of the organization itself. These goals will give an indication of the organizational climate in which the behaviour takes place (Forehand and Gilmer, 1964), and will exert an influence on the ways in which the individual regulates his own behaviour and perceives the behaviour of others.

There may be a formally stated policy which outlines the goals of the organization; this may not correspond too closely with the goals towards which the organization appears to move in its actual operation. Such discrepancies can arise from a variety of causes. They may, for example, reflect the fact that organizations often develop additional goals of a kind which are not a part of their explicit policy but seem to have arisen as a function of the organizational process itself. In some situations the preservation of the *status quo* can become a goal towards which much organizational activity is directed; in this case any form of change or innovation can be seen as a threat.

Conflict between organizational and individual goals can have considerable effects upon the direction or limitation of action within the organization (Simon, 1964). Any sub-unit leader can influence in some degree the ways in which goals are interpreted, modifying them in terms of his own approach either consciously or unconsciously.

In a drug trial conducted in a psychiatric hospital (Jacobs and Glen, 1964) in which sisters and charge nurses were asked to report changes in patients' behaviour, one charge nurse reported adverse changes much more frequently than his colleagues. On enquiry it was found that he rated increased activity in mute and withdrawn patients as an adverse change because their increased responsiveness to their environment disrupted the smooth running of his ward.

It is less easy than it might appear to define the organizational goals of a hospital. Blau and Scott (1963) suggested a system of classification of organizations in terms of who benefits from their activities. Morris (1969) has suggested that, although it might be natural to assume that hospitals are service organizations in that they exist for the benefit of their clientele, subnormality hospitals could be regarded more readily as commonweal organizations in exercising a custodial function for the benefit of society. It could be argued that the latter classification could be applied at least in part to the activities of some hospitals which care for psychiatric patients or the chronic sick.

It has been suggested that some aspects of general hospitals are 'legacies from the era of charity and custodial care' (Cartwright, 1964). She suggests that this is reflected in such factors as a failure to recognize the patient's need for explanation, clinical teaching which takes no account of the patient's feelings in the situation, attitudes of condescension and lack of consideration by consultants who keep patients waiting.

Titmuss (1958) foresaw a danger that hospitals 'may tend increasingly to be run in the interests of those working in and for the hospital rather than in the interests of the patients'. While it is accepted that the two interests need not be incompatible, some aspects of current ward management are unlikely to be seen by the patients as being for their benefit. In one female surgical ward the normal preparation for a consultant's round is that by 30 minutes before the time of the round all patients should be in readiness; no books, magazines or knitting should be visible and bedclothes should be neatly arranged. This state is maintained until the consultant arrives, possibly more than 30 minutes after the appointed time. It might be considered that it would take some courage for a patient to request a bed pan during this period!

An objective evaluation of organizational goals, and the ways in which they are interpreted within the hospital, can be an effective way of identifying and examining a wide range of working practices. If the goals of an organization can be identified and shown to be appropriate, the effect of a particular activity can be evaluated as beneficial or otherwise in terms of these goals. As in therapy, it may be necessary to balance eventual benefit against adverse side effects, but it should be possible to justify the existence of any activity if it is to continue as a part of the organizational system.

It is not a question of establishing a definite system of rules for all organizational activities. Organizations show high degrees of individuality both as a function of the balance of interpersonal and group processes within them, and of the need for each organization to adapt to the particular conditions under which it operates. The validity of observations based on individual and group behaviour can only be fully assessed in the context of the organizational setting in which the observations are made.

Effects of change

Change is an emotive word in most organizations. The immediate reaction to the suggestion that change is to be introduced may be one of interest, anxiety, resistance or apathy even before the nature of the change is specified. Such reactions may reflect the individual's past experience of change situations, his degree of interest and involvement in his role, his rigidity, general apathy, frustration or feelings of inadequacy.

Random and inconsistent changes in the working of any organization can have a markedly disruptive effect, prejudicing the attitude of the members of the organization to change in general. Unplanned change, even when well-intentioned, can be a damaging experience in its long-term effects. It is not unusual for a medical administrator, who would normally insist upon establishing the underlying cause of a patient's symptoms before committing himself to a course of treatment, to ignore the diagnostic process when dealing with symptoms of malfunction in the organization for which he is responsible. Not infrequently the result of such an approach is to obscure the causes and exacerbate the condition.

The possible effects of any change upon the functioning of an organization and upon its members should be thoroughly considered before it is introduced. Following its introduction it is necessary to monitor its effects, both in order to determine whether the expected result has been achieved and also to identify, as soon as possible, any unexpected consequences.

Although some degree of resistance is to be expected when change is suggested, the extent to which it is perceived as a threat can be reduced by adequate information about the change and effective communication of this information. Such communication should extend to include not only those who must implement the change but also those who would be affected by it or might reasonably be interested in it. When information is not given directly to the individuals concerned it is generally necessary to ensure that it has not been re-interpreted with consequent distortion by those responsible for passing it on.

When a change has been adequately planned and the problems of its implementation have been considered, the fact that it is initially unwelcome need not unduly influence its success and eventual acceptance. In a study of the effect of unrestricted visiting in a psychiatric hospital, the nursing staff were asked to forecast possible difficulties and later asked to report on difficulties which had arisen in practice (Barton, Elkes and Glen, 1961). Initially 34 per cent of the nursing staff were in favour of the suggested change. The follow-up questionnaire six months' later, after the experiment had proved to be successful, asked whether they had been in favour of the change when it was first suggested — 74 per cent stated that they had supported it. It is suggested that the discrepancy of 40 per cent does not so much reflect a misrepresentation of the previous answer as an initial reluctance to express a definite view favouring change. The fact that this nursing staff were consulted before, during and after the introduction of changes in the hospital organization had a beneficial effect, both upon the ease with which change could be introduced and upon the level of interest and participation of the majority of the nurses themselves. They seemed to respond favourably to the idea of active consultation in planned change, seeing themselves as participants rather than as victims.

Unless one assumes that an organization is both perfect and static, examination of processes of change must be seen as a continuous aspect of the study of behaviour in the organization. This applies both to the natural processes of change which are a function of the internal dynamics of an organization, and to planned changes whether generated within the organization itself or imposed upon it by external pressures. Both at the level of planning and of implementation this is a study which can be facilitated or inhibited by the communication processes of the organization. It is often these processes which must first be assessed in approaching problems of change.

Implications for research and training

Hospitals are a highly specialized type of organization, unusual in that they can include both the most advanced and the most anachronistic elements within the same system. This applies both to the actual work situation and to the behavioural concepts which may exist within the organization.

Factors of size and organizational complexity are such that management problems within the hospital system are necessarily complex but, until comparatively recently, it seems to have been generally assumed that promotion in the nursing and medical hierarchies would somehow be associated with an increasing competence in the non-clinical skills associated with the promoted role. This assumption seems to have been made even in settings where there was little or no opportunity for acquiring such skills through training, or where the individuals concerned did not avail themselves of such opportunities as existed.

This is not to say that highly competent managers did not emerge. Any industrial organization can cite examples of self-made men who achieved considerable success without the benefit of the conventional training usually associated with their function. Certainly, many of the skills of management can be acquired, to greater or lesser degree, through experience.

There are comparatively few complex organizations, however, which would be inclined to rely on learning through experience as the preferred method of developing management skills, particularly in individuals who entered the organization for reasons other than a wish to succeed in management and who may have mixed feelings about the management aspect of their role.

This problem has been highlighted by the reactions of nursing staff seconded to attend first- and second-line management courses following the implementation, in Scotland, of the recommendations of the Salmon Commission. Many of them see the exercise as being one which will tend to separate them from the nursing role which is their main source of work satisfaction. They express resentment of a situation in which promotion in their chosen career is seen as necessitating a movement away from the nurse–patient relationship. Even when the relevance of the content of the training course is accepted, doubt is expressed about its practical value in situations where their superiors do not seem inclined to use or accept the implications of the training. Each course produced almost identical comments in its final sessions to the effect that Matron X or Dr Y should have been the first people to attend.

There may well have been some justification for the comments as Matron X had expressed the view that she would second the sisters who could best be spared rather than the ones who were most useful, and Dr Y had given his opinion that the exercise was a waste of time but at least it gave the nurses a bit of a break!

The situation illustrates organizational problems which require considerable study. Change imposed from outside the organization is unlikely to succeed when it lacks the support of the senior members of the organization itself. Further, when one has reached a senior level in a highly traditional organizational structure by subscribing to its rigid value system, innovations which seem to criticize the traditional structure of the organization are likely to be perceived as a threat.

In a sense the sisters who attended the courses were right. The senior members of the organization should have preceded them, if not in the same training situation at least in one in which their resistance to the implied changes could have been discussed with a view to allaying their anxieties and gaining a sufficient degree of co-operation to give the training exercise a better chance of success.

The illustration serves to emphasize the point made above. That change can only be implemented effectively when its effects upon the total organization are taken into account. In order to do this it is necessary to study not only change and techniques in isolation but the total area of organizational behaviour.

In this connection the need will arise to study traditional roles in the hospital service, their interrelationship and their appropriateness to the demands of current hospital administration in both its clinical and social context. In addition, the significance of new roles within the hospital service might be examined. Such roles are not readily assimilated within the hospital organization as they frequently fail to fall within any of the three traditional hierarchies. They may even be resented as potentially impinging in some way upon the proper function of existing roles. It is suggested that a re-appraisal of the organizational structures of the hospital services could lead to the emergence of a more effectively structured organization both in terms of its internal efficiency and its role in society.

The study of behaviour in organizations is one of the approaches which can contribute to such a re-appraisal. Although not a tool of management in the conventional sense it can make available to the hospital services systems of analysis and evaluation which have been shown to be effective in other fields.

References

Anderson, T. and Warkov, S. (1961). 'Organisational Size and Functional Complexity: A Study of Administration in Hospitals.' *Am. Sociol. Rev.* **26**, 23

Barton, R. (1959). *Institutional Neurosis.* Bristol; John Wright

– Elkes, A. and Glen, F. (1961). 'Unrestricted Visiting in Mental Hospitals.' *Lancet* **1**, 1220

Blau, P. and Scott, W. (1963). *Formal Organisations: A Comparative Approach.* London; Routledge and Kegan Paul

Brown, G. and Wing, J. (1962). 'A Comparative Clinical and Social Survey of Three Mental Hospitals.' *Sociol. Rev.* Monog. 5

Cartwright, Ann (1964). *Human Relations and Hospital Care.* London; Routledge and Kegan Paul

Forehand, G.A. and Gilmer, B.V.H. (1964). 'Environmental Variation in Studies of Organisational Behaviour.' *Psychol. Bull.* **62**, 361

Hall, R. (1963). 'The Concept of Bureaucracy: An Empirical Assessment.' *Am. J. Sociol.* **69**, 32

Jacobs, H. and Glen, F. (1964). 'A Clinical Trial of CI-383 and CI-384 in Psychiatric Patients.' *J. Neuropsychiat.* **5**, 235

Kahn, R.L., Wolfe, D.M., Quinn, R.P., Snoeck, J.D. and Rosenthal, R.A. (1964). *Organisational Stress: Studies in Role Conflict and Ambiguity.* New York; Wiley

Leavitt, H.J. (Ed.) (1964). *The Social Science of Organisations: Four Perspectives.* Englewood Cliffs, N.J.; Prentice-Hall

Mechanic, D. (1964). 'Some Considerations in the Methodology of Organisational Studies.' In *The Social Science of Organisations* (Ed. by H.J. Leavitt). Englewood Cliffs, N.J.; Prentice-Hall

Morris, Pauline (1969). *Put Away: A Sociological Study of Institutions for the Mentally Retarded.* London; Routledge and Kegan Paul

Porter, L.W. and Lawler, E.E. (1965). 'Properties of Organisational Structure in Relation to Job Attitudes and Job Behaviour.' *Psychol. Bull.* **64**, 23

Revans, R.W. (1962). 'Hospital Attitudes and Communications.' *Sociol. Rev.* Monog. 5, 117

Roby, T.B., Nicol, E.H. and Farrell, F.M. (1963). 'Group problem solving under two types of executive structure.' *J. abnorm. soc. Psychol.* **67**, 530

Schein, E.H. (1965). *Organisations Psychology.* Englewood Cliffs, N.J.; Prentice-Hall

Simon, H.A. (1964). 'On the Concept of Organisational Goals.' *Admin. Sci. Quart.* **9**, 1

Titmuss, R.M. (1958). *Essays on the Welfare State.* London; Allen and Unwin

13—Research in Organization Structure and Behaviour

David M. Boswell

Personal Service in Community Services

The community services provided by the health departments of local authorities in Britain have developed by processes of *ad hoc* accumulation, and have been modified by specific statutory orders and the reorganization of local authority responsibilities. The particular experience underlying this section is that of the mental health services in the north west of England. In 1965 a research project was established, by the erstwhile Ministry of Health, under the direction of the Department of Social and Preventive Medicine at Manchester University, to evaluate the new system of residential care for the mentally disordered which was being provided by Lancashire County Council. This large local authority had responded dramatically to the encouragement of the Royal Commission on Mental Health and the permissive clauses of the Mental Health Act of 1959. I acknowledge, with gratitude, the assistance given by the County Medical Officer of Health and all the staff and residents in the mental health service. Previous reports on this research have already been published by Dr Alison Campbell (now Mrs A.C. Rosen) the research psychologist, in the *Medical Officer,* the *British Journal of Social and Preventive Medicine* and the *British Journal of Social Psychiatry.* As the research sociologist, I should also like to acknowledge the advice and opportunities for discussion availed me by the Department of Sociology and Social Anthropology at Manchester University. However, the points made here are of general application to the administration and provision of all personal services with fieldwork staff.

It is particularly important that this should be understood because, at the time of writing (March, 1970), measures are before Parliament which will lead to the creation of a very different more closely integrated system of health provision and welfare services within a system of local government that completely departs from the division of town and country central to the last era of reform in the nineteenth century.

The present responsibilities of local authorities are summarized in the Annual Report of the County Medical Officer of Health for Lancashire County Council for 1968 (Lancashire County Council, 1969). 'The duties of the County Council under the National Health Service Act, 1946, and the Mental Health Act, 1959, include the provision of junior and adult training centres, special care units and social clubs for mentally disordered persons and residential accommodation for juniors and adults who are suitable to live in the community at large but who, for one reason or another, cannot live in their own homes. These are embraced within wider responsibilities for the prevention of mental illness and the care and after-care of persons who are suffering or have suffered from mental disorder. The Council's powers in relation to prevention, care and after-care in all forms of illness, under section 28 of the former Act, had been more specifically detailed, so far as the mentally disordered were concerned, in the Act of 1959. Section 12 of the Health Services and Public Health Act, 1968, is intended to put beyond doubt the power of local health authorities to provide residential accommodation, training centres and other ancillary or supplementary services for the prevention of all types of illness, including mental disorder, and for the care and after-care of persons suffering from illness. Consolidating with amendments sections 28 (1) and (2) of the National Health Service Act, 1946, and sections 6 and 7 of the Mental Health Act, 1959, this section came into force on the 9th September, 1968.'

From the Tables in this section it can be seen how the local authorities in the north west of England have responded to these permissive powers and what their plans officially intend. I have selected only those services that cater most directly for those adults classified as mentally subnormal, but it is of course a fact that most of the work of the mental welfare officers is concerned with those who are mentally ill (Rehin and Martin, 1968; a). The scale of a local authority's undertaking in the field of mental health is relative to the size of its population

TABLE 13.1

Area	Population in 1965	Places for the mentally subnormal per 1,000 population in adult hostels		
		1965	1971	1976
MANCHESTER REGION				
Westmorland C.C.	66,950	–	–	–
Barrow-in-Furness C.B.C.	64,600	–	0·18	0·18
Blackpool C.B.C.	150,440	–	–	–
Preston C.B.C.	109,030	–	0·17	0·17
Blackburn C.B.C.	103,070	0·09	0·15	0·15
Burnley C.B.C.	78,680	–	–	–
Lancashire C.C.	2,326,890	0·09	0·31	0·29
Bolton C.B.C.	157,990	0·14	0·29	0·29
Salford C.B.C.	148,260	0·13	0·48	0·69
Wigan C.B.C.	77,690	0·08	0·08	0·08
Bury C.B.C.	62,710	–	0·46	0·44
Manchester C.B.C.	638,360	0·04	0·26	0·43
Oldham C.B.C.	111,480	0·23	0·33	0·38
Rochdale C.B.C.	86,490	–	–	0·57
Stockport C.B.C.	141,770	–	0·17	0·17
Cheshire C.C.	1,004,730	0·04	0·16	0·22
LIVERPOOL REGION				
Bootle C.B.C.	82,750	–	0·16	0·15
Liverpool C.B.C.	722,010	0·11	0·21	0·21
Southport C.B.C.	79,980	–	0·22	0·22
St. Helens C.B.C.	104,440	–	–	0·24
Warrington C.B.C.	74,720	0·16	0·57	0·58
Birkenhead C.B.C.	143,660	–	0·18	0·18
Chester C.B.C.	59,800	–	–	0·15
Wallasey C.B.C.	103,090	–	–	–
National averages	47,762,800	0·03	0·14	0·17

C.C. – County Council   C.B.C. – County Borough Council
(Source. *Ministry of Health* (1966b), *reproduced by courtesy of H.M.S.O.*)

343

and the prevalence of the physical or mental condition under considera-tion. It is therefore to be expected that some should provide more than others. Nevertheless, the ratio of places or staff per 1,000 of the population indicates the true level of acceptance of responsibility in each area.

Three events could dramatically alter the organization and operation of the mental health services in the next few years. First, social service departments are recommended to be set up under their own local authority committees, with officers trained in social work as their directors (*see* Report, 1968). Secondly, local government boundaries are to be redrawn and grouped. In the north west of England those suggested closely resemble the existing county councils and incorporate boroughs and county areas. Other areas are grouped round main urban areas as Metropolitan districts. For a brief description of the develop-ment of local authority responsibilities in the north west of England in the nineteenth century' *see* Midwinter (1969)*. Thirdly, Area Health Boards are to localize the provision of hospital and personal health services under central government direction for areas corresponding to those of local government (Department of Health and Social Security, 1970), which will continue to be responsible for public health and personal social services.

Two things have happened to the mental health service. One follows on the implementation of the Local Authority Social Services Act 1970. The hostels and training centres of health divisions and the adjacent boroughs are brought together as one section of the social services departments, under the direction of a social worker trained in social administration with an administrative staff. However, it would be naïve to suppose that the social workers' charter will necessarily produce greater understanding, as perceived by field workers in the service, than direction by medical officers. As is discussed in this section, bureau-cratic administration makes its own demands by virtue of the situation of the office of responsibility. However, this reorganization could allow for the clearer articulation of the service and the projection of more socially developmental goals for it.

The other direction in which some services have gone would be towards a functional integration with the work of other departments implying the dismemberment of a mental health service as such. The junior training centres are already designated for transfer to the Department of Education and Science. The adult training centres could logically be placed in the Department of Employment and Productivity, particularly those that approximate to sheltered workshops and eschew the tasks of

---

*Map 1, p. 6 may be compared with maps of the Maud Report.

TABLE 13.2

Area	Area (square miles)	Mental health social workers per 1,000 population		
		1965	1971	1976
MANCHESTER REGION				
Westmorland C.C.	789·0	0·02	0·02	0·02
Barrow-in-Furness C.B.C.	17·2	0·05	0·06	0·06
Blackpool C.B.C.	16·7	0·03	0·06	0·05
Preston C.B.C.	9·9	0·04	0·05	0·05
Blackburn C.B.C.	12·6	0·04	0·04	0·05
Burnley C.B.C.	7·3	0·05	0·05	0·05
Lancashire C.C.	1614·0	0·03	0·04	0·04
Bolton C.B.C.	23·9	0·03	0·05	0·06
Salford C.B.C.	8·1	0·06	0·08	0·09
Wigan C.B.C.	7·9	0·05	0·07	0·07
Bury C.B.C.	11·6	0·05	0·06	0·06
Manchester C.B.C.	42·6	0·03	0·04	0·05
Oldham C.B.C.	10·0	0·05	0·07	0·08
Rochdale C.B.C.	14·9	0·05	0·05	0·05
Stockport C.B.C.	13·2	0·02	0·04	0·05
Cheshire C.C.	972·0	0·03	0·04	0·04
LIVERPOOL REGION				
Bootle C.B.C.	4·8	0·04	0·03	0·03
Liverpool C.B.C.	43·5	0·04	0·04	0·05
Southport C.B.C.	14·7	0·04	0·06	0·06
St. Helens C.B.C.	13·9	0·04	0·06	0·06
Warrington C.B.C.	7·2	0·03	0·07	0·10
Birkenhead C.B.C.	13·5	0·03	0·03	0·03
Chester C.B.C.	7·3	0·03	0·05	0·05
Wallasey C.B.C.	9·3	0·04	0·05	0·05
National averages		0·03	0·05	0·05

C.C. – County Council   C.B.C. – County Borough Council
(Source. *Ministry of Health* (1966b), *reproduced by courtesy of H.M.S.O.*)

education and social training. Trainees could then be paid a wage reflecting their labour output and 'out-work' regularized. But there remains a place for those centres that will try to train and educate young adults who are mentally handicapped.

Hostels are unlikely to go to the Area Health Boards as providing 'residential accommodation for those needing continuing medical supervision and not ready to live in the community' (Department of Health and Social Security, 1970; *a*) for this would represent a total reversal of all mental health policy since 1959. However, it is likely that these boards will provide a similar type of accommodation *in lieu* of new residential blocks in mental hospitals. The Wessex and Sheffield Regional Hospital Boards are already implementing such plans. It is conceivable that the provision of residential accommodation for special categories of the population may be seen as the responsibility of housing departments; there has already been some acceptance of the provision of special flats for elderly people by local authorities.

Whichever type of service results from the administrative reforms of this decade, the mental health social workers in the social service departments will have an increased administrative and social work function to play in the co-ordination and personalization of the services provided for the mentally disordered. The wide variation in the aims of local authority departments of health to develop this part of their service is apparent in Table 13.2. It is of critical significance because it indicates the apparent intention of the two largest in population and area, Lancashire and Cheshire, to provide fewer mental health social workers per 1,000 population than all but three local authorities in the north west. It is the purpose of the next section to consider this type of formal organization which ostensibly exists to offer a range of personal services to clients who, often through multiple disadvantages, have become dependent on other people.

Bureaucratic Characteristics of Formal Organizations

It would appear axiomatic that an organization established in relation to some particular social phenomenon should be structured according to the requirements best suited to fulfil this function. Such an organization has formal aims for its existence which are usually explicitly stated or generally acknowledged. It has an authorized staff of officers to carry out its work and a set pattern of procedures usually involving written records (Gerth and Mills, 1948).

Once established, however, such a bureaucracy generates its own aims and rules of procedure, and its staff act upon priorities that relate as much to their position in the hierarchy and to the continuity of the structure as to the desires and needs of the persons for whom it was apparently established. Whereas other formal organizations may be orientated to the production of things, those orientated towards the direct needs of people, usually significantly termed services, face the acute dilemma of balancing the interests of the organization and its staff with those of its willing or unwilling users. For a further discussion of the nature of 'people—work' within total institutions, *see* Goffman (1961).

It is the aim of this section to raise some of the issues inherent in this situation, because they have to be faced and understood by all concerned in working with people in situations structured in this sort of way. Although the groundwork for the section lies in research into the provision of community services for the mentally disordered, the analysis is generally applicable to all situations in which relatively long-term and face-to-face relationships form the basis of the work involved in the services provided.

Partly because of its reference as a popular term of abuse, bureaucracy has tended to give way to that of formal organization, which also has more general applicability (Blau and Scott, 1963). Both, however, imply a regular and regulated system of running affairs. Whatever the ideal type of the formal organization as a goal-directed structure, it is in just the sort of personal services considered here that the most serious accusations have been levelled against formalism, inhumanity, unassailable faceless hierarchies and self-protective humbug by those claiming to represent the common man, the humble user and the human rights of individuals. Any provider of such services has to meet both these accusations and the requirement for the provision of a service which may be evaluated as effective in achieving its formal aims, that is meeting a public need, and rational, that is equitable and straightforward, in its means of achieving them.

Public services are liable to receive this form of value-laden criticism because of the monolithic strength which is their characteristic. This is also because of their particular relationship with individuals, who are often in acute distress, in a situation that accords them inferior status. When faced with descriptions of what has actually taken place in their organization, officials find difficulty in accepting the evidence. To the public, they may appear to be the custodians of virtually impregnable bastions who are isolated from the reactions of consumers to the product of their services. The officials then find that good intentions are not enough in the face of unacceptable practice.

It is usually assumed that, although an organization may present an array of formal aims or goals, other interests and forces are at work within the organization which cause a displacement of goals (Merton, 1968), so that self-perpetuation and equanimity replace innovation and forceful activity, and a set of informal goals underlie its actual workings. However, given the present formal structure of health administration, it is quite possible for a service to exist without even the formal expression of goals, and for apparently conflicting aims to be presented by different or even the same parts of the Health Service at one and the same time.

PSYCHIATRIC IDEOLOGIES

Different psychiatric ideologies (Strauss and colleagues, 1964; *a*) operate simultaneously within the mental health services, so there is no single approach to the provision of such services. *Somatic* forms of treatment lay stress upon particular symptoms and the alleviation or masking of these by chemotherapy, that is drugs. I have used the term 'chemotherapy', rather than somatotherapy because drugs, rather than a variety of electric shock and other forms of treatment, are more commonly administered to mentally subnormal adults. *Psychotherapy,* which is less common in Britain than in other countries such as the United States of America, places supreme importance on the actual confrontation of doctor and patient, which is left to diagnosis by the former. Here I am referring to therapeutic programmes rather than to routine contacts. Various forms of *sociotherapy,* on the other hand, lay emphasis upon the precipitating factors in the environment of the mentally disordered, and upon the community relations of the latter when in care.

It is possible for the same regional hospital board to encourage the development of small-scale psychiatric units in general hospitals for the care of the mentally ill on a short-term basis, whilst the few large-scale institutions for the mentally subnormal continue to remain central to this part of the board's provision, with their out-patient clinics inevitably orientated to the geographically isolated long-stay hospitals. For an assessment of the work of the psychiatric units in general hospitals of the north west of England, *see* Hoenig and Hamilton (1969).

The Department of Health and Social Security encourages the provision of local authority hostel and training services, although their goals are not clearly expressed. As the Department's powers are mainly advisory, it is, in fact, quite possible for local authorities to pay little attention to its general policies (Ministry of Health, 1962; 1966b)*. The difference between this collection of local authority plans, with its brief commentary, and the Hospital Plan for England and Wales, with its clear assessment of needs and policy, determines the role and function of the Ministry in the two cases. However, this second set of plans does indicate the extent to which local authorities had or had not responded to the implied criticism and encouragement to greater activity in the introduction to the first set of plans (Ministry of Health, 1963). On the other hand, local authorities which have responded to the spirit of the Royal Commission on Mental Health (*see* Report, 1957), rather than to the mere administration of the Mental Health Act, 1959, may have implemented a policy of residential care differing considerably from the expectations of the central government Department of Health. As seems not infrequent, the goals of the new policy are relatively clearly expressed in relation to the separate Scottish Department (Department of Health for Scotland, 1957).

It is one thing to provide long-stay homely accommodation for the more amenable of the severely subnormal who need not be incarcerated in what local councillors call 'the Bastilles'†. It is quite another to provide short-stay hostel accommodation for the mentally ill or more able of the mentally subnormal, whose problems are rather those of social adaptation to work and independent living in the community itself (Mountney, 1968).

It seems to be the case that community care officially means 'paid for and administered by' the local authority rather than a central government agency. One might assume that it implied the acceptance by ordinary people of responsibility for the personal care of some of society's deviants. In the case of the mentally ill who attend the psychiatric units, this is expected of their relatives (Hoenig and Hamilton, 1969). In the case of the more able of the mentally subnormal, this is just the category that has the greatest difficulty finding acceptance in either the community or in local authority hostels, and even in the hospitals they

---

*In Circular 28/59 *Mental Health Services* (para. 6., 'Residential Accommodation B') the Department of Health was relatively specific in indicating that:

'The intended developments should state the type of case to be provided for, an estimate of the number of places and whether the intention is that the residents should attend a training centre or work in ordinary or sheltered employment.'

†Alderman H. Davies, deputy Chairman of the Mental Health Sub-committee of Lancashire County Council, at the opening of the new hostel in Padiham, June, 1969.

TABLE 13.3

Area	Places for the mentally subnormal in adult training centres per 1,000 population			Social centres and clubs for the mentally subnormal run by local authorities		
	1965	1971	1976	1965	1971	1976
MANCHESTER REGION						
Westmorland C.C.	0·22	0·30	0·30	–	–	–
Barrow-in-Furness C.B.C.	–	0·31	0·30	–	1	1
Blackpool C.B.C.	0·21	0·44	0·43	1	1	1
Preston C.B.C.	0·28	0·75	0·75	2	2	2
Blackburn C.B.C.	0·78	0·78	0·79	1	1	1
Burnley C.B.C.	1·08	1·40	1·42	2	2	2
Lancashire C.C.	0·35	0·84	0·79	15	19	19
Bolton C.B.C.	0·44	0·44	0·44	–	–	–
Salford C.B.C.	0·67	0·88	0·97	1	1	1
Wigan C.B.C.	0·90	0·94	0·96	–	–	–
Bury C.B.C.	0·21	0·61	0·59	–	–	–
Manchester C.B.C.	0·29	0·97	1·31	–	–	–
Oldham C.B.C.	0·72	1·03	1·06	–	–	–
Rochdale C.B.C.	–	0·46	0·46	–	1	1
Stockport C.B.C.	0·54	0·72	0·70	–	–	–
Cheshire C.C.	0·54	0·65	0·59	5	7	10
LIVERPOOL REGION						
Bootle C.B.C.	–	1·53	1·42	–	1	1
Liverpool C.B.C.	0·33	0·62	0·86	–	–	–
Southport C.B.C.	0·31	0·56	0·55	–	–	–
St. Helens C.B.C.	0·48	0·48	0·71	1	1	1
Warrington C.B.C.	0·27	0·68	0·69	–	–	–
Birkenhead C.B.C.	0·35	0·47	0·46	–	–	–
Chester C.B.C.	0·84	0·79	0·76	–	–	–
Wallasey C.B.C.	0·49	0·46	0·45	–	1	1
England and Wales	0·32	0·59	0·65	142	207	230

C.C. – County Council   C.B.C. – County Borough Council
(Source. *Ministry of Health* (1966b), *reproduced by courtesy of H.M.S.O.*)

are castigated as a collection of deviant delinquents referred to as 'the fly-boys'. The more amenable of these often disappear into the ranks of the normal population, married and in work*.

Continuity and Change

Two basic dilemmas underlie the planning of any new service, or the introduction of innovations within existing administrative structures. First, to what extent should established patterns and forms of organization be used and taken as models for the new service? Secondly, how much may these innovations demand new ways of doing things and an abandonment or replacement of past authority boundaries, official hierarchial structures, and departmental forms of administration? For whatever the nature of the service provided, it will assume some organizational form and formal rationale, whether it be initially planned or arise out of the way in which its instigators carry on their activities (Michels, 1949).

To the extent that continuity is preserved, so innovations are appended to formal organizations which have already developed their routines and priorities and hence become subordinate to these. Different services, such as those for the provision of residential care for the elderly may have been taken as general background experience for the accommodation of the mentally disordered. The transfer of existing staff to new duties may take the form rather of the accumulation of additional duties, based on totally different aims and values, as the responsibilities of existing staff. This may mean that an officer, no longer designated duly authorized officer but called Mental Welfare Officer, has a range of roles calling for a fundamental reworking of his occupational image as well as his operational activities. However, the sort of demands made on him may remain much as before, so that his old expectations of the role may also remain.

ADMINISTRATION AREAS

The present local health authority boundaries in the north west of England bear a close resemblance to the nineteenth century poor law unions, with the county boroughs excised from their midst as autonomous authorities (Midwinter, 1969). It is because these are based on a re-allocation of the same parochial areas around the same

---

*Personal communications from Mr M.J. Bailey and Dr T. Fryers relating to their analysis of the 'dormant' case files of the mental welfare officers in Sheffield and Salford County Boroughs respectively.

administrative centres and capital services. A system that provided the existing distribution of hospital services is, for example, bound to continue to form the basis of subsequent systems using those same services. Hence, although hospitals are now grouped under the regional boards their catchment areas may remain similar to those of which they were once an administrative part. However, the District General Hospitals are increasingly taking over the functions of the smaller hospitals which are being used for less acute cases (Ministry of Health, 1962).

On the other hand, innovations in the provision of services may add functions and activities that are totally new and for which no direct reference already exists. The building and staffing of adult training centres for the mentally subnormal is such an enterprise. The recruitment of instructors and superintendents drawn from the ranks of skilled tradesmen in industry, and a potential conflict of aims over the educational or occupational *raison d'etre* of the establishments, are radical innovations in the administrative experience of medical officers of health.

Other services have been taken over by central government departments whose boundaries and points of reference to authority are totally different from those of the community services provided by local authorities. It was, indeed, to try to ensure the continuity of viable regional authorities with a locally responsible reference to authority that local government reforms have been recommended*. An alternative would be the assumption by central government departments of all responsibility for health, welfare and educational services. As the present provision of community services by local authorities is a policy that is advised but not enforced by statute, their withdrawal can lead to critical difficulties arising from the reduction of staff and even services hitherto provided. Reference is specifically to the two incidents that followed attempts by the newly elected Salford County Borough Council to reduce expenditure in its health department. This was on the grounds that other local authorities spent less and provided less. In the first case, March–April 1969, notice was given of a decision

---

*Sir Peter Mursell in a letter to *The Times* (January 12, 1970) gave the following warning:

'If these changes go on, and they will if local government is not made an apt organization to meet today's immensely complicated and costly problems, we shall in twenty years or so be left with only the pomp and circumstance and the smaller albeit important, community services in local government.

It is immensely important that local people should have some say in how local affairs are run; should be able to air grievances and put right wrongs and abuses.' (Reproduced with permission.)

to close the hostel for the mentally disordered. A public outcry in the national press and the organization of a conference on 'Comprehensive Community Mental Health Services', by Dr Hugh Freeman, helped to effect a reconsideration of this decision. However, a further decision not to fill two of every three vacancies occurring in the health department, which had already resulted in the closing of the public analyst's section, led to a second case relating this time, January–February 1970, to the staff of mental health social workers. A comparison of the provision of local authorities relating to both parts of the services can be seen in Tables 1, 2 and 3 Rehin and Martin (1968; *b*) note that:

'Some authorities provided more than five mental health social workers per 100,000 population, which was the standard as a goal for local authorities by the Younghusband Committee. In this light, Salford's provision of staff was not exceptionally high.'

The increased scale of provision of social workers was anticipated and encouraged in a White Paper published by the Ministry of Health (1968b; *a*).

RESEARCH

Because of the importance of ways of introducing innovations into existing structures, and of implementing new policies, it is as well to emphasize the place of evaluation and research into the operation of formal organizations. If new policies and services are to be evaluated from evidence of their working, it is essential that implementable aims should exist. These may be: (1) to provide less deprived and more humane conditions of living; (2) to train in skills, to present new opportunities of independence; (3) to rehabilitate to normal living; and (4) to shelter from the normal world.

Where, however, no agreement exists upon the aims, and several either conflict or are regarded as futile by those delegated with the responsibility of executing the policy, it is natural that evaluation, in simple terms, may be rendered impossible. For further discussion of these principles underlying the practice of residential care, *see* Campbell (1971). For the residential care of children, *see* King and Raynes (1968). It should also be obvious that basic demographic and epidemiological data should be ascertained for the population for whom such services are planned. Need is often determined merely by scarcity or resources. It is only now that health authorities are beginning to use registers which provide the necessary data for planning and monitoring their services (Tizard, 1964; Kushlick and Cox, 1967; Susser, 1968).

For the same reason innovations in policy and structure cannot be called experimental unless specific aims and methods are tried out in relation to some end and found relatively more or less successful than others. Trying not to repeat the greatest mistakes or avoiding the most embarrassing situations may be a way of achieving uneventful continuity rather than development. The maintenance of the *status quo* is convenient to the system. But it is only by enforced risk taking that new strategies can be attempted and achievments made. It is, for example, possible to ensure the incompetence of the mentally disordered by depriving them of the opportunities of learning and the company of more competent people. It is as easy within a training centre workroom as within the apparent impersonality of a large-scale formal organization, to let expectations fall and derive satisfaction from lassitude and an ecological harmony instead of from planned achievement. For the situation of education, training and other specialist services in mental subnormality hospitals, *see* Morris (1969).

PROBLEMS ARISING FROM LONG-TERM CONTACTS

Problems arising from long-term contacts are inherent in community services. Unlike children who grow up and leave school and home at will, and unlike elderly people who sicken and die, the physically and mentally handicapped may be chronically impaired in their functions. Although attempts can be made to meet their disabilities, for many the development or opportunity provided may remain within a context of enduring dependency. It is therefore understandable that the sort of activities and relationships that make for harmonious continuity should appear of paramount importance to those in face-to-face relationships with them.

Equally, tolerance of disability or bizarre behaviour which enables them to be accepted in this environment, but not outside, may remove the possibility of introducing yardsticks by which development may be assessed. Nevertheless it is apparent that if their own work is to have any meaning to the staff, they must have grounds for feeling that they are achieving something. It is interesting to observe how quickly new staff assume an essentially self-protective role of *laissez-faire* practice with minimal expectations.

RECORDS

A characteristic of most formal organizations is the keeping of records which, first, may be kept for the working use of whoever is keeping them and as a means of directing observation at the time. Secondly, they may be intended to provide information for others at the time or at subsequent times. Thirdly, they may be kept in a standardized form to allow for general analysis and accumulation such as for research purposes. Lastly, they may be used to provide an ongoing assessment of achievments by individuals.

Ideally, records are capable of fulfilling all these functions at the same time. In fact they usually perform only some of them. However, it is possible for them not to be kept at all, so that disciplined observation is never maintained and the criteria for assessment of achievement never worked out or applied. In such a situation work assumes a purposelessness, and the crudest features of bureaucracy are achieved in face-to-face relationships; this is quite different from another situation with which it may be confused. When research is done the findings may have certain implications which are ignored because the *status quo* exists for political and administrative reasons which have been granted priority.

Structured Roles in Formal Organizations

Reference has already been made to two characteristics of formal organizations. (1) They are established with specific goals. (2) Once established, their perpetuation of themselves and judgement of the goals of others, in relation to their security, may lead to a displacement of these goals in favour of others more strictly related to the organization's cohesion and continuity. This process may operate to reduce the effects of innovation. For a perceptive analysis of bureaucracy and social change, *see* Blau (1963; *a*).

FORMAL ROLES

Within any such formal organization the holding of office implies some formal role relationship. *Formal roles* within an organization represent the allocation of duties and responsibilities and therefore the behaviour expected of their holders as it relates to the organization in question. Two features govern the relationship of these roles within the structure.

(1) The principle of *authority,* implying some form of hierarchy, provides one structural dimension.

(2) There may be an *equivalence of status* between the roles of those responsible for the several functioning parts that make up the whole organization. This is particularly so in the sort of organization which has several different functional aspects, such as a community mental health service.

Reference has already been made to the goals governing the establishment of organizations, and the lack of direction implied in their absence or obscurity. This apparent aimlessness may be felt and expressed by various parts of the formal organization concerned with fieldwork in the services. It may also be consciously expressed, however, by those holding authoritative positions in the administrative hierarchy. There are several reasons for this, one of which I have already enumerated; for example, the way in which those in a position to establish goals may stall in taking an overt decision until they can utilize the experience of their subordinates in achieving something which may then be claimed as a general goal.

The structure of the National Health Service and services provided by local government in Britain at present is such that clear lines of authority and policy creation and execution may not be apparent to those working in them. The two-tier system, which in some of the larger local authorities may become a three-tier system, leaves scope for local decision making as to the priorities for and scale of expenditure on community services. Once implemented, powers over loan sanction and other matters may place the central government department in an influential position at the planning stage. It is at this stage also that the county office departments may exert their influence on the general form to be taken by the Service. Thereafter, it is in the hands of those responsible for implementing the policy by running the services provided. These points are discussed more fully in a paper by Boswell (1969b).

It can be seen that significant breaks can exist in the formal structure of an organization, which become central to the negotiative nature of administration and policy implementation. Not only is there a parallel structure of committees and councils made up of various elected representatives and co-opted experts from the general population, whose wielding of power may be considerable and whose final decision is mandatory, but there may, within the official hierarchy, be a fragmentation of the service into multiple hierarchical structures such as health and welfare divisions of a county council area whose composition is general rather than specialized.

Although the specialized parts that go to make up those divisional units may also come under the direction of specialist sections at the centres of local government or regional planning, this relationship may be obscure or conflict with the other general and more immediate divisional hierarchy. One result may be the derivation of satisfaction from the apparent autonomy given to the latter; but this confusion also engenders a feeling of isolation. It mitigates against development and innovation, because these require financial backing which is subject to the ultimate positive sanction of the highest most relevant authority. It may be difficult to find the centre of responsibility in the working arrangement of this form of organization, regardless of what the constitutional formalities may appear to be.

FORMAL ORGANIZATIONS

Through their role structures and forms of hierarchy, formal organizations generate a range of related status positions which have certain characteristics in common, as well as an affinity with the evaluation of social status and the form of social class structure of the wider society in which they are established. These positions owe their status partly to their level in the hierarchy, but also to the functional part of the service to which they belong. Seeing that occupation, income and education are closely related, it is to be expected that those filling these status positions will also draw conclusions and take their stand according to their estimation of their position within the hierarchy and within the wider society. For consideration of a crucial section of modern British society, *see* Goldthorpe and colleagues (1969). So important is this for understanding the dynamic aspects of bureaucracy that considerable emphasis will be placed upon it here and in the next section.

It is when the industrial economy is based upon private capital that it is usual to draw a distinction between management and worker, but this distinction is of general application. Within all formal organizations, in most forms of industrial society, there is a differentiation in function between management staff and others who may be on the production line or in specialized departments peripheral to this powerful hierarchy. Burns and Stalker (1966) have analysed the situation of research innovation, in relation to the management of industrial plants. It is a fact that although they are no more part of the management than the factory operatives, the clerical workers have to a great extent related their role to that of the management with whom they are in face-to-face contact. Hours, the timing of their salary payments, and reflected status refer to their superiors, whilst their processing functions place them in a powerful situation as intermediaries in relation to those outside the administrative core, such as those running the actual productive processes. For an analysis of the status of the clerical worker in Britain, *see* Lockwood (1958). In the case of community services these latter processes are represented by the fieldwork services.

This is a central feature of the formal organizations with which we are concerned, particularly because all local government officials are salaried and the activities of their departments are concerned with the provision and administration of services financed from other sources than the profits from products (Blau, 1963; *b*). At the level of the general administrative unit of the services, whether it be a centralized authority or a divisional health office, a medical officer is, at present (March, 1970) the senior officer in charge, with a central core of administrative officers and their clerical staff, as well as medical officers in departments and the other fieldwork personnel.

CONFLICT OF AUTHORITY

The controller of the administrative machine has the ability to determine priorities and the general tenor of policy. It is for this reason that conflict is bound to arise between the specialists who staff the fieldwork services and the professional values of the directors of the whole service, which often differ from the former and which determine the nature of decisions taken. The demand of social workers to run their own departments indicates the most clearly expressed rejection of the present system under medical authority but it is also present in the incipient manoeuvres of the training centre instructors and hostel wardens in the mental health services.

Some of these, such as that of the social workers, represent a professional challenge to management in order to obtain control of the administration (*see* Report, 1968)*. When the salary scales of administrative officers are related to the quantity of clerical work done by those under them, it is not surprising that the administrative core holds together and maintains its autonomy. Others, such as the hostel wardens may seek the formation of an association that campaigns more for their interests to be heard than their control to be extended (Society for Mental Health Hostel Officers, 1969). Their role is never likely to be other than functional within a larger service managed by others. What is happening is that the sorts of conflicts that led to the implementation of the Bradbeer and Salmon Reports by the hospital service are to be seen in the much more fragmented community services (Ministry of Health, 1964; 1966a).

In the sort of community services under consideration, it is not only significant that some form of official hierarchy exists placing some in positions of authority over others, it is also the case that certain branches

---

*Particularly relevant here are Chap. 7, 'A Social Service Department', para. 139–169; Chap. 12, 'Future of the Local Authority Health Department', para. 381–386 and Chap. 19, para. 611–636, which advocate a separate committee, the choice of a head of the department 'professionally qualified in social work' , and mandatory enforcement of the new structure on local authorities. The aim of the Government is to implement the central recommendation through the Local Authority Services Act 1970.

of the services may be more prestigious as a whole, and more central to the determination of policy and running of affairs. But it is also the case that the formal structuring of the service and allocation of roles with special functions is bound to provide the basis for some form of structural opposition. Where different establishments are responsible for different aspects of the same persons, in this example trainees who are also residents and cases, conflicts are bound to arise that require an arbiter. The normal incidence of conflict between the staff of training centres, hostels and mental welfare officers, is only one case in point. Herein lies the strength and managing power of the administrative core. There is a horizontal relationship between the functional parts of a service, as well as a vertical relationship with authority.

It is common to place the blame for conflict in formal organizations upon a failure of communication or a clash of personalities. One, of course, represents the opposite of the other, for a failure of communication is usually taken as implying a lack of personal contact, whereas a clash of personalities results from the effects of such contact. These are illuminating central legends in the myth that harmony and peaceful coexistence are the normal state of affairs.

It is hoped that this has indicated the ways in which the structure of a formal organization, such as that for the provision of community services, may reflect any indecision and obscurity in the setting of goals for the service; an administrative emphasis on placid continuity rather than innovation and, still less, experimentation; and the presence of interested parties structurally opposed in the functions and responsibilities of their parts of the service. I have hitherto been concerned to discuss the formal structure of community services, because this must logically come before a consideration of the personalization of roles and the actual face-to-face relations implicit in working with people.

Personal Attributes and Role Performance

In previous sections two assumptions have been made of formal organizations; that they have a formal structure, and that roles are allocated according to the goals for which the organization is established. Reference has also been made to the way in which such organizations operate as hierarchies and tend to a form of practice ensuring their quiet continuity. For an analysis of the impact of a change of personnel and policy in a formal organization *see* Gouldner (1954).

However, persons who fill roles related to the formal structure simultaneously fulfil other roles and functions within their families and community and assume an identification with others of similar general social status, age or categorical affiliation. These statuses and experiences, outside their work, impinge on that of their work role, because they provide references and interests by which meaning is given to interaction and relationships formalized. For an introduction to the concept of social roles, *see* Banton (1965).

Although it is often the case that what appear to be personal conflicts coincide with points of tension in the articulation of a formal organization or the structural opposition of its parts, it is also the case that what may loosely be categorized as clashes of personality is a central feature of formal organizations established to deal with persons. Face-to-face relationships are not only an essential feature of the work, but what the work is all about.

This is not to suggest that the same factors do not affect other forms of work situation. The differences between administrative structures indicate not only the implementation of different procedural forms, but also the relative weight and significance of the incumbents of office. Medical officers, senior administrative officers, elected representatives, and even clerks or secretaries in crucial positions, assume status and powerful negotiative positions in relation to one another, which endures as a system so long as its dominant members can make it work. This is as true of so-called open and democratic methods of co-operation as it is of closed, autocratic forms of domination. But the nature of the work in personal services places these relationships at the centre of every interaction and negotiated arrangement.

Personal services directed to the alleviation of acute crises and curing of serious conditions must show successful or unsuccessful results. For elaboration of the concept of the sick role, *see* Parsons (1951) and Kassebaum and Baumann (1965). By the nature of the processes of selection, those coming into the care of community mental health services may have been classed as chronic dependants. Caring for a certain proportion of long-stay residents is bound to result in the orientation of staff to the more permanent residents, so that those coming for short periods, or of greater ability than most, appear to be deviants and have difficulty in finding acceptance in any available role. Similarly those whose behaviour is for some reason unacceptable to staff or the other residents find such roles withdrawn from them, with the result that they can be reclassified and downgraded (Strauss and colleagues, 1964; *b*).

LEVELS OF AUTHORITY

Within any one community service, and I have in mind the mental health services as now constituted, principles operate which are similar to those already discussed in connection with the whole formal organization. Staff hierarchies are more clearly demonstrated in costume and status-defining activities, because these all work in close proximity to one another. The persons for whom the service exists take their place beneath, but apart from, this hierarchy. Although some, by reason of their abilities, usefulness, or self-estimation, may take on other roles more specifically related to the staff or to those in the wider community. Certain sociotherapeutic philosophies may espouse and even practice other more egalitarian, libertarian, or communitarian social relations, but such ideas are not part of the normal experience of staff. *See*, for example, the analysis of the results of residents in a therapeutic community (Rapaport, 1960). For a more conventional but specifically rehabilitative regimen for long-stay patients *see* Morgan, Cushing and Morton (1965). In personnel management these hostel regimens take their reference from the large, mother-dominated family, or the *laissez-faire* authoritarian forms of institutional life. Because of the face-to-face relationships deviance is taken as a demonstration of insubordination, and inevitably represents a challenge to staff authority because of the social significance attached to social distance between staff and residents, and the lack of intermediaries to cushion the effects.

REORGANIZATION

It is in fact impossible to practise some of the tenets of sociotherapy and, still less, psychotherapy in the context of group organization unless the roles of so-called staff and others are drastically reallocated and restructured. This can only be done by practical training, with a strong emphasis on social dynamics, and the provision of greater emotional security and status for the staff through this. If staff are left to their own devices and the only reference they have is to an official hierarchy with other values, they can only fall back on available referants within their experience; for example, the parental and other authority roles such as the school-teacher, foreman and nurse. The various viewpoints of this situation are discussed elsewhere (Scheff, 1961; Strauss and colleagues, 1964; c; National Health Service, 1969).

Faced with implied criticism from outside, those in authority inside large- or small-scale total institutions feel challenged and threatened by those whom they feel have neither the will to participate in their experience, nor the social grace to understand their lowly position and the directness of face-to-face encounters. To an observer it may seem difficult to believe that staff placed in positions of such total authority should feel so vulnerable. They seem to have all the sanctions on their side and all the room for manoeuvre. But, because of the directness of confrontation, they stand to demean themselves and to lose face; and in face-to-face relationships this matters (Goffman, 1956). This of course is the fundamental weakness of this form of authoritarian regimen. Its existence can be evaded by straight forward denial or ignorance of its existence, whereas the other techniques of man-management are more subtle, although also essentially manipulative.

Authority in this situation exists only in so far as it is acknowledged. But the social and emotional experience which staff and residents bring to their roles determines the form these may take and the resulting social character of group relations. The possible lines of action open to either, that is, the options available to them to plan and choose, are strictly limited by these factors, as well as by the formal functional expectations of their roles within the formal structure (Krause, 1965; Boswell, 1969a).

These factors not only reduce, or rather channel, the possible variations in planning and action, but also determine the social meaning that staff and residents give to their own behaviour and to that of others. Any discussion of roles implies not formal requirements but people's expectations of each other's behaviour, and the interpretation that can be made of their actions.

Depending on the interpretation and the actions that ensue from it, so social relations are generated and the social structure given the particular form, which outsiders often refer to as 'its atmosphere'. The behaviour of persons to one another is justified in terms of their image of themselves and its relationship to the estimation that others appear to hold of them. To this extent, an understanding of the social situation is assisted by an understanding of the social personalities interacting within the structure of the formal organization.

Management of Community Services and Staff Selection

In this section considerable reference is made to conflict. This is because it is inherent in the plurality of functions and the hierarchy of statuses that make up any formal organization. In the sort of face-to-face relationships that form the working lives of the staff in the fieldwork agencies and personal services provided in community health services it plays a direct part in the challenge to authority expressed in most regimens. It is conflict which disturbs staff and others, whereas harmony is, for some reason, assumed. But moral norms may not represent statistical norms.

Given the present formal hierarchical structure, the balancing of parts of the service in favour of the administrative core, the lack of clear aims and the lack of developmental practices, it is most unlikely that great developments will be made. The activity of services will reflect their structure and the morale and relations of their personnel. This observation has led to the closely related styles of the recommendations for local government regions, for the co-ordination of social work authority, and the regrouping of area health services, with which other sections of this book are concerned and which underlie present national discussion of the health and welfare services.

INTERVIEWING FOR STAFF SELECTION

It may be worth considering here, however, the selection of fieldwork staff, because by their performance the *raison d'etre* of any social service stands or falls. All sorts of combinations exist in the composition of interviewing panels. The elected representatives on the Health Committee, the Medical Officer and his senior administrative officer, with or without the presence of the elected chairman of the Health Committee, and with or without senior staff from the fieldwork agency or establishment for which staff are being selected — all are possible combinations, and many conceptions exist of the nature of the work and the goals of the service for which staff are being selected.

Nevertheless it should be possible to systematize the technique of selection so that it is more related to the work situation for which applicants are to be selected. If what counts in personnel services is a flexibility and individuality of approach to persons and a way of dealing with, and reacting to, awkward situations that reduce their scale and impact, then procedures should be followed which test the applicants' qualities of reaction to this sort of situation. It is probably of little consequence what other formal training has been given, because the situations are ones that demand immediate, not considered, political action. Interviews establish the *rapport* of the applicant with the selection panel, but if they are not the people with whom future interaction will take place in the work situation this may be of less consequence than interacting with the mentally disordered. Other formal organizations in industry and government, have devised techniques designed to select personnel with qualities considered relevant to the task. It should be worth considering such personnel for selection for personal community services. But it does assume a considerable degree of attention, and respect for staff and the roles they are to fulfil.

Morale appears to be low in many parts of the Health Service, and the salaries paid to those responsible for personal care and face-to-face relationships reflect their position in the hierarchy and the lack of esteem associated with their work. At the same time their authority over others is very considerable although not reflected in their own status. This situation generates most of the characteristics of total institutions, which the present trend in the provision of community services is supposed to modify. One must therefore look to a clear expression of policy and the formal organization of services whose hierarchy are informed of the policy, and whose fieldstaff can secure the authority to implement it and attempt innovation, having been selected according to relevant criteria for their role in action.

Conclusions

In this section an attempt has been made to indicate the main features of the formal organization of personal services. Inherent in the social interaction that is, the *raison d'etre* of these services, lie conflict situations. However, the form that these take, the impact that they make and the use to which they are put, are closely related to the formal structure according to which the services are organized and authority distributed. This analysis is relevant to all forms of personal service, although I have taken the mental health service for the case study because it is most familiar to me. Other community services such as the welfare services for the elderly or the children's department would have raised similar problems, although with particular points of reference.

In the bibliographic references official policy statements and documents have been cited, as well as the most relevant work on industrial sociology. In Britain, as in the United States of America, the analytical study of the working of formal organizations has concentrated on industrial structures. No analysis of other forms of management and work situation could ignore these studies; nor could any student of public and personal service administration ignore them. The insights to be gained from situations that have much in common, although they are functionally or just customarily considered to be distinctly different, can be illuminating. It is to be hoped that by raising issues normally played down or set aside, a greater understanding may be achieved of the working of the personal services and of their different levels of organization and social interaction.

ADDENDUM

The 1970 General Election has resulted in the alteration of reorganization plans for local government and the N.H.S. (Department of the Environment, 1971; Department of Health and Social Security, 1971). By these plans the Government retains the N.H.S. regional structure. Although Area Health Boards are related to the new local authority boundaries, the latter are based on existing county or conurbation boundaries. These are therefore much larger than those recommended by the Maud Report and perpetuate many characteristics of the present two-tier administration. The long awaited White Paper (1971) has also been published, enabling local authorities to work for specific targets, presumably with a rate support grant.

Bibliography and References

Apte, R.Z. (1968). *Halfway Houses.* Occasional Papers in Social Administration. No. 18. London; Bell

Benton, M. (1965). *Roles: An Introduction to the Study of Social Relations.* London; Tavistock

Blau, P.M. (1963). *The Dynamics of Bureaucracy. A Study of Interpersonal Relations in Two Government Agencies* (*a,* p. 231; *b,* p. 260). Chicago; University of Chicago Press

— and Scott, W.R. (1963). *Formal Organizations. A Comparative Approach.* (p. 7). London; Routledge and Kegan Paul

Boswell, D.M. (1969a). 'Orders of Analysis and Conflict in Structured Situations: The Case of the Mental Health Service.' In *A.S.A. Conference on Social Change and Conflict Theory.* Ed. by P.C. Lloyd. In press

— (1969b). 'Structural Relationships within the Mental Health Service.' Annual Conference of Medical Sociology Group, B.S.A. In press

Burns, T. and Stalker, G.M. (1966). *The Management of Innovation* (2nd edn.) London; Tavistock

Campbell, A.C. (1968a). 'Characteristics of 352 Residents and 119 ex-Residents of 14 Lancashire County Council Hostels for Mentally Disordered Adults.' *Med. Offr.* **119,** 1, 3

— (1968b). 'The Preventive Use of Mental Health Hostels.' *Med. Offr.* **120,** 10, 137

— (1971). 'Aspects of Personal Independence of Mentally Subnormal and Severely Subnormal Adults in Hospitals and Local Authority Hostels.' *Br. J. Soc. Psychiat.* In press

Department of the Environment (1971). *Local Government in England.* Cmnd. 4584. London; H.M.S.O.

Department of Health for Scotland (1957). *The Welfare Needs of Mentally Handicapped Persons.* Edinburgh; H.M.S.O.

Department of Health and Social Security (1959a). *Mental Health Service.* Circular 9/59
– (1959b). *Mental Health Service.* Circular 28/59
– (1966). *Hostels for the Mentally Ill.* LHAL 10/66
– (1970). *National Health Service. The Future Structure of the National Health Service. (a,* p. 11). London; H.M.S.O.
– (1971). *Consultative Document: The Reorganization of the National Health Service*
Durkin, E. (1971). *Hostels for the Mentally Disordered.* Young Fabian Pamphlet No. 24. London; Fabian Society
Gerth, H.H. and Mills, C.W. (Eds.) (1948). *From Max Weber* (p. 196). London; Routledge and Kegan Paul
Goffman, E. (1956). 'The Nature of Deference and Demeanour.' *Am. Anthrop.* **58,** 473
– (1961). *Asylums: Essays on the Social Situation of Mental Patients and Other Inmates.* (p. 79). New York; Doubleday
Goldthorpe, J.H., Lockwood, D., Bechofer, F. and Platt, J. (1969). *The Affluent Worker in the Class Structure.* Cambridge; University Press
Gouldner, A.W. (1954). *Patterns of Industrial Bureaucracy.* New York; Free Press
Hoenig, J. and Hamilton, M.W. (1969). *The Desegregation of the Mentally Ill. (a,* p. 96). London; Routledge and Kegan Paul
Kassebaum, G.G. and Baumann, B.O. (1965). 'Dimensions of the Sick Role in Chronic Illness.' *J. Health Hum. Behav.* **6,** 16
King, R.D. and Raynes, N.V. (1968). 'An Operational Measure of Inmate Management in Residential Institutions.' *Soc. Sci. Med.* **2,** 1
Krause, E.A. (1965). 'Structured Strain in a Marginal Profession: Rehabilitation Counselling.' *J. Health Hum. Behav.* **6,** 55
Kushlick, A. (1967). 'A Method of Evaluating the Effectiveness of a Community Health Service.' *Soc. Econ. Adm.* **1,** 4, 29
– and Cox, G. (1967). 'The Ascertained Prevalence of Mental Subnormality in the Wessex Region on 1st July 1963.' *Proceedings of the First Congress of the Interantional Association for the Scientific Study of Mental Deficiency* (p. 161). National Association for Mental Health
Lancashire County Council (1969). Report of the Medical Officer of Health for the Year 1968. (p. 88). Preston
Local Authority Social Services Act 1970. c. 42. London; H.M.S.O.
Lockwood, D. (1958). *The Black-coated Worker. A Study in Class Consciousness*
Mental Health Act 1959. c. 72. (Part 2, paras. 6–13). London; H.M.S.O.
Merton, R.K. (1968). *Social Theory and Social Structure.* (p. 253). New York; Free Press

Michels, R. (1949). *Political Parties*. (p. 31). Glencoe; Free Press

Midwinter, E.G. (1969). *Social Administration in Lancashire 1830–1860. Poor Law, Public Health and Police*. Manchester; University Press

Ministry of Health (1962). *A Hospital Plan for England and Wales*. Cmnd. 1604. London; H.M.S.O.

– (1963). *Health and Welfare*. (pp. 23, 46). Cmnd. 1973. London; H.M.S.O.

– (1964). *Report of the Committee on the Internal Administration of Hospitals*. London; H.M.S.O.

– (1966a). *Report of the Committee on Senior Nursing Staff Structure*. London; H.M.S.O.

– (1966b). *Health and Welfare. The Development of Community Care*. (*a*, paras. 53–55). Cmnd. 3022. London; H.M.S.O.

Mittler, P. (1966). *The Mental Health Services*. Fabian Research Series, 252. London; Fabian Society

– (1968). *Mental Health Services in the Community*. Fabian Occasional Paper 4. London; Fabian Society

Morgan, R., Cushing, D. and Morton, N.S. (1965). 'A Regional Psychiatric Rehabilitation Hospital.' *Br. J. Psychiat.* **111**, 955

Mountney, G.H. (1968). 'Adjusting to the Environment – Transitional Accommodation.' *Conference on Psychiatric Care in the Community* (p. 20). London; The Royal Society for the Promotion of Health

Morris, P. (1969). *Put Away* (p. 131). London; Routledge and Kegan Paul

National Health Service (1969). *Report on the Committee of Enquiry into Allegations of Ill-treatment and Other Irregularities at the Ely Hospital, Cardiff*. Cmnd. 3975. London; H.M.S.O.

Parsons, R. (1951). *The Social System*. (Ch. 10). New York; Free Press

Rapaport, R.N. (1960). *Community as Doctor – New Perspectives on a Therapeutic Community*. London; Tavistock

Rehin, G.F. and Martin, F.M. (1969). *Patterns of Performance in Community Care*. (*a*, p. 138; *b*, p. 139). London; Oxford University Press for Nuffield Provincial Hospitals Trust

Report of the Committee on Local Authority and Allied Personal Social Services (1968). Chairman: Sir Frederick Seebohm. Cmnd. 3703. London; H.M.S.O.

Report of the Royal Commission on the Law Relating to Mental Illness and Mental Deficiency (1957). Cmnd. 169 (paras. 601–625). London; H.M.S.O.

Report of the Royal Commission on Local Government in England 1966–69 (1969). Chairman: Lord Redcliffe-Maud. Cmnd. 4039, 4040. London; H.M.S.O.

Scheff, T.J. (1961). 'Control over Policy by Attendants in a Mental Hospital.' *J. Health Hum. Behav.* **2**, 93

Society for Mental Health Hostel Officers (1969). *The Key to the Door. The Aims of the Society*

Strauss, A., Schatzman, L., Bucher, R., Ehrlich, D. and Sabshin, M. (1964). *Psychiatric Institutions and Ideologies.* (*a*, p. 54; *b*, p. 109; *c*, pp. 94, 118). New York; Free Press

Susser, M. (1968). *Community Psychiatry: Epidemiologic and Social Themes.* (Part 4, Mental Subnormality in the Community: a Medical Care Paradigm, p. 272). New York; Random House

Tizzard, J. (1964). *Community Services for the Mentally Handicapped* (Part 1, p. 15). London; Oxford University Press

White Paper (1971). *Better Services for the Mentally Handicapped.* Cmnd. 4683. London; H.M.S.O.

Index